Ambulatory Care

**CLINICAL
SKILLS
PROGRAM**

Type 2 Diabetes Mellitus Management Module

Mary Lynn McPherson

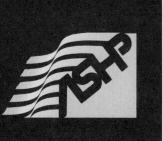

American Society of Health-System Pharmacists

Any correspondence regarding this publication should be sent to the publisher, American Society of Health-System Pharmacists®, 7272 Wisconsin Avenue, Bethesda, MD 20814, attn.: Cynthia Reilly, Pharmacist Editor/Project Manager, Special Publishing. Produced in conjunction with the ASHP Publication Production Center (Bill Fogle, Technical Editor). Cover and page design by David Wade.

The information presented herein reflects the opinions of the contributors and reviewers. It should not be interpreted as an official policy of ASHP or as an endorsement of any product.

Drug information and its applications are constantly evolving because of ongoing research and clinical experience and are often subject to professional judgment and interpretation by the practitioner and to the uniqueness of a clinical situation. The author and ASHP have made every effort to ensure the accuracy and completeness of the information presented in this book. However, the reader is advised that the publisher, author, contributors, editors, and reviewers cannot be responsible for the continued currency of the information, for any errors or omissions, and/or for any consequences arising from the use of the information in the clinical setting.

The reader is cautioned that ASHP makes no representation, guarantee, or warranty, express or implied, that the use of the information contained in this book will prevent problems with insurers and will bear no responsibility or liability for the results or consequences of its use.

ISBN: 1-879907-93-3

Contents

Preface

Pharmacists practicing in ambulatory care settings are increasingly responsible for designing, recommending, and managing patient-specific pharmacotherapy regimens. Patients in the ambulatory care setting usually present with chronic conditions; thus, pharmacists in this setting develop long-term relationships with patients. Patients are the most important members of the health care team and are increasingly involved in their own health care. Patients should take a primary role when the pharmacist begins to design a care plan. An important element of care is developing a professional relationship with the patient. The pharmacist in the ambulatory care setting learns many things from the patient through interviewing, but the pharmacist is also in a position to help educate the patient about the importance of adhering to a therapeutic plan.

To make the best decisions possible, you must learn to identify relevant information and format it into a patient-specific database. Much of the information to be included in an Ambulatory Pharmacist's Patient Database is obtained from patient interview, assessment of vital signs and general appearance, laboratory data, and a patient's ambulatory care medical record.

After patient-specific information is collected, you must be able to develop an Ambulatory Pharmacist's Care Plan. The process of designing a care plan includes assessing therapy, identifying the patient's health care needs, and identifying pharmacotherapeutic and related health care goals with the patient.

Once the Ambulatory Pharmacist's Care Plan is designed, the pharmacist must implement the plan and evaluate outcomes; the pharmacist may have to redesign the care plan if goals are not met or new goals are identified.

The *Ambulatory Care Clinical Skills Program: Type 2 Diabetes Mellitus Management Module* will teach you what information is needed, how to collect it, and how to design and manage the Ambulatory Pharmacist's Care Plan for a patient with type 2 diabetes.

Writer

Mary Lynn McPherson, Pharm.D., BCPS, CDE
Associate Professor
University of Maryland School of Pharmacy
Baltimore, Maryland

Contributors

ASHP wishes to acknowledge the following people who contributed their time and expertise to the development of this text:

Elliot D. Bleicher
Dawnelle Borkey
Bill Boyce
Peter Chen
Sandra Oh Clarke
Lourdes M. Cuellar
Scott Evans
Kerri Eye
Nancy T. Fong
Patricia Fung
William C. Gong
Karen A. Grace
David R. Gray
Laurel M. Janney
Leslie Dotson Jaggers
Milica Jovic
Michael W. Kelly
Teresa Klepser
Sherri L. Konzem
Con Ann Ling
Azita Mavandadi
Patricia A. Montgomery
Anthony P. Morreale
Leigh Anh Nguyen
Stephanie H. Pihl–Leggett
Charles D. Ponte
Patricia Racioppi
Cynthia Reilly
Jane S. Ricciuti
My-Trang Robinson
Sheila Ann Salamunovich
Beata Saletnik
Maria C. Sciame
Naomi M. Schultheis
Michael L. Simeone
Marie A. Smith
Paula G. Sondergeld
Jane Tran
Shelly Van Note
Holli Wetzler
Winston Wong
Helen S. Yee
Sue Y. Yim

Pharmacy Continuing Education Program

By successfully completing the three CE tests for the *Ambulatory Care Clinical Skills Program: Type 2 Diabetes Mellitus Management Module*, you can earn 1.15 CEU. The ACPE numbers for the *Ambulatory Care Clinical Skills Program: Type 2 Diabetes Mellitus Management Module* are: Part I, Collecting and Organizing Patient-Specific Information for Patients with Type 2 Diabetes, 204-000-99-046-H01; Part II, Developing an Ambulatory Pharmacist's Care Plan for Patients with Type 2 Diabetes, 204-000-99-047-H01; and Part III, Managing an Ambulatory Pharmacist's Care Plan for Patients with Type 2 Diabetes, 204-000-99-048-H01. The tests and answer sheets are bound separately from this book.

The American Society of Health-System Pharmacists is approved by the American Council on Pharmaceutical Education as a provider of continuing pharmaceutical education.

Copyright Information

Introduction

Who Can Benefit From Using the *Type 2 Diabetes Mellitus Management Module*?

ASHP created the *Ambulatory Care Clinical Skills Program: Type 2 Diabetes Mellitus Management Module* as part of a profession-wide effort to increase pharmacy's involvement in clinical practice and pharmaceutical care in the ambulatory care setting. Both pharmacists and pharmacy students can enhance their clinical skills by engaging in these self-study activities. Current staff pharmacists, pharmacists experiencing a career change, recent graduates wishing to sharpen their skills, and pharmacy students involved in clinical clerkships can benefit from this program, working either alone or as part of a staff development plan.

The skills referred to in the title are problem-solving skills. Before you can begin to solve a problem, however, you must have content knowledge related to the problem area. To achieve the objectives of the *Type 2 Diabetes Mellitus Management Module*, you should have a solid foundation in the following knowledge areas as they relate to type 2 diabetes:
- pathophysiology
- clinical pharmacology and therapeutics
- clinical laboratory data interpretation
- clinical pharmacokinetics
- medical terminology and abbreviations

The *Type 2 Diabetes Mellitus Management Module* presumes that participants have current mastery of these areas and makes no effort to reteach fundamental knowledge gained in pharmacy school. Instead, these modules help you to apply these pharmacy knowledge areas in solving drug therapy problems. Participants should take the self-assessment test found on pages xvii–xxii before beginning work on this module. A score of less than 90% indicates that the participant requires additional didactic preparation prior to beginning coursework. Your self-assessment test results will also demonstrate specific areas in which reinforcement of content is required.

What to Do If You Need Didactic Preparation

You may feel uneasy about your didactic preparation for this program. Perhaps it has been some time since you were a pharmacy student and your didactic preparation is outdated. Perhaps you went to a pharmacy school that did not emphasize one of the content areas required by the *Type 2 Diabetes Mellitus Management Module*. Or perhaps your job has been focused on distribution, so you have forgotten some of the therapeutic concepts you learned. If so, use the clinical library noted in the Preface to the *Ambulatory Care Clinical Skills Program: Core Module* to refresh or enhance your knowledge. These include basic medical texts, physical assessment texts, pharmacotherapeutic texts, pharmacokinetic applications texts, and other valuable resources.

Your colleagues in pharmacy are also potential sources of help. Your department director, clinical coordinator, staff development coordinator, or professor at the local college of pharmacy may assist you in developing a plan of reading assignments.

There are additional references specific to diabetes mellitus that you may find useful in working through this module and in future practice. Several recommendations include:

1. Funnell MM, Hunt C, Kulkarni K, Rubin RR, et al., editors. *A Core Curriculum for Diabetes Education*. 3rd ed. Chicago, IL: American Association of Diabetes Educators; 1998.
2. Lebovitz HE, editor. *Therapy for Diabetes Mellitus and Related Disorders*. 3rd ed. Alexandria, VA: American Diabetes Association; 1998.
3. Kelley DB, editor. *Medical Management of Type 2 Diabetes*. 4th ed. Alexandria, VA: American Diabetes Association; 1998.
4. Holler HJ, Pastors JG. *Diabetes Medical Nutrition Therapy*. Chicago, IL: American Dietetic Association; 1997.

How This Program is Organized

The *Ambulatory Care Clinical Skills Program* is organized into two tracks of instruction. The first track covers the problem-solving skills you need to design, recommend, and manage patient-specific pharmacotherapy. These skills are taught in three sections of the *Ambulatory Care Clinical Skills Program: Core Module* that cover the following topics:

1. Collecting and Organizing Patient-Specific Information
2. Developing an Ambulatory Pharmacist's Care Plan
3. Managing an Ambulatory Pharmacist's Care Plan

Participants are encouraged to complete the coursework found in the *Core Module* and accompanying videotape before beginning work on this module. As you work through this module, you may wish to return to the *Core Module* to review unfamiliar concepts.

The *Type 2 Diabetes Mellitus Management Module* is a component from the second track of instruction that teaches the problem-solving skills you need to provide pharmaceutical care to patients with specific disease states in the ambulatory care setting.

All modules are print-media–based, but may employ other media as well. Some modules have a video component to demonstrate specific skills.

The Best Way to Use the Ambulatory Care Clinical Skills Program

When using the *Type 2 Diabetes Mellitus Management Module*, you can work either alone or as part of a group. If you are working alone, you may want to ask your practice site supervisor to help you practice the clinical skills you learn. To gain competence in assessment of vital signs and general appearance, you must participate in an educational environment that includes repetitive hands-on demonstration and practice with trained educators.

The units of the *Type 2 Diabetes Mellitus Management Module* should be studied in sequential order. The *Type 2 Diabetes Mellitus Management Module* is a carefully structured, systematic approach to acquiring drug therapy and drug information problem-solving skills.

Finally, each module offers ACPE-approved continuing education (CE) credit to those students who successfully pass the CE test. Directions are enclosed with each module.

How to Study

Successful completion of this self-study module may require that you adopt some different approaches than those you customarily use for classroom learning. If you have never used a self-study text before, you will quickly discover that learning can be difficult when you do not have a teacher answering your questions, demonstrating the relationships between ideas, setting deadlines, or evaluating your work. A good self-instruction program guides you through the text as if a teacher were presenting the material and supplies you with study aides. Make this module an effective self-study tool by following these suggestions:

1. Set a goal for completing the module and establish a schedule for studying without interruption or distraction. A library may be an ideal place for this project.
2. Read the introduction and learning objectives of each unit. These sections will tell you why the unit is important, what specific information you will be expected to learn for answering the self-study questions, and how the unit is organized.
3. Scan the unit, noting the subject headings.
4. Read the unit, keeping the learning objectives in mind. Underline or highlight important passages and make notes in the margins.
5. Read the summary to review the main points of the unit. Review anything that still seems unclear.
6. Answer the self-study questions to evaluate your understanding of the information and preparedness for the CE test questions.
7. Review information pertaining to the questions that you answered incorrectly.
8. Expand your knowledge by referring to the suggested readings that follow the module. Although you will not be tested on this information, independent learning will add depth and detail to your understanding.

Determining the Role of Pharmaceutical Care

Pharmaceutical care cannot be accomplished within the confines of the pharmacy. Probably the most important influence on pharmaceutical care is the personal relationship between the pharmacist and patient. However, this relationship requires that you assume responsibility for appropriate drug therapy outcomes.

You also need to establish positive, cooperative relationships with a patient's other health care providers. You must clearly communicate your purpose to the patient and these providers for them to benefit from such collaboration.

Remember, too, that pharmaceutical care cannot be provided without considering the *individual* patient. A typical example is when a health care provider asks you for the dose of a drug. If you provide only the "usual dose," you exclude that patient's health care needs.

The "ASHP Statement on Pharmaceutical Care" provides a thorough discussion of pharmaceutical care. The Principal Elements section of this document details the relationship of the pharmacist with the patient and other health care providers as follows.

The principal elements of pharmaceutical care are that it is *medication related*; it is care that is *directly provided* to the patient; it is provided to produce *definite outcomes*; these outcomes are intended to improve the patient's *quality of life*; and the provider accepts personal *responsibility* for the outcomes.

Medication related. Pharmaceutical care involves not only medication therapy (the actual provision of medication) but also decisions about medication use for individual patients. As appropriate, this includes decisions *not* to use medication therapy as well as judgments about medication selection, dosages, routes and methods of administration, medication therapy monitoring, and the provision of medication-related information and counseling to individual patients.

Care. Central to the concept of care is caring, a personal concern for the well-being of another person. Overall patient care consists of integrated domains of care including (among others) medical, nursing, and pharmaceutical care. Health professionals in each of these disciplines possess unique expertise and must cooperate in a patient's overall care. At times, they share in the execution of the various types of care (including pharmaceutical care). To pharmaceutical care, however, the pharmacist contributes unique knowledge and skills to ensure optimal outcomes from the use of medications.

At the heart of any type of patient care, there exists a one-to-one relationship between a caregiver and a patient. In pharmaceutical care, the irreducible "unit" of care is one pharmacist in a direct professional relationship with one patient. In this relationship, the pharmacist provides care directly to the patient and for the benefit of the patient.

The health and well-being of a patient are paramount. The pharmacist makes a direct, personal, caring commitment to the individual patient and acts in the patient's best interest. The pharmacist cooperates directly with other professionals and the patient in designing, implementing, and monitoring a therapeutic plan intended to produce definite therapeutic outcomes that improve the patient's quality of life.

Outcomes. It is the goal of pharmaceutical care to improve an individual patient's quality of life through achievement of definite (predefined), medication-related therapeutic outcomes. The outcomes sought are:

1. cure of a patient's disease,
2. elimination or reduction of a patient's symptomatology,
3. arresting or slowing of a disease process, and
4. prevention of a disease or symptomatology.

This, in turn, involves three major functions:

1. identifying potential and actual medication-related problems
2. resolving actual medication-related problems
3. preventing potential medication-related problems

A medication-related problem is an event or circumstance involving medication therapy that actually or potentially interferes with an optimum outcome for a specific patient. There are at least the following categories of medication-related problems:

Untreated indications. The patient has a medical problem that requires medication therapy (an indication for medication use) but is not receiving a medication for that indication.

Improper drug selection. The patient has a medication indication but is taking the wrong medication.

Subtherapeutic dosage. The patient has a medical problem that is being treated with too little of the correct medication.

Failure to receive medication. The patient has a medical problem that is the result of not receiving a medication (e.g., for pharmaceutical, psychological, sociological, or economic reasons).

Overdosage. The patient has a medical problem that is being treated with too much of the correct medication (toxicity).

Adverse drug reactions. The patient has a medical problem that is the result of an adverse drug reaction or adverse effect.

Drug interactions. The patient has a medical problem that is the result of a drug–drug, drug–food, or drug–laboratory test interaction.

Medication use without indication. The patient is taking a medication for no medically valid indication.

Patients may possess characteristics that interfere with the achievement of desired therapeutic outcomes. Patients may be nonadherent to prescribed medication use regimens, or there may be unpredictable variations in patients' biological responses. Thus, intended outcomes from medication-related therapy are not always achievable. Patients bear a responsibility to help achieve the desired outcomes by engaging in behaviors that will contribute to—and not interfere with—the achievement of desired outcomes. Pharmacists and other health professionals have an obligation to educate patients about behaviors that will contribute to achieving desired outcomes.

Quality of life. Some tools now exist for assessing a patient's quality of life. These tools are still evolving, and pharmacists should maintain familiarity with the literature on this subject. A complete assessment of a patient's quality of life should include both objective and subjective (e.g., the patient's own) assessments. Patients should be involved, in an informed way, in establishing quality of life goals for their therapies.

Responsibility. The fundamental relationship in any type of patient care is a mutually beneficial exchange, in which the patient grants authority to the provider and the provider gives competence and commitment to the patient (accepts responsibility).

Responsibility involves both moral trustworthiness and accountability.

In pharmaceutical care, the direct relationship between an individual pharmacist and an individual patient is that of a professional covenant, in which the patient's safety and well-being are entrusted to the pharmacist, who commits to honoring that trust through competent professional actions that are in the patient's best interest. As an accountable member of the health care team, the pharmacist must document the care provided. The pharmacist is personally accountable for patient outcomes (the quality of care) that ensue from the pharmacist's actions and decisions.

An Ambulatory Care Pharmacist's Flow of Decisions

This section will give an introductory overview of the flow of decisions you go through when providing therapy to patients in the ambulatory setting. A flow diagram of these steps is presented in **Figure 1** (page xvi). A detailed description of how to make the decisions in each step will be given later in the module.

The first step in the flow of decisions is establishing a professional relationship with the patient. This relationship lays the foundation on which the other steps are built. If you do not establish this relationship properly, the rest of the process can be negatively affected. For example, if a professional relationship is not established, a patient may be reluctant to share information you need to make accurate decisions, or a patient may not trust you enough to be adhere to the therapeutic recommendations you make.

With a professional relationship established, you must then decide what information is needed to address the patient's problems. The module will give guidelines and practice in determining the information needed as well as how to gather the information and assess its reliability.

Next, you must decide what pharmacotherapeutic and related health care problems this patient has. An organized approach for ensuring that all possible types of problems are considered will be presented. After identifying the patient's problems, you should step back to look at the whole picture. How do these problems fit in with the patient as a whole? How do they relate to the patient's overall therapy from other members of the health care team? This process helps you process the next decision: the patient's health care needs.

Having determined the patient's problems and needs, you can proceed to determine appropriate pharmacotherapeutic and related health care goals for the patient. The module will cover factors that may influence goal setting in the ambulatory care setting.

Following the definition of goals, you must determine how the goals will be reached. What is an appropriate therapeutic regimen for the patient? In addition, how is the therapeutic regimen to be monitored?

Implementation decisions must be made next. How is the regimen to be implemented? The module will describe key considerations, steps, and skills needed for effective implementation of a patient's therapeutic regimen.

Once the patient's regimen has been implemented, its effectiveness must be assessed. Did the regimen meet its goals? If the goals haven't been met, why not? Based on answers to these questions, as well as changes in the patient's status and other factors, you must decide if the therapeutic regimen needs to be redesigned. Factors to consider when redesigning a regimen will be covered in detail in the module.

The flow of decisions described above provides you with a systematic and comprehensive approach to providing therapy to patients in the ambulatory setting.

Module Organization

The *Type 2 Diabetes Mellitus Management Module* is divided into three parts:
1. Collecting and Organizing Patient-Specific Information for Patients with Type 2 Diabetes
2. Developing an Ambulatory Pharmacist's Care Plan for Patients with Type 2 Diabetes
3. Managing an Ambulatory Pharmacist's Care Plan for Patients with Type 2 Diabetes

You should study these units in the order presented because each unit builds on understanding gained from the prior unit. Each unit begins with an introduction explaining the relevance of what you will learn, the objectives you will attain, and the organizational structure of the material. At the end of each unit summary are self-study questions you can use to check your mastery of the objectives. Three separate CE tests cover the objectives of each unit. If you can successfully answer the self-study questions at the end of each unit, you should also do well on the CE tests. You may submit the CE answer sheets for continuing education credit.

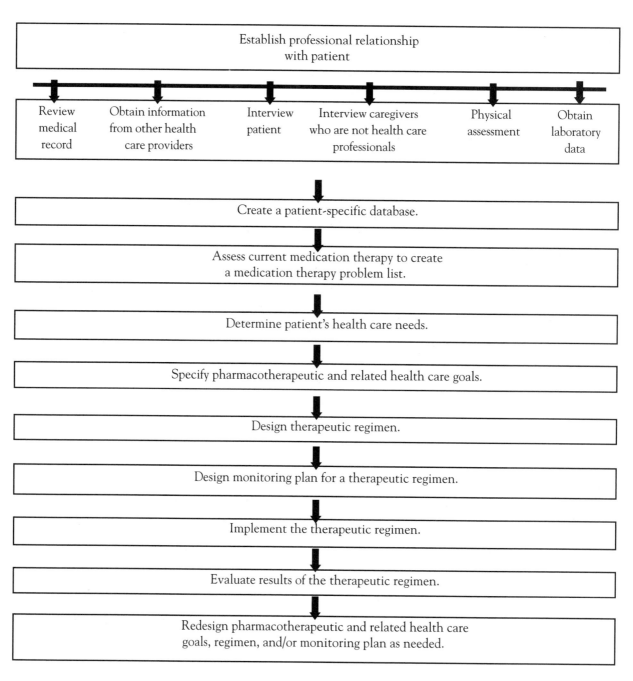

Figure 1. Flow of decisions

Type 2 Diabetes Mellitus Self-Assessment Test

1. Circle all of the following that are signs or symptoms of uncontrolled type 2 diabetes.
   A. Polyphagia
   B. Polydipsia
   C. Shakiness
   D. Hypotension
   E. Palpitations
   F. Polyhydrosis
   G. Polyuria
   H. Blurred vision
   I. Sweating

2. Which of the following best describes why hyperglycemia may cause polyuria?
   A. Excess glucose is renally excreted, causing polyuria due to an osmotic effect that pulls water into the urine.
   B. Excess glucose is renally excreted, which causes an irritation of renal parenchymal cells that results in increased urination.
   C. Excess glucose is renally excreted, resulting in a urinary tract infection, with one symptom being increased urination.
   D. Excess glucose is renally excreted, thus altering urine pH and resulting in increased urination.

3. Which of the following best describes the occurrence of transient blurred vision (unrelated to retinopathy) with diabetes?
   A. The blurred vision is caused by hypoglycemia.
   B. The blurred vision is caused by hyperglycemia.
   C. The blurred vision is unrelated to blood glucose control.
   D. Blurred vision is a warning sign of an impending stroke.

4. Diabetes occurs most frequently in which of the following populations?
   A. Caucasians
   B. African Americans
   C. Hispanic Americans
   D. Pima Indians

5. Which of the following best describes the incidence of type 2 diabetes?
   A. It is increasing.
   B. It is decreasing.
   C. The incidence is relatively stable.
   D. We are unable to determine this statistic.

6. Which of the following best estimates the number of people in the United States with diabetes (types 1 and 2)?
   A. 4 million
   B. 8 million
   C. 16 million
   D. 32 million

7. Circle all of the following that are risk factors for developing type 2 diabetes (as defined by the American Diabetes Association).

   A. A diet rich in sweets

   B. Obesity

   C. Male sex

   D. Female sex

   E. <30 years old

   F. Family history of type 1 diabetes

   G. >45 years of age

   H. Family history of type 2 diabetes

   I. Delivery of a large-birth-weight baby

   J. Living with someone who has type 2 diabetes

8. Which of the following best explains why obesity is a risk factor for type 2 diabetes?

   A. Obese people cannot exercise as well, therefore they have slowed metabolism.

   B. Obese people generally maintain a diet high in sweets.

   C. Obesity causes insulin resistance.

   D. Obesity causes decreased insulin secretion.

9. Patients with concurrent diabetes and hypertension have a higher incidence of all of the following complications of diabetes, except:

   A. Cardiovascular disease

   B. Renal disease

   C. Retinopathy

   D. Coagulation defects

10. Which of the following best describes the pathogenesis of type 2 diabetes?

    A. Patients produce endogenous insulin receptor antagonists.

    B. Islet cell antibodies attack the pancreatic β cells.

    C. Insulin resistance develops, and there is inadequate insulin secretion to compensate for this resistance.

    D. Patients are absolutely insulinopenic.

11. Which of the following best describes the pathogenesis of type 2 diabetes?

    A. The insulin level is reduced by the presence of insulin autoantibodies.

    B. Insulin may be present in normal, lower, or higher than normal levels, but the insulin is not acting correctly.

    C. The C-peptide level is greatly reduced at the time of type 2 diabetes diagnosis.

    D. Insulin levels are very high in type 2 diabetes, causing down-regulation of the insulin receptors.

12. Which of the following best describes the pathogenesis of diabetes?

    A. Patients with type 2 diabetes inactivate their endogenous insulin.

    B. There is no test that can distinguish between type 1 and type 2 diabetes; the clinician must be guided by clinical presentation.

    C. Patients with type 2 diabetes are generally below ideal body weight, causing insulin deficits.

    D. Patients with advanced, progressive type 2 diabetes may have pancreatic β cell function similar to a patient with type 1 diabetes.

13. Which of the following best explains the clinical course of type 2 diabetes?

   A. Patients have subclinical symptoms for 1–2 months, then present with increasing polydipsia, polyuria, and polyphagia.

   B. Patients may be asymptomatic at the time of diagnosis.

   C. When patients are diagnosed with type 2 diabetes and begin therapy, they experience a "honeymoon" phase during which little or no insulin is required.

   D. Patients with type 2 diabetes are generally diagnosed around age 30.

14. Which of the following best explains the clinical course of type 2 diabetes?

   A. Type 2 diabetes may be present on average for 6.5 years prior to clinical identification and treatment.

   B. Type 2 diabetes that is clinically silent is less likely to be associated with the development of complications.

   C. The major cause of death in patients with type 2 diabetes is cerebrovascular disease.

   D. Patients with type 2 diabetes develop frequent episodes of hypoglycemia 15–20 years after diagnosis.

15. Which of the following is not consistent with the clinical course of type 2 diabetes?

   A. Macrovascular complications associated with diabetes include increased cardiovascular disease, cerebrovascular disease, and peripheral vascular disease.

   B. Microvascular complications associated with diabetes include an increased incidence of retinopathy and nephropathy.

   C. Neuropathic complications associated with diabetes include autonomic and peripheral complications.

   D. Foot and leg ulcers associated with diabetes are frequently caused by combined peripheral neuropathy and microvascular changes.

16. Circle all of the following that describe an accepted treatment for diabetes.

   A. Insulin

   B. Glyburide

   C. Metformin

   D. Chromium

   E. Insulin lispro

   F. Rosiglitazone

   G. Repaglinide

   H. Acarbose

   I. Medical nutrition therapy

   J. Exercise plan

17. Which of the following best describes why metformin is an effective treatment for type 2 diabetes?

   A. It reduces hepatic glucose production.

   B. It stimulates insulin release from pancreatic β cells.

   C. It decreases insulin activity in the periphery.

   D. It blocks the alpha-glucosidase enzyme in the gut.

18. Which of the following best describes why repaglinide is an effective treatment for type 2 diabetes?

A. It reduces hepatic glucose production.

B. It stimulates insulin release from pancreatic β cells.

C. It blocks the alpha-glucosidase enzyme in the gut.

D. It decreases glucose utilization and uptake into muscle cells.

19. Circle all of the following that are contraindications or precautions for the use of metformin.

   A. Pregnancy

   B. Hepatic dysfunction

   C. Renal dysfunction

   D. Retinopathy

   E. History of alcoholism

   F. History of flatulence

20. Which of the following diabetes medications may cause hypoglycemia when used alone?

   A. Metformin

   B. Troglitazone

   C. Repaglinide

   D. Acarbose

21. Which of the following best explains why an alanine aminotransferase (ALT) of 120 IU/L is a contraindication for troglitazone therapy?

   A. Troglitazone has been associated with renal toxicity, and the ALT is a marker of renal function.

   B. Troglitazone has been associated with hepatic toxicity, and the ALT is a marker of liver function.

   C. Troglitazone may cause pulmonary infiltrates, and the ALT is a marker of respiratory function.

   D. Troglitazone may cause brain cancer, and the ALT is a marker of malignant cells.

22. Which of the following best explains the mechanism of action of acarbose?

   A. It reduces hepatic glucose production.

   B. It stimulates insulin release from pancreatic β cells.

   C. It blocks the alpha-glucosidase enzyme in the gut.

   D. It enhances glucose utilization and uptake into muscle cells.

23. Which of the following best explains the mechanism of action of glyburide?

   A. It reduces hepatic glucose production.

   B. It stimulates insulin release from pancreatic β cells.

   C. It blocks the alpha-glucosidase enzyme in the gut.

   D. It enhances glucose utilization and uptake into muscle cells.

24. Which of the following best explains the pharmacokinetics of repaglinide?

   A. Insulin levels begin to increase within 15 minutes of repaglinide administration.

   B. Insulin levels begin to increase within 45 minutes of repaglinide administration.

   C. Insulin levels begin to increase within 1 hour of repaglinide administration.

   D. Insulin levels begin to increase within 3 hours of repaglinide administration.

25. Which of the following agents has the longest half-life?

   A. Chlorpropamide

   B. Glipizide

   C. Repaglinide

   D. Tolbutamide

26. Which of the following insulin preparations has the shortest duration of effect?

   A. Regular

   B. Lispro

   C. NPH

   D. Semi-lente

27. Which of the following diabetes regimens is most expensive?

   A. Acarbose 25 mg by mouth three times daily.

   B. Metformin 500 mg by mouth three times daily.

   C. Troglitazone 400 mg by mouth each day.

   D. Insulin 10 units NPH each morning, 5 units each evening.

28. Which of the following best describes an appropriate diabetes regimen?

   A. Acarbose 25 mg by mouth three times daily after meals.

   B. Repaglinide 25 mg by mouth three times daily before meals.

   C. Glyburide 25 mg by mouth each morning.

   D. Metformin 850 by mouth three times daily.

29. Circle all of the following that describe possible drug interactions when treating patients with diabetes.

   A. Hydrochlorothiazide in a 48-year-old female with type 2 diabetes

   B. Aspirin 325 mg by mouth every 4–6 hours as needed in a 62-year-old male with type 2 diabetes

   C. Cimetidine and metformin

   D. Ciprofloxacin and glyburide

30. Which of the following best explains why pharmacists should be aware of the interaction of furosemide and glipizide when treating patients with diabetes?

   A. Furosemide can cause volume depletion, enhancing the effect of glipizide.

   B. Furosemide can cause hyperglycemia, partially negating the effect of glipizide.

   C. Furosemide can cause hyperuricemia, which increases glipizide renal excretion.

   D. Furosemide can cause metabolic alkalosis, which increases glipizide toxicity.

31. With which diabetes medication is the disulfiram effect most prominent?

   A. Repaglinide

   B. Glyburide

   C. Chlorpropamide

   D. Acarbose

32. Circle all of the following that describe common adverse reactions with oral sulfonylurea agents.

   A. Hyperglycemia

   B. Rash

C. Weight gain

D. Hypoglycemia

E. Excess antidiuretic hormone secretion (SIADH)

F. Weight loss

G. Hirsutism

33. Which of the following diabetes therapies is not associated with weight gain?

A. Insulin

B. Glyburide

C. Metformin

D. Repaglinide

34. Which of the following explains why acarbose generally does not cause hypoglycemia when used as monotherapy?

A. It only affects sucrose levels, not glucose.

B. It is not systemically absorbed to any great degree.

C. It is inactivated when it crosses the gastrointestinal wall into the systemic circulation.

D. It does not cause hypoglycemia because it is administered before meals, rather than after.

Self-Assessment Answers

1. A, B, G, H
2. A
3. B
4. D
5. A
6. C
7. B, G, H, I
8. C
9. D
10. C
11. B
12. D
13. B
14. A
15. D
16. A, B, C, E, F, G, H, I, J
17. A
18. B
19. A, B, C, E
20. C
21. B
22. C
23. B
24. A
25. A
26. B
27. C
28. D
29. A, C, D
30. B
31. C
32. B, C, D, E
33. C
34. B

Part I

Collecting and Organizing Patient-Specific Information for Patients with Type 2 Diabetes

Establishing a Collaborative Relationship with Ambulatory Type 2 Diabetes Patients

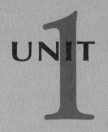

UNIT 1

Despite its prevalence, type 2 diabetes mellitus often goes undiagnosed, and undiagnosed or uncontrolled diabetes may cause significant morbidity and mortality. The best defense against the development of diabetes-related complications is early diagnosis and treatment. Ambulatory care pharmacists are in an excellent position to identify patients with type 2 diabetes early in their disease process, particularly asymptomatic patients, who could potentially remain undiagnosed for years. Ambulatory care pharmacists are also well suited to work with diabetes patients, serving as self-management coach, diabetes educator, and pharmacotherapy specialist.

Suppose you are working in your community pharmacy when a patient, Mrs. Gonzalez, approaches the counter.

MRS. GONZALEZ:

"Hello, my name is Mrs. Gonzalez. I just talked to my physician, Dr. Thompson, and he said I have diabetes. He said I should come see you, and together you, he, and I will sort it all out. Can you help me?"

After completing this unit, through discussion and case application, you will gain the knowledge and skills necessary to develop a pharmacist-patient relationship with Mrs. Gonzalez, as well other patients in your practice with type 2 diabetes.

Unit Objectives

After you successfully complete this unit, you will be able to:

- explain emotional and physical characteristics of ambulatory patients with type 2 diabetes that may affect the establishment of a collaborative patient-pharmacist relationship,
- describe the rationale and opportunities for establishing collaborative professional relationships with patients with type 2 diabetes, and
- design an effective strategy for establishing collaborative professional relationships with patients with type 2 diabetes.

Unit Organization

To begin, this unit will discuss the physical and emotional characteristics commonly found in patients with type 2 diabetes that affect the pharmacist-patient relationship. We will explore the rationale behind establishing a mutually beneficial alliance between an ambulatory diabetes patient and a pharmacist, as well as how best to establish this professional relationship. This unit concludes with example cases of pharmacist-patient relationships pertinent to type 2 diabetes management.

Patient Emotional and Physical Characteristics Affecting the Establishment of a Collaborative Relationship

Type 2 diabetes is a chronic, progressive disease that requires patient participation for proper management and prevention of long-term complications, including blindness and renal, nerve, and heart disease. When caring for patients with type 2 diabetes, it is important to realize that patients may exhibit strong emotional characteristics that can affect how they manage their disease, as well as the pharmacist-patient relationship.

A patient's reaction to the diagnosis of type 2 diabetes may range from complete denial to complete acceptance of the disease. Some patients may feel defeated by the possibility of developing long-term complications. This may lead to feelings of denial or even anger. Other patients accept their ability to control disease progression and are able to actively participate in disease management from the time of diagnosis. Regardless of the response, it will affect the patient's willingness to establish a relationship with a pharmacist and other health care providers. As a member of the health care team, you must acknowledge these emotions and enable patients to take an active role in their disease management.

Patient Empowerment

Health care providers frequently lose sight of the fact that nearly all of the care provided in diabetes management is furnished by the patient.[1] When the patient has all the necessary information, he or she will make an informed decision about daily diabetes self-care. Anderson *et al.*[1] describe two major responsibilities of the health care professional working with diabetes patients that empower patients to make appropriate decisions regarding their self-care:

- provide the knowledge and skills required for the development of an effective diabetes self-care plan, and
- provide the support and encouragement necessary for patients to make and sustain behavioral changes designed to improve their diabetes care and quality of life.

This model credits the significant emotional component of diabetes. Although the medications we have available to treat diabetes are invaluable, behavioral change (e.g., change in diet, exercise, or adherence to medication therapy) is the backbone of diabetes management. Few adults will change their behavior (in some cases, life-long behaviors) unless they feel a strong motivation (e.g., the prospect of negative consequences). The empowerment approach described by Anderson *et al.* helps patients:

1. realize they are responsible for and in charge of the daily treatment of their diabetes,
2. prioritize their diabetes-related problems and identify situations they want to improve,
3. experience the emotional and psychological commitment necessary to make and sustain behavioral changes, and
4. develop a behavioral change plan.

The Anderson *et al.* protocol includes a series of questions the practitioner may use to guide the patient to developing and committing to a behavioral change that would be beneficial in the management of diabetes:

- What part of living with diabetes is the most difficult or unsatisfying for you?
- How does that (the situation described above) make you feel?
- How would the situation have to change for you to feel better about it?
- Are you willing to take action to improve the situation for yourself?
- What are some steps that you could take to bring you closer to where you want to be?
- Is there one thing that you will do when you leave here to improve things for yourself?

Which of the following two examples do you think will most likely result in success?

Example 1

Mrs. Rosen is a 74-year-old-woman newly diagnosed with type 2 diabetes mellitus. She is ~75 lb overweight. She is meeting with the pharmacist to discuss her meal plan.

PHARMACIST:
  "Mrs. Rosen, you are quite overweight. You know that losing weight is a very important part of your diabetes management. You must start a diet immediately."

MRS. ROSEN:
  "Well, I can try, but I've been eating this way all my life. I don't think I even know how to cook any other way. Plus, I have to cook for my son and his three children, too. They don't want me to change the way I cook either."

PHARMACIST:
  "Well, your family will just have to start cooking their own meals. This is for your own good. Here's a sheet describing a 1500-calorie diet. Follow this diet and come back to see me in a month. You should lose at least 10 pounds by then."

Example 2

PHARMACIST:
  "It's quite common for people diagnosed with type 2 diabetes to be overweight, Mrs. Rosen. Weight loss, even in small amounts, has been shown to be very beneficial in controlling glucose levels."

MRS. ROSEN:
  "I know you're right. But it's too hard having to cook the way I'm supposed to, and my family still expects me to cook the same way I always have for them."

PHARMACIST:
  "How does that make you feel, trying to cook two different meals?"

MRS. ROSEN:
  "Well, I try hard not to get mad at my son and his children, but I'm getting pretty resentful. After all, I've worked hard all my life, and now that I've got diabetes I need to think about myself, but they don't see that."

PHARMACIST:
  "Do you think there's room for a compromise? Have you explained to your family that a diet for people with diabetes is really a heart-healthy diet that is beneficial for everyone?"

MRS. ROSEN:
  "Well, no, they think my diabetes diet will be pretty restrictive."

PHARMACIST:

"Perhaps you could educate them. Do you think you could work with your family so they will see your side of things, so you'll be getting closer to eating the way you know is better for you, without your family getting upset with you?"

MRS. ROSEN:

"I see your point. Yes, I could explain that this is a meal plan that is good for everyone in the family. My boy has gained quite a few pounds since his wife left him, and I don't want the children to develop bad habits either."

PHARMACIST:

"That's great. Is there one change you would be willing to make over the next few weeks to improve your diet?"

MRS. ROSEN:

"Yes, I've been thinking that, because I was raised in the South, I've always fried a lot of my foods. But the doctor said my cholesterol was pretty high, and that increases my risk for a heart attack. I think instead of frying food three or four nights a week, I'm going to cut back to no more than once a week, and it will be good for all of us!"

In Example 2, the pharmacist led Mrs. Rosen through the decision-making process, and her behavioral change is one she decided on, not one mandated by her pharmacist. It is important to note that while Mrs. Rosen has not yet achieved a perfect diet, she is agreeable to making small changes toward attainment of the ultimate goal.

Opportunities for Collaborative Practice in Type 2 Diabetes

The needs of the patient with type 2 diabetes and the skills that the ambulatory care pharmacist possesses are an excellent fit. There are many roles pharmacists can play in the care of this patient population.

As discussed earlier, a significant portion of patients with diabetes in this country remain undiagnosed. There are several possible reasons for this, including the slow and insidious onset of type 2 diabetes and the tendency toward asymptomatic presentation. Many patients with type 2 diabetes are diagnosed only after a blood glucose test included in routine laboratory work shows an abnormality. But

we do know there are major risk factors for the development of type 2 diabetes (**Table 1**).[2] Pharmacists can keep an eye open for patients at increased risk for the development of diabetes and screen those patients. Early detection and prompt treatment of type 2 diabetes may reduce complications associated with diabetes and the economic burden as well. The American Diabetes Association (ADA) has developed a questionnaire entitled "Take the Test. Know the Score" (**Figure 1**). An on-line version is available at the ADA Web site (www.diabetes.org). Patients who have been determined to be at risk for diabetes, as well as patients who present with classic signs and symptoms of diabetes, should be referred to their physician for further evaluation.

In addition to diabetes screening, the ambulatory care pharmacist has several other opportunities for collaborative practice with the type 2 diabetes patient. As stated earlier, diabetes is largely a self-managed disease. To this end, pharmacists can serve as diabetes educators. The ADA recommends that an educational program be capable of offering instruction in fifteen content areas, which will be covered in greater detail in unit 8. Beyond simply educating patients about their diabetes medications, ambulatory care pharmacists can address each content area, such as selection and utilization of a

Table 1. Major Risk Factors for Type 2 Diabetes

- Family history of diabetes (i.e., parents or siblings with diabetes)
- Obesity (i.e., $\geq 20\%$ over desired body weight or body mass index [BMI] ≥ 27 kg/m²)
- Race/ethnicity (e.g., African American, Hispanic American, Native American, Asian American, or Pacific Islander)
- Age ≥ 45 years
- Previously identified impaired fasting glucose or impaired glucose tolerance
- Hypertension ($\geq 140/90$ mmHg)
- HDL cholesterol ≤ 35 mg/dl (0.90 mmol/l) and/or a triglyceride level ≥ 250 mg/dl (2.82 mmol/l)
- History of gestational diabetes or delivery of babies over 9 lb

Could You Have Diabetes and Not Know It?

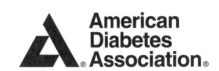

American Diabetes Association®

Take the Test. Know the Score.

Sixteen million Americans have diabetes – and one-third of them doesn't even know it! Take this test to see if you are at risk for having diabetes. Diabetes is more common in African Americans, Hispanics/Latinos, American Indians, Asian Americans, and Pacific Islanders. If you are a member of one of these ethnic groups, you need to pay special attention to this test.

To find out if you are at risk, write in the points next to each statement that is *true* for you. If a statement is *not true*, put a zero. Add your total score.

1. My weight is equal to or above that listed in the chart.   **Yes   5**   _____

2. I am under 65 years of age **and** I get little or no exercise.   **Yes   5**   _____

3. I am between 45 and 64 years of age.   **Yes   5**   _____

4. I am 65 years old or older.   **Yes   9**   _____

5. I am a woman who has had a baby weighing more than nine pounds at birth.   **Yes   1**   _____

6. I have a sister or a brother with diabetes.   **Yes   1**   _____

7. I have a parent with diabetes.   **Yes   1**   _____

| | **TOTAL** | |

Scoring 3-9 points

You are probably at low risk for having diabetes now. But don't just forget about it—especially if you are Hispanic/Latino, African American, American Indian, Asian American, or Pacific Islander. You may be at higher risk in the future. **New guidelines recommend everyone age 45 and over consider being tested for the disease every three years. However, people at high risk should consider being tested at a younger age.**

Scoring 10 or more points

You are at high risk for having diabetes. Only your health care provider can determine if you have diabetes. See your health care provider soon and find out for sure.

At-Risk Weight Chart

Height	Weight
feet/inches without shoes	pounds without clothing
4' 10"	129
4' 11"	133
5' 0"	138
5' 1"	143
5' 2"	147
5' 3"	152
5' 4"	157
5' 5"	162
5' 6"	167
5' 7"	172
5' 8"	177
5' 9"	182
5' 10"	188
5' 11"	193
6' 0"	199
6' 1"	204
6' 2"	210
6' 3"	216
6' 4"	221

If you weigh the same or more than the amount listed for your height, you may be at risk for diabetes. This chart is based on a measure called the Body Mass Index (BMI). The chart shows unhealthy weights for men and women age **35 or older** at the listed heights. At-risk weights are lower for individuals under age 35.

Diabetes Facts You Should Know

Diabetes is a serious disease that can lead to blindness, heart disease, strokes, kidney failure, and amputations. It kills more than 193,000 people each year.

Some people with diabetes have symptoms. If you have any of the following symptoms, contact your doctor:

extreme thirst • frequent urination • unexplained weight loss

For more information on diabetes, call the American Diabetes Association at **1-800-DIABETES (1-800-342-2383).**

Order Code: 3020.08 1999

Figure 1. Diabetes Risk Test
Source: reprinted with permission from the American Diabetes Association.

blood glucose meter; prevention, detection, and treatment of acute complications; behavioral change strategies; use of health care systems; community resources; and more. Because ambulatory patients interact significantly more with their pharmacist than with any other member of the health care team, having pharmacists provide diabetes education is an ideal solution.

A significant portion of caring for patients with diabetes is ensuring their adherence to recommended standards of care, such as blood glucose monitoring and monitoring of diabetes-related complications. In this case also, the pharmacist is the health care team member best suited to ensure that patients adhere to recommended standards of care, such as an annual dilated retinal exam, a podiatric exam, etc. Records of such care can easily be incorporated into the pharmacist's record keeping.

The objective of this module is to facilitate the ambulatory pharmacist's development of pharmaceutical care plans for patients with type 2 diabetes. As more diabetes medications become available, the medication regimens used to control blood glucose become complex, often involving two (or even three) diabetes medications in combination. The pharmacist is well suited to collect a database for diabetes patients, assess their current regimen for drug therapy problems, and make recommendations to prescribers.

Pharmacists can also make a significant impact by counseling patients on the selection of nonprescription medications and diabetes-related supplies as well as by providing them (if appropriate).

Establishing a Professional Relationship

In the core module you read several suggestions for developing a working patient-pharmacist relationship. Some strategies included acknowledging the patient promptly and making an effort to establish trust; introducing yourself and clarifying your role, responsibilities, and accessibility; working in a quiet, safe, and private environment; maintaining patient confidentiality; and encouraging the patient to express his or her needs and views. With diabetes management specifically, it is important to let patients know you are interested in helping them manage their diabetes in any way possible, and that you would like to be a supporting member of their

health care team. Patients like to hear that you have specialized in diabetes and have experience dealing with patients with similar problems. You serve as coach, educator, and medication management consultant, but don't forget that the patient is the locus of control and decision-making in the daily treatment of diabetes.

Cipolle, Strand, and Morley[3] discuss the concept of "caring through a therapeutic relationship." They define a *therapeutic relationship* as "an alliance between a practitioner and a patient . . . [that] is formed for the very specific purpose of meeting the patient's health care needs." They cited many characteristics of caring behavior and the vital components of the therapeutic relationship (**Table 2**).

Case Study

Let's consider the case of Mrs. Gonzalez. As you recall, Mrs. Gonzalez approached the pharmacy counter to speak to the pharmacist.

Mrs. Gonzalez:
"Hello, my name is Mrs. Gonzalez. I just talked to my physician, Dr. Thompson, and he said I have diabetes. He said I should come see you and together you, he, and I will sort it all out. Can you help me?"

Pharmacist:
"Hello, Mrs. Gonzalez. I would be glad to help you. My name is Jane Radcliffe. I work with many people with diabetes in our practice, and I would be happy to work with you as well. Do you have a few minutes now to meet?"

Mrs. Gonzalez:
"Of course."

Pharmacist:
"Let's meet in our counseling room. It will be more private, and we can both sit down and take notes." They proceed to the counseling room. Pharmacist Radcliffe unlocks a filing cabinet and removes a blank folder. "First, could you tell me when you met with Dr. Thompson and what he told you?"

Mrs. Gonzalez:
"Well, I saw him last week for my yearly physical, and he drew blood to just make sure everything was OK. Then he called me a few days ago and said my sugar was high and that he wanted to check it again. I went in first thing yesterday morning before breakfast, and he took

Table 2. Characteristics of a Caring and Therapeutic Relationship

- Mutual respect
- Honesty/authenticity
- Open communication
- Cooperation
- Collaboration between patient and practitioner
- Empathy
- Sensitivity
- Promotion of patient independence
- Seeing the patient as a person
- Exercising patience and understanding
- Trust
- Competence
- Putting the patient first
- Offering reassurance
- Confidence
- Paying attention to the patient's physical and emotional comfort
- Supporting the patient
- Offering advocacy
- Assuming responsibility for interventions
- Being willing to be held accountable for all decisions made and recommendations given

more blood. Then he called me this morning and said I had diabetes. I was so upset, but he said that if I came to see you, the three of us would work together to straighten it all out. Am I going to die?" Mrs. Gonzalez is getting quite tearful. "I don't know why I got this; am I eating too much sugar?"

PHARMACIST:

"No, you're not going to die. At least, not for a long time. It's true that diabetes is a serious disease, but we have a lot of evidence that controlling your blood glucose, or sugar, as you called it, greatly reduces the risk of complications. I'm here to teach you about living with diabetes, and you can call me anytime you'd like. Did Dr. Thompson give you any instructions?"

MRS. GONZALEZ:

"Well, he said not to eat any more sweets, and to schedule an appointment with you. Oh, he also said he wants me to get one of those machines that checks my blood sugar."

PHARMACIST:

"Well, why don't we talk about how we should address this. I would like to suggest that if you have about an hour today, we can talk for a while about what diabetes is. We'll cover some basic dietary instructions, and we can select a blood glucose meter. Then, if you're comfortable with continuing today, I can show you how to use your blood glucose meter, and we can schedule a follow-up appointment for next week. In the meantime, I'd also like to give you some literature to read about diabetes. What do you think about this plan?"

MRS. GONZALEZ:

"Oh, I feel much better. I was so alarmed when Dr. Thompson called, but it sounds like we're going to get along fine, and I think I can handle this now."

You can easily identify the elements of this encounter that helped the pharmacist establish a professional relationship with Mrs. Gonzalez. The pharmacist was friendly, introduced herself, and clarified her role, responsibilities, and accessibility. The patient was led to a quiet, safe, and private environment and encouraged to express her views. The patient could observe that the pharmacist unlocked a filing cabinet to begin a folder for record keeping and could take comfort that her records would be treated with confidentiality. As the pharmacist-patient relationship progresses, Pharmacist Radcliffe may request that Mrs. Gonzalez sign an informed consent form allowing the pharmacist to obtain critical laboratory and other data necessary to follow Mrs. Gonzalez's progress. The pharmacist suggested a plan and sought the patient's agreement, rather than dictating the course of events. A patient who agrees with a plan is more likely to participate.

Practice Example

Read the following case, and think about how you would handle this patient inquiry and begin to establish a professional relationship.

Mr. Jones approaches the pharmacy counter and asks to speak to the pharmacist. The pharmacist comes forward and observes an elderly, overweight African American man.

PHARMACIST:

"Hello, I'm the pharmacist. How can I help you?"

MR. JONES:

"Well, I just got these pills refilled," he gestures to his newly refilled bottle of furosemide tablets. "When I first started taking these pills I would take one every evening, even though my doctor said to take them in the morning. But I like to go to the race track in the morning, and I kept running to the bathroom. But taking them in the evening meant I was going to the bathroom all night, so I switched back to taking them in the morning. Everything has been fine for the past couple years, but over the past two or three weeks I notice that I have to get up to go the bathroom two or three times a night. I'm still taking these pills in the morning; do you think it's related to this medicine?"

How would you respond to Mr. Jones? What would you do to establish a professional relationship with this patient? When you have finished designing your approach, compare it with the scenario described below.

Obviously this is a discussion of some sensitivity, so the pharmacist should either invite Mr. Jones to step aside or into the counseling room. The pharmacist should also be prepared with a printout of Mr. Jones' medication refill history to evaluate possible drug-induced causes. The pharmacist will also need to collect, at the minimum, a problem-oriented database (i.e., a database pertinent to the patient's chief complaint) so the pharmacist can assess the patient's complaint and decide to make a recommendation or to triage the patient. In running through a mental checklist of precipitating causes of nocturia, the pharmacist must formulate a list of questions, some of which may be sensitive in nature.

One possible scenario is as follows:

PHARMACIST:

"I can see that this is really of concern to you, Mr. Jones. Why don't we step over here so we can both be seated and have a little privacy. Please have a seat while I pull up your medication profile so I can review it while we talk."

MR. JONES (moving to the semiprivate counseling area):

"OK, thanks."

PHARMACIST (returning with profile and pad in hand):

"Mr. Jones, so that I can evaluate your problem, I'd like to ask you for some additional information. Once I have that information we can decide on the best plan to treat this issue. Does that sound acceptable to you?"

MR. JONES (nodding):

"Sure, Doc, let's go. I'm anxious to get this cleared up."

Using sensitive, direct, open-ended questions, as described in unit 3, Interviewing, in the *Ambulatory Care Clinical Skills Program: Core Module*, the pharmacist asks questions to more fully evaluate Mr. Jones' chief complaint. On concluding this line of questioning, the pharmacist feels fairly certain that Mr. Jones' complaint is not related to his medications, a urinary tract infection, or prostatic hypertrophy. It occurs to the pharmacist that Mr. Jones may be at risk for type 2 diabetes, given his age, weight, and race.

PHARMACIST:

"Mr. Jones, did either of your parents have diabetes, or do any of your sisters or brothers?"

MR. JONES:

"Oh yes, my mother had diabetes; she got it when she was about 50 years old, and three of my four sisters have it. I thought I was lucky because I'm a man and never got it."

PHARMACIST (pulling out the ADA "Take the Test" risk assessment sheet):

"Well, let's look at your risk status for developing diabetes."

The pharmacist completes the risk test and determines that Mr. Jones is at high risk for developing diabetes.

PHARMACIST:

"Mr. Jones, I think you should see your physician in the next week to ten days. You have several risk factors that are seen in people who develop diabetes. You also have increased urination, which is a symptom of diabetes. Regardless, you should have this checked out. What do you think of this plan?"

This encounter illustrates how the pharmacist efficiently collected data to evaluate the patient's complaint, in an empathetic and confidential manner.

Summary

Type 2 diabetes is a serious chronic disease that is becoming increasing prevalent in the United States. There are many chronic complications associated with type 2 diabetes, and management of this disease is quite costly. Because most of the management associated with type 2 diabetes is carried out by the patient, what is left for health care providers is to provide diabetes expertise as well as support and encouragement for the patient's behavioral changes.

There are many opportunities for pharmacists to establish collaborative relationships with type 2 diabetes patients: identifying patients at risk for developing diabetes and serving as diabetes coach, educator, and pharmaceutical care provider.

As with any disease, the pharmacist should embrace strategies that put the patient at ease and pave the way for a mutually beneficial relationship.

References

1. Anderson RM, Funnell MM, Arnold MS. Using the empowerment approach to help patients change behavior. In: Anderson BJ, Rubin RR, editors. *Practical Psychology for Diabetes Clinicians*. Alexandria, VA: American Diabetes Association; 1996. p. 163–72.

2. American Diabetes Association. Screening for type 2 diabetes. *Diabetes Care* 1999;22(*Suppl* 1):S20–3.

3. Cipolle RJ, Strand LM, Morley PC. *Pharmaceutical Care Practice*. New York:McGraw-Hill; 1998. p. 19–26.

Self-Study Questions

Objective

Explain emotional and physical characteristics of ambulatory patients with type 2 diabetes that may affect the establishment of a collaborative patient-pharmacist relationship.

1. Explain emotional characteristics of ambulatory patients with diabetes that may affect the establishment of a collaborative patient-pharmacist relationship.

2. Explain a physical characteristic of ambulatory patients with diabetes that may affect the establishment of a collaborative patient-pharmacist relationship.

3. Explain how a patient's reluctance to make lifestyle changes affects the establishment of a collaborative patient-pharmacist relationship.

Objective

Describe the rationale and opportunities for establishing collaborative professional relationships with patients with type 2 diabetes.

4. Describe the rationale for establishing collaborative patient-pharmacist relationships with diabetes patients, and list three areas where patients would benefit from such relationships.

5. Mrs. Johnson is a 58-year-old African American female, 5'4", 185 lb, with a history of diabetes during pregnancy (which resolved postdelivery) and gout. What are her risk factors for developing type 2 diabetes?

6. Mr. Thomas is a 62-year-old male who was recently diagnosed with diabetes. His medication regimen is as follows: niacin for hypercholesterolemia, captopril for hypertension, and Robitussin DM for cough. How can Mr. Thomas benefit from a collaborative relationship with his pharmacist?

Objective

Design an effective strategy for establishing collaborative professional relationships with patients with type 2 diabetes.

Questions 7–9 refer to Mrs. Stonsifer.

The pharmacist is meeting with Mrs. Stonsifer, a 62-year-old female with diabetes. Her physician has asked that the pharmacist instruct Mrs. Stonsifer on beginning insulin therapy. Mrs. Stonsifer and her pharmacist meet in a private examination room.

PHARMACIST:
"Hello Mrs. Stonsifer. I am Joan Redding, the pharmacist for this clinic. Dr. Smith asked that I meet with you to teach you how to begin insulin therapy. Are you ready to begin?"

MRS. STONSIFER:
"Well, I can't say I'm crazy about the idea."

PHARMACIST:
"Don't worry, no one is crazy about the idea, but there's nothing to it. Do you want to learn to inject in your thigh or abdomen?"

7. How can the pharmacist assure the patient is in a quiet, safe, private environment?

8. What strategy could the pharmacist use to offer reassurance and support the patient?

9. How could the pharmacist facilitate a trusting relationship with a patient, which would hopefully optimize the patient's adherence to therapy?

Self-Study Answers

1. Because diabetes is largely a self-managed disease, a major goal of diabetes therapy is the need for patients to accept responsibility for their disease management and decide to change the behaviors that adversely affect disease outcomes. Most adults change behavior only when they feel a strong need to do so, not because someone tells them they must do so.

2. Diabetes is associated with significant morbidity and mortality, such as blindness, renal disease, nerve disease, heart disease, and death. The pharmacist continually strives to work with the patient to improve blood glucose control to minimize the development of these complications.

3. If a patient is unwilling to make lifestyle changes, the pharmacist's efforts are less likely to be successful. Diabetes is largely a self-managed disease.

4. A patient-pharmacist relationship can be mutually beneficial, given the pharmacist's skills and the potential benefits the patient can realize. Situations in which the patient could benefit from this relationship include identification of risk factors for diabetes, diabetes education to assure the patient follows the recommended standards of care for patients with diabetes, medication management, and nonprescription medication/diabetes-related supply counseling and/or provision.

5. age, race, obesity, and history of gestational diabetes

6. The pharmacist would discover during drug regimen review that niacin may cause hyperglycemia, a pharmacodynamic drug interaction; captopril may be causing the patient's cough. If the captopril were not the cause of Mr. Thomas' cough, and he required a cough suppressant, the pharmacist would ensure that the patient received a sugar and alcohol free cough suppressant product.

7. The educational session could be conducted in a private room, with the door closed. Teaching a patient to inject insulin can be a tense educational moment, and privacy is absolutely necessary.

8. The pharmacist could sympathize with the patient's concerns about injecting insulin, which did not occur in this case, as the pharmacist dismissed her concerns. It would be useful to allow the patient to express her needs or views. This also did not occur; the pharmacist limited the patient's participation to simply indicating her choice of injection site.

9. It is useful for the pharmacist to share his or her background in diabetes management with the patient at the beginning of an encounter. This facilitates the development of trust and ultimately enhances the patient's adherence to therapy. In this case, the pharmacist just stated that the physician asked her to meet with Mrs. Stonsifer. For all the patient knew, she was the first patient the pharmacist ever instructed to inject insulin.

Creating a Patient-Specific Database
Part 1: Specific Physical Assessment Skills

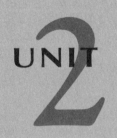

UNIT 2

Type 2 diabetes is a chronic illness that requires continuing physical and laboratory assessment to prevent and detect complications. This information is used to monitor patients' responses to medication therapy, including efficacy and adverse effects. Traditionally, pharmacists have obtained information about patients' vital signs, general appearance, and other physical assessment measurements from other health care professionals' assessments. Pharmacists taking expanded roles in ambulatory care settings are now performing physical assessment of patients.

In the *Ambulatory Care Clinical Skills Program: Core Module* you learned how to assess patients' vital signs and general appearance. In this unit you will learn physical assessment procedures important in the care of ambulatory diabetic patients, including how to perform a limited skin exam and a foot assessment. Although not covered in this unit, keep in mind the relationship between the patient's current pharmacologic treatments and physical findings.

After completing this unit, you may want to look through unit 4 of the *Ambulatory Care Clinical Skills Program: Core Module* and view the videotape again to review the techniques taught in that module. To gain further competence in assessment of physical parameters such as those taught in this unit, you must participate in an educational environment that includes repetitive hands-on demonstration and practice with trained educators.

Unit Objectives

After you successfully complete this unit, you will be able to:

- state which physical assessment procedures are routinely conducted for ambulatory patients with type 2 diabetes,
- explain the role of physical assessment information in planning for the pharmaceutical care of patients with type 2 diabetes,
- describe the correct technique for a skin exam,
- describe the correct technique for a foot exam, and
- accurately interpret the results of a physical assessment of an ambulatory patient with type 2 diabetes.

Unit Organization

To begin, this unit will review the physical assessment recommendations set forth by the American Diabetes Association. The technique for each physical assessment procedure, the information provided by each procedure, and its relevance to the pharmacist's pharmaceutical care planning process will be explained. We will focus on how the pharmacist can perform a limited skin exam, as well as a foot exam. Finally, you will learn how to accurately interpret results from the physical assessment of an ambulatory patient with diabetes.

Recommended Physical Assessment Procedures

Diabetes is associated with multiple complications whose presence can only be detected by a comprehensive physical assessment. The American Diabetes Association has made recommendations for both the initial and continuing care visits for the physical assessment of patients with diabetes (**Table 1**).[1]

Foot and skin screening will be covered in this unit; thyroid palpation, and the cardiac, neurological, and oral examinations are generally completed by other members of the health care team.

Weight and Height

You learned how to accurately assess a patient's weight and height in the *Ambulatory Care Clinical Skills Program: Core Module*. This assessment is very important and should be performed at every visit for patients with type 2 diabetes. Eighty to ninety percent of patients with type 2 diabetes are obese. Consequently, weight loss is an important goal in the management of the majority of cases of type 2 diabetes. Modest weight loss, even as little as 5–10% of body weight, will lead to improved insulin sensitivity and glucose uptake. Type 2 diabetes is caused by insulin resistance, which is usually a genetically determined insensitivity to insulin-mediated glucose disposal in peripheral tissues.[2] As the patient becomes more sedentary and his or her weight increases, there is less exercise-mediated carbohydrate disposal, and the body becomes more dependent on insulin-mediated glucose disposal. This increased dependence requires higher insulin levels to maintain glucose homeostasis. Eventually,

Table 1. Physical Assessment Recommendations for the Patient with Diabetes Mellitus

Initial Visit	Continuing Care Visit (Annual)	Continuing Care Visit (Every Visit)
Height and weight	Physical examination	Weight
Blood pressure	Dilated eye examination	Blood pressure
Ophthalmoscopic examination	Foot examination	Previous abnormalities on the physical exam
Thyroid palpation		Foot screening
Cardiac examination		
Evaluation of pulses		
Foot examination		
Skin examination		
Neurological examination		
Oral examination		
Sexual maturation (if peripubertal)		

Source: adapted from reference 1.

however, the ß cells of the pancreas become exhausted and fail, leading to decreased insulin secretion.

Weight loss will also have a positive impact on the patient's blood pressure and serum lipid levels. Exercise and medical nutrition therapy (MNT) are usually the first step in treating type 2 diabetes, with weight loss as a primary treatment goal. Even if a patient requires pharmacologic treatment to control blood glucose, exercise and MNT should be continued.

Perhaps as important as the patient's absolute weight is the distribution of adipose tissue. Patients who have more visceral than subcutaneous fat accumulation have a higher risk for insulin resistance as well as the entire constellation of findings commonly associated with type 2 diabetes, known as *cardiovascular dysmetabolic syndrome* (previously known as *Syndrome* X, the *Deadly Quartet*, and the *Insulin Resistance Syndrome*).[3] The cardiovascular dysmetabolic syndrome describes a set of findings that includes insulin resistance, obesity, glucose intolerance, hypertension, and dyslipidemia. Other abnormalities that may be associated with this syndrome include elevated serum uric acid, elevated plasminogen activator inhibitor 1 (PAI-1) levels, and atherosclerosis (especially coronary artery disease).

Obesity type can be determined by measuring the waist-to-hip ratio. Patients with increased visceral fat accumulation have more of an "apple" build if the circumference at the umbilicus (the narrowest point) divided by that at the pubic symphysis (widest point) is greater than 0.8 for women and 0.95 for men.[2]

The body mass index (BMI) is the measurement of choice to determine obesity. The BMI accounts for both the patient's height and weight (BMI = weight [kg]/height squared [m^2] = kg/m^2). **Table 2** illustrates how to determine a patient's BMI, based on his or her height and weight. In general, a person ≥ 35 years old is considered obese if he or she has a BMI ≥ 27. The BMI does not take into consideration a patient's body fat distribution.

Blood Pressure

An estimated 2.5 million Americans have both diabetes mellitus (types 1 or 2) and hypertension, with prevalence increasing with age.[4] The combination of hypertension and diabetes is highly significant because it is directly linked to increased morbidity and mortality. The risk of death from cardiovascular disease is approximately doubled with concomitant hypertension and diabetes, and the rates of strokes, transient ischemic attacks, and peripheral vascular disease are increased as well. Hypertension is associated with acceleration of diabetic retinopathy, the progression of which has been shown to slow with effective treatment of

Table 2. Determining Body Mass Index (BMI) from Height and Weight

Height (in.)	BMI (kg/m^2)

	19	20	21	22	23	24	25	26	27	28	29	30	31	32	33	34	35	36	37	38	39	40
58	91	95	100	105	110	114	119	124	129	133	138	143	148	152	157	162	167	172	176	181	186	191
59	94	99	104	109	114	119	124	129	134	139	144	149	154	159	164	269	174	179	184	188	193	198
60	97	102	107	112	117	122	127	132	138	143	148	153	158	163	168	173	178	183	188	194	199	204
61	101	106	111	117	122	127	132	138	143	148	154	159	164	169	175	180	185	191	196	201	207	212
62	103	109	114	120	125	130	136	141	147	152	158	163	168	174	179	185	190	196	201	206	212	217
63	107	113	119	124	130	135	141	147	152	158	164	169	175	181	186	192	198	203	209	214	220	226
64	111	117	123	129	135	141	146	152	158	164	170	176	182	187	193	199	205	211	217	223	228	234
65	114	120	126	132	138	144	150	156	162	168	174	180	186	192	198	204	210	216	222	228	234	240
66	118	124	131	137	143	149	156	162	168	174	180	187	193	199	205	212	218	224	230	238	243	249
67	121	127	134	140	147	153	159	166	172	178	185	191	198	204	210	217	223	229	236	242	248	255
68	125	132	139	145	152	158	165	172	178	185	191	198	205	211	218	224	231	238	244	251	257	264
69	128	135	142	149	155	162	169	176	182	189	196	203	209	216	223	230	236	243	250	257	263	270
70	133	140	147	154	161	168	175	182	189	196	203	210	217	224	231	237	244	251	258	265	272	279
71	136	143	150	157	164	171	179	186	193	200	207	214	221	229	236	243	250	257	264	271	279	286
72	140	148	155	162	170	177	185	192	199	207	214	221	229	236	244	251	258	266	273	281	288	295
73	143	151	158	166	174	181	189	196	204	211	219	226	234	241	249	257	264	272	279	287	294	302
74	148	156	164	171	179	187	195	203	210	218	226	234	242	249	257	265	273	281	288	296	304	312
75	151	159	167	175	183	191	199	207	215	223	231	239	247	255	263	271	279	287	294	302	310	318
76	156	164	172	181	189	197	205	214	222	230	238	246	255	263	271	279	287	296	304	312	320	328

Weight (lb.)

Body mass index (BMI) is the measurement of choice to determine obesity. BMI is a formula that takes into account both a person's height and weight. The unit of measure of BMI is kilograms divided by height in meters squared (BMI = kg/m^2). The table above has already done the conversions. To use this table, find the appropriate height (in inches) in the left-hand column. Move across that row to the given weight. The number at the top of that column is the BMI for that height and weight.

In general, a person age 35 or older is obese if he or she has a BMI ≥27. For people age 34 or younger, a BMI ≥25 indicates obesity. Obesity is an indication for further clinical evaluation.

The BMI measurement poses some of the same problems as weight-for-height tables. BMI does not provide information on a person's percentage of body fat or take into account the person's body fat distribution.

Source: adapted with permission from American Diabetes Association (ADA). ADA 1998 Clinical Practice Recommendations At-a-Glance, Tri-fold Pocket Chart. Catalog number, 5905-02; Alexandria, VA: American Diabetes Association; 1998

hypertension.[4] Control of hypertension has also been shown to reduce the rate of progression of diabetic nephropathy.[1]

Unit 4 of the *Ambulatory Care Clinical Skills Program: Core Module*, as well as the accompanying videotape, gives a very effective overview of the procedures used to assess a patient's blood pressure. Some considerations in assessing the blood pressure of a diabetic patient include:

- Blood pressure should be assessed at every patient encounter.

- Blood pressure may be labile in patients with diabetes, so multiple readings should be obtained over several weeks.
- Ambulatory 24-hour blood pressure measurements may help detect the absence of a nocturnal fall in blood pressure in elderly patients or patients who have developed diabetic autonomic neuropathy. Ambulatory 24-hour blood pressure assessment is performed using a noninvasive monitor that measures blood pressure at intervals over a

Table 3. JNC VI Classification of Blood Pressure (BP)

Category	Systolic BP (mmHg)		Diastolic BP (mmHg)
Optimal[a]	<120	and	<80
Normal	<130	and	<85
High normal	130–139	or	85–89
Hypertension[b]			
Stage 1	140–159	or	90–99
Stage 2	160–179	or	100–109
Stage 3	≥180	or	≥110

These categories apply when the patient is not taking antihypertensive drugs and is not acutely ill. When systolic and diastolic blood pressures fall into different categories, the higher category should be selected to classify the individual's blood pressure status. For example, 160/92 mmHg should be classified as stage 2 hypertension, and 174/120 mmHg should be classified as stage 3 hypertension. Isolated systolic hypertension is defined as systolic blood pressure ≥140 mmHg and diastolic blood pressure <90 mmHg and staged appropriately (e.g., 170/82 mmHg is defined as stage 2 isolated systolic hypertension). In addition to classifying stages of hypertension on the basis of average blood pressure levels, clinicians should specify presence or absence of target organ disease and additional risk factors. This specificity is important for risk classification and treatment.

[a]Optimal blood pressure with respect to cardiovascular risk is <120/80 mmHg. However, unusually low readings should be evaluated for clinical significance.
[b]Based on the average of two or more readings taken at each of two or more visits after an initial screening.

Source: reference 5.

period of time. The purpose of ambulatory blood pressure monitoring is to obtain data that reflect the cardiovascular state of the patient under conditions of everyday life. The blood pressure readings are stored in the monitor's memory and can be down-loaded to computer software for data analysis, creation of graphic representations, and printing.

- A thorough history and physical exam should be completed when hypertension is diagnosed to assess end organ damage from hypertension and to identify secondary causes of hypertension.[4]

The Joint National Committee on Prevention, Detection, Evaluation, and Treatment of High Blood Pressure published its sixth report in late 1997 (JNC VI). The blood pressure classification described in that report is shown in **Table 3**.[5] The goal for adults with diabetes is to decrease blood pressure to <130/85 mmHg.[1,5]

Ophthalmoscopic Examination

Diabetic retinopathy is a microvascular complication associated with diabetes mellitus, with prevalence strongly related to duration of disease. After 20 years of diabetes, >60% of patients with type 2 diabetes have some degree of retinopathy, which poses a serious threat to the patient's vision.[6] Because many patients have had diabetes for years before it is diagnosed, the American Diabetes Association recommends that all patients with type 2 diabetes should have an initial dilated and comprehensive eye examination by an ophthalmologist (or an optometrist knowledgeable and skilled in diagnosing diabetic retinopathy) shortly after being diagnosed.[6] Subsequent examinations should be repeated annually by an ophthalmologist or optometrist who is knowledgeable and experienced in diagnosing diabetic retinopathy and is well-versed in its management. The frequency of examinations may need to be increased as the retinopathy progresses.

Table 4. Dermatological Definitions

bullae: large vesicles, usually ≥ 2 cm in diameter

carbuncle: a necrotizing infection of skin and subcutaneous tissue composed of a cluster of boils (furuncles), usually caused by *Staphylococcus aureus*, with multiple formed or incipient drainage sinus

erysipelas: a contagious disease of skin and subcutaneous tissue caused by infection with *Streptococcus pyogenes* and marked by redness and swelling of affected areas, with constitutional symptoms

erythema: a name applied to redness of the skin produced by congestion of the capillaries, which may result from a variety of causes

furuncle: a painful nodule formed in the skin by circumscribed inflammation of the corium and subcutaneous tissue, enclosing a central slough or "core." Also known as a *boil.*

induration: an abnormally hard spot or place

macule: a general term for an area distinguishable by color or otherwise from its surroundings; a discolored spot on the skin that is not elevated above the surface

maculopapular: both macular and papular, as an eruption consisting of both macules and papule

morbilliform: resembling the eruption of measles

papule: a small circumscribed, superficial, solid elevation of the skin

pruritus: itching

Stevens-Johnson syndrome: the severe form of erythema multiforme in which, in addition to other symptoms, there is involvement of the oronasal and anogenital mucosa, the eyes and viscera. It may be fatal.

Skin Examination

Many skin disorders are associated with diabetes. These skin disorders fall within four categories: cutaneous markers of diabetes, cutaneous manifestations of diabetic complications, cutaneous complications of diabetic treatment, and cutaneous manifestations of associated endocrine and metabolic conditions.[7] Dermatological conditions commonly found in type 2 diabetic patients are defined in **Table 4**.[8]

The physical examination techniques used to assess the skin are primarily inspection and palpation. As discussed in the *Ambulatory Care Clinical Skills Program: Core Module*, begin your observation of the skin and related structures during the general survey. While inspecting the skin, note its color, presence of moisture or dry skin, the temperature (use the backs of your fingers to make this assessment), texture (roughness or smoothness), turgor, and lesions (anatomical location, grouping or arrangement, type [such as macule, papule, or vesicle], and color).

Cutaneous Markers of Diabetes

This category includes dermatological conditions that occur with a greater incidence among patients with diabetes, although they occur in the general population as well. Examples in this category include diabetic dermopathy ("shin spots"), diabetic erythema and rubeosis (rosy discoloration of the face), acanthosis nigricans (a velvety, papillomatous overgrowth of the epidermis, which is usually hyperpigmented), and vitiligo (patchy depigmentation of the skin, which is often symmetrical). An in-depth description of these conditions is beyond the scope of this unit, but the pharmacist should be alert for skin discoloration on any part of the body. As discussed in unit 4 of the *Ambulatory Care Clinical Skills Program: Core Module*, if any lesions are present, the pharmacist should identify their color, type (primary or secondary; macule, papule, or vesicle), configuration (e.g., clustered, linear, or annular [ring-like]), anatomical distribution (e.g., localized or generalized), and consistency (e.g., soft or firm). These findings should be reported to the patient's primary care physician.

Cutaneous Manifestations of Diabetic Complications

These dermatological abnormalities are associated with the chronicity of diabetes and include cutaneous infections (bacterial and fungal), autonomic neuropathy, peripheral neuropathy, and vascular and ischemic changes.

Glucose disposition from the skin is slowed in patients with chronic hyperglycemia, and this excess glucose serves as a medium for microbial growth. Additional abnormalities associated with chronic hyperglycemia include impaired leukocyte chemotaxis, phagocytosis, and bacterial killing. Bacterial infections that are seen to a greater extent among patients with diabetes include furuncles, carbuncles, styes, erysipelas, malignant otitis externa, and *Pseudomonas* infections in toe-web spaces or secondarily in a venous ulcer.

Candida infections are commonly associated with poorly controlled diabetes and may be a presenting symptom in undiagnosed patients. One of the most common manifestations is vulvovaginal candidiasis. Women complain of vulvular itching, an erythematous vulva, and a white, cottage-cheese-type vaginal discharge. This infection frequently either fails to respond to antifungal treatment or relapses until the diabetes is controlled. Another *Candida* infection is Candidiasis intertrigo, which occurs in intertrigonous skin folds, such as under the breasts, in the groin and axillae, or in the folds of abdominal skin.

Dermatophyte infections (most commonly caused by the pathogen *Trichophyton rubrum*) occur in both the diabetic and the general populations and respond well to traditional therapy (e.g., a topical imidazole antifungal cream, or systemic therapy if extensive). The infection is typically an erythematous lesion, often annular with a scaly edge. Common sites include the scalp, face, flexures, and interdigital web spaces.

Patients with diabetes may experience autonomic neuropathy as a complication. One of the manifestations of this is anhidrosis, a condition in which little or no perspiration is produced by the sweat glands of the feet and legs, leading possibly to drying and cracking of the skin. Acute or chronic hyperglycemia can also cause dehydration and subsequent dry skin if the patient develops severe or persistent polyuria.

Additional diabetes-related complications include peripheral neuropathy and peripheral vascular disease. When present in combination, the patient has impaired blood flow to the extremities as well as impaired sensation. If the patient loses protective sensation and develops an injury or ulcer subsequent to impaired perfusion, he or she is less likely to feel the associated pain, which can lead to undetected foot and leg ulcers that may be difficult to heal, cold feet, hair loss, and skin atrophy. Foot

and leg ulcers will be discussed to a greater degree in Foot Examination, later in this unit.

Cutaneous Complications of Diabetic Treatment

This category includes dermatologically adverse effects associated with insulin or oral antidiabetic therapy. Insulin allergy, characterized by generalized urticaria or bullae, dyspnea, wheezing, hypotension, tachycardia, diaphoresis, angioedema, and anaphylaxis, has been reported, although mostly with impure animal source preparations. Modern insulin administration of human insulin and lispro has made insulin allergy rare; allergic reactions most often occur after intermittent insulin therapy or in patients with increased circulating insulin antibodies.[9] As with insulin allergy, generalized reactions (such as pruritus, erythema, urticaria and angioedema) are also rare. Generalized reactions may occur soon after injection, may be delayed up to 24 hours after injection, or may be a combination of immediate and delayed reactions. Insulin-dependent patients who exhibit one of these responses should be referred to a specialist in diabetes and immunology.

More commonly, patients may experience local reactions to insulin administration, particularly during the first months of therapy. These reactions may include erythema, induration, and, occasionally, ulceration at the insulin injection site. Patients who experience local reactions should be switched to a purer form of insulin, have their injection technique reviewed, or, if the reaction persists, be referred to a specialist.

Patients receiving insulin should have their injection sites examined for lipoatrophy, which is loss of subcutaneous fat at the injection site that gives it a "hollowed-out" appearance. Lipoatrophy was more common with older, less-purified insulins and is rarely seen with today's purified and human insulins. Injection of purified insulin into the edges of the lipoatrophic area has been shown to reduce subcutaneous fat loss.

Lipohypertrophy, an increase in the amount of subcutaneous fat, can also be seen at the injection site. This increase is generally caused by repeated insulin injections at the same site, which cause a local lipogenic reaction. It is best treated by reviewing the patient's injection technique and recommending injection site rotation.

Improper injection technique may cause small, scar-type lesions at the injection site. If insulin is injected superficially (intradermally rather than

Table 5. Endocrine and Metabolic Conditions Associated with Diabetes and Their Cutaneous Findings

Endocrine or Metabolic Condition	Example Cutaneous Finding
acromegaly	thickened skin increased sweating
Cushing's syndrome	skin atrophy striae hirsutism
glucagonoma syndrome	necrolytic migratory erythema
hemochromatosis	"bronzed" pigmentation cutaneous signs of liver disease
hyperlipidemia	eruptive xanthomata
lipodystrophy (partial and total)	absence of subcutaneous fat
polycystic ovarian disease	acanthosis nigricans hirsutism

subcutaneously), a wheal may rise with each injection and result in scarring. The patient's injection technique should be reviewed and corrected (e.g., injection should occur at a 45–90° angle to the skin).

All patients who monitor their blood glucose should also have their fingertips examined for callus formation, or signs of infection, such as inflammation, redness, or drainage.

Oral sulfonylurea agents have been available for many years, and their ability to cause dermatological reactions are well known. The incidence of dermatological reactions is slightly higher with the first-generation oral sulfonylurea agents, particularly chlorpropamide (incidence, ~3%). Allergic or idiosyncratic dermatological reactions associated with the oral sulfonylurea agents include pruritis; erythema; and urticarial, morbilliform, or maculopapular eruptions. Erythema multiforme may progress to its most severe form, Stevens-Johnson syndrome. Photosensitivity reactions have also been reported with the oral sulfonylurea agents. These dermatological reactions may be transient and subside with continued administration, or they may require discontinuing the agent.[7,9]

The newer oral agents, including the α-glucosidase inhibitors, the thiazolidiones, metformin, and repaglinide, either have no significant dermatological reactions reported, or they occur at an incidence similar to patients in the placebo group in clinical trials.

Cutaneous Manifestations of Associated Endocrine and Metabolic Conditions

Although these manifestations will not be discussed in detail, some dermatological conditions are seen with endocrine and metabolic conditions associated with diabetes. These conditions are described in **Table 5**.[7]

Foot Examination

Foot ulcers and other problems are a significant cause of morbidity, mortality, and disability among patients with diabetes. According to National Institutes of Health (NIH) statistics, 67,000 people undergo diabetes-related lower limb amputation each year, costing the health care system $268 million annually.[10]

Three major abnormalities represent primary risk factors for the development of foot ulcers and amputation in patients with diabetes: peripheral vascular disease, foot deformities, and peripheral neuropathy. Patients with peripheral vascular disease have impaired perfusion of their extremities. Bone and joint deformities may cause abnormal distribution of pressure over bony prominences and increase the risk of ulcer formation. Finally, concomitant neuropathy may leave the patient unaware of any injuries or trauma to the extremities, possibly resulting in worsened ulceration and amputation.

Interventions to prevent this disease progression range from a simple foot inspection and patient education to complicated vascular surgery. The American Diabetes Association recommends that all patients with diabetes receive a thorough foot examination at least annually to identify high-risk foot conditions.[11] This examination should include an assessment of protective sensation, foot structure and biomechanics, vascular status, and skin integrity. Patients with one or more high-risk foot conditions should be evaluated more frequently to assess the development of additional risk factors. This evaluation can be performed by a skilled diabetes primary care provider or deferred to another qualified health care professional (e.g., a podiatrist). The American Diabetes Association also recommends that patients with diabetes have frequent foot screenings; this is one area the pharmacist may participate in. The foot screen consists of obtaining a history and performing physical assessment to evaluate the three risk factors for ulcers and amputation.

There are many excellent resources available for developing a foot screening and education process, but a particularly useful one has been developed by the National Institute of Diabetes and Digestive and Kidney Diseases (NIDDK), a branch of the NIH. The "Feet Can Last a Lifetime: A Health Care Provider's Guide to Preventing Diabetes Foot Problems" can be ordered by telephone (1-800-GET-LEVEL, or 1-800-438-5383), or the text and an order form can be downloaded from the NIDDK Web site at **http://www.niddk.nih.gov**, under "Health Information."

Objectives of the foot screen are to:
- quickly identify patients with current foot problems or those with a risk of developing foot problems;
- obtain information needed to diagnose a foot problem, develop a treatment plan, identify referral point, and schedule follow-up;
- document the level of foot deformity and/or disability;
- determine the need for therapeutic footwear;
- refer for or perform diabetes education; and
- compare future examinations with this baseline information.[12]

The NIDDK program provides a "Screening Form for Diabetes Foot Disease" (see **Figure 1**).

The first part of the foot screen is to obtain a good medical history of foot problems. The pharmacist should ask several questions to assess the patient's history of foot problems, including:
- Any changes in the foot since the last evaluation?
- Do you have a foot ulcer now or a history of foot ulcers?
- Do you have pain in the calf muscles when walking (e.g., pain occurring in the calf or thigh when walking less than one block that is relieved by rest)?[12]

The pharmacist should next observe the patient's feet. Are the nails thick, too long, ingrown, or infected with fungal disease? Does the pharmacist observe any obvious foot deformities, such as toe deformities (e.g., hammer toes or claw foot), bunions, or any bony prominences?

Using the pads of your index and middle fingers, palpate for pedal pulses, both the dorsalis pedis and the posterior tibial pulses. (**Figure 2**).[13] To palpate the dorsalis pedis pulse, feel the dorsum of the foot (not the ankle) just lateral to the extensor tendon of the great toe. If you cannot feel a pulse, explore the dorsum of the foot laterally. To palpate the posterior tibial pulse, curve your fingers behind and slightly below the medial malleolus (ankle bone) of the ankle. This pulse may be hard to feel in an overweight or edematous ankle.[12] Pulses may be described as normal, diminished, or absent. A numerical scale[12] may be used, from 0 to 4, as follows:

 0—completely absent
 1—markedly impaired
 2—moderately impaired
 3—slightly impaired
 4—normal

Be sure to palpate pulses in both feet and compare the intensity.

Some tips for taking pulses include:
- Keep your own body and examining hand comfortable. Being in an uncomfortable or awkward position decreases your tactile sensitivity.
- Place your hand in the proper location to palpate the pulse and linger there, varying the pressure of your fingers to pick up weak pulsation. If you cannot find the pulse, explore in the approximate area of where the pulse should be located.
- Do not confuse the patient's pulse with your

SCREENING FORM FOR DIABETES FOOT DISEASE

Name: _____

Date: _____

ID #: _____

I. Medical History

Check all that apply.

_____ Peripheral neuropathy
_____ Nephropathy
_____ Retinopathy
_____ Peripheral vascular disease
_____ Cardiovascular disease

For Sections II & III, fill in the blanks with an "R," "L," or "B" for positive findings on the right, left, or both feet.

II. Current History

1. Any change in the foot since the last evaluation?
_____ Yes _____
_____ No

2. Current ulcer or history of a foot ulcer?
_____ Yes _____
_____ No

3. Is there pain in the calf muscles when walking that is relieved by rest?
_____ Yes _____
_____ No

Figure 1. Screening Form for Diabetes Foot Disease

III. Foot Exam

1. Are the nails thick, too long, ingrown, infected with fungal disease?

_____ Yes _____

_____ No

2. Note foot deformities

_____ Toe deformities

_____ Bunions (hallus valgus)

_____ Charcot foot

_____ Foot drop

_____ Prominent metatarsal heads

_____ Amputation (specify date, side, and level) _____

3. Pedal Pulses *(Fill in the blanks with a "P" or an "A" to indicate present or absent.)*

Posterior tibial:

_____ Left

_____ Right

Dorsalis pedis:

_____ Left

_____ Right

4. Skin Condition (*Measure, draw in, and label the patient's skin condition, using the key and the foot diagram below.*)

C = Callus   PU = Pre-ulcerative lesion

U = Ulcer   F = Fissure

R = Redness   S = Swelling

W = Warmth   D = Dryness

M = Maceration

IV. Sensory Foot Exam

Label sensory level with a "+" in the five circled areas of the foot if the patient can feel the 5.07 Semmes-Weinstein (10-gram) nylon filament and "−" if the patient cannot feel the filament.

Notes

Right Foot

Left Foot

Notes

Figure 1. Screening Form for Diabetes Foot Disease (cont.)

V. Risk Categorization

Check appropriate item.

_____ Low-Risk Patient
All of the following:
Intact protective sensation
Pedal pulses present
No severe deformity
No prior foot ulcer
No amputation

_____ High-Risk Patient
One or more of the following:
Loss of protective sensation
Absent pedal pulses
Severe foot deformity
History of foot ulcer
Prior amputation

VI. Footwear Assessment

Fill in the blanks.

Does the patient wear appropriate shoes?
_____ Yes
_____ No

Does the patient need inserts?
_____ Yes
_____ No

Should therapeutic footwear be prescribed?
_____ Yes
_____ No

VII. Education

Fill in the blanks.

Has the patient had prior foot care education?
_____ Yes
_____ No

Can the patient demonstrate appropriate self-care?
_____ Yes
_____ No

Figure 1. Screening Form for Diabetes Foot Disease (cont.)

VIII. Management Plan

Check all that apply.

_____ Provide patient education for preventive foot care.

Date: _____

Diagnostic studies:
_____ Vascular laboratory
_____ Other: _____

Footwear recommendations:
_____ None
_____ Athletic shoes
_____ Accommodative inserts
_____ Custom shoes
_____ Depth shoes

Refer to:
_____ Primary care provider
_____ Diabetes educator
_____ Orthopedic foot surgeon
_____ RN foot specialist
_____ Orthotist
_____ Podiatrist
_____ Pedorthist
_____ Endocrinologist
_____ Rehab. specialist
_____ Vascular surgeon
_____ Other: _____
_____ Schedule follow-up visit

Date: _____

Provider Signature: _____

Figure 1. Screening Form for Diabetes Foot Disease (cont.)
Source: http://www.niddk.nih.gov/health/diabetes/feet/feet2/screenfo.htm

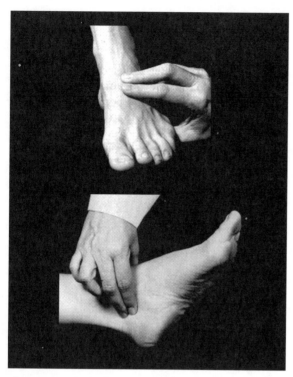

Figure 2. Palpation of dorsalis pedis and posterior tibial pulses
Source: reference 13

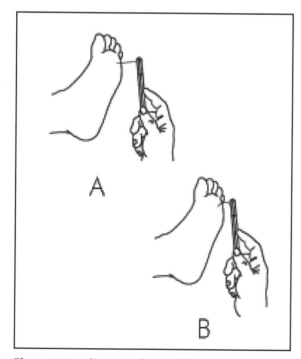

Figure 3. Application of monofilament.
A: Perpendicular application.
B: Application of sufficient pressure to cause filament to bend or buckle.

own pulsating fingertips. If you can't tell the two apart, count your own heart rate and compare it with the patient's (they are usually different). Your carotid pulse is convenient for this comparison.[12]

Next, the pharmacist should examine the skin condition of each foot.[12] If you observe any abnormalities, record each by drawing or labeling the condition on the foot diagram. Take note of calluses, pre-ulcerative lesions (such as blisters or hematomas), or open ulcers. Label areas that are significantly red, warmer that other areas, dry, or macerated (friable, moist, soft tissue).

For the next part of the exam, you will need a 10-gram sensory testing device (5.07 Semmes-Weinstein). This nylon filament is mounted on a holder that has been standardized to deliver a 10-gram force when properly applied. Patients who can feel the 10-gram filament when applied to selected sites on the foot have a reduced risk of developing ulcers. The foot screening instructions from the "Feet Can Last a Lifetime Kit" guide[12] are as follows:

1. The sensory exam should be done in a quiet and relaxed setting. The patient must not watch while the examiner applies the filament.
2. Test the monofilament on the patient's hand so he or she knows what to anticipate.
3. The five sites to be tested are indicated on the screening form (**Figure 1**).
4. Apply the monofilament perpendicular to the skin's surface (**Figure 3A**).
5. Apply sufficient force to cause the filament to bend or buckle (**Figure 3B**).
6. The total duration of the approach, skin contact, and departure of the filament should be approximately 1.5 seconds.
7. Apply the filament along the perimeter and *not* on an ulcer site, callus, scar, or necrotic tissue. Do not allow the filament to slide across the skin or make repetitive contact at the test site.
8. Press the filament to the skin so that it buckles at one of two times as you say "time one" or "time two." Have patients identify at which time they were touched. Randomize the sequence of applying the filament throughout the examination.

If you order the "Feet Can Last a Lifetime" kit from NIDDK, a monofilament device will be included. **Table 6** lists other sources from which monofilament devices can be purchased.

Table 6. Sources of Monofilament Device

Center for Specialized Diabetes Foot Care
P.O. Box 373
405 Hayden Street
Belzoni, MD 29038
(800) 543-9055
Single 5.07 (10-g) monofilament: $10.00

North Coast Medical, Inc.
187 Stauffer Blvd.
San Jose, CA 95125-1042
(408) 283-1900
Set of six assorted sizes: $124.95
Single 5.07 (10-g) monofilament: $24.95

Smith & Nephew, Incorporated
P.O. Box 1005
Germanton, WI 53022-8205
(800) 558-8633 or (800) 228-3693
Set of five assorted sizes: $99.75
Single 5.07 (10-g) monofilament: $18.95

Curative Health Services
14 Research Way, Box 9052
East Setauket, NY 11733-9052
(516) 689-7000
Single 5.07 (10-g) monofilament: $10.00

Sensory Testing Systems
1815 Dallas Drive, Suite 11A
Baton Rouge, LA 70806
(504) 923-1297
Single 5.07 (10-g) monofilament: $10.00

National Institute of Diabetes and Digestive
   and Kidney Diseases (NIDDK)
National Diabetes Information Clearinghouse
   (NDIC)
1 Information Way
Bethesda, MD 20892-3560
(800) 438-5383
http://www.niddk.nih.gov or
ndic@info.nih.gov

Based on these findings, the patient's risk of foot ulcers and amputation can be assessed. Patients are defined as low risk or high risk, and NIDDK has provided management guidelines based on these categories.

Low-risk patients are those who have none of the following: loss of protective sensation, absent pedal pulses, severe foot deformity, history of foot ulcer, or prior amputation. These patients should have a foot exam at least once a year, be instructed to purchase appropriate footwear, and receive appropriate education on preventive foot self-care.

High-risk patients have one of the five risk factors described above. These patients should have a foot exam every 3 months, be able to demonstrate preventive foot self-care, be under the care of a foot care specialist, be instructed to purchase appropriate footwear, receive appropriate education on preventive foot self-care, receive therapeutic shoe benefits from Medicare if appropriate, and have a "High-Risk Feet" sticker placed in their medical record.

You will learn more about educating patients about preventive foot self-care in unit 8.

Case Study

Let's revisit the case of Mrs. Gonzalez. On her follow-up appointment to your pharmacy, you complete your database of information and collect some physical assessment data. Physical findings include:

General appearance: Patient is a well-developed, overweight, Hispanic female who appears her stated age of 55 years old. She is alert and oriented to person, place, and time, although somewhat anxious. Patient has normal posture and gait, neat personal presentation, and normal affect and speech.

Height: 5'5"

Weight: 228 pounds

Waist: 40"   *Hips*: 42"

Waist/Hip Ratio = 0.95

BMI = 38

Blood pressure, left arm, seated: 152/100 mmHg

Heart rate: 92 beats per minute, regular rate and rhythm

Respiratory rate: 18 breaths per minute and regular

Temperature: 98.6°F with electronic thermometer

Skin exam: Skin normal color (Hispanic), texture, and turgor. No evidence of abnormalities, lesions, or edema, but patient reports three cases of vaginal candidiasis within the past year, of similar presentation.

Foot screen: Patient denies any foot problems or ulcers. She denies pain on walking. On exam, her toenails are normal in appearance and no foot deformities are noted. Dorsalis pedis and posterior tibial pulses are both normal. Skin of both feet appears to be normal. Patient had normal sensation on both feet in all areas assessed.

Based on the patient's general appearance, she is cognitively intact and mildly anxious subsequent to her conversation with her physician. No gross abnormalities are noted from general observation.

Given Mrs. Gonzalez's height, she is above ideal body weight. Her BMI of 38 indicates that she is obese, as she is over 35 years of age. Because she is obese, she probably has some degree of insulin resistance. She has an "apple build," which further supports the probability that she is insulin resistant and at risk for cardiovascular dysmetabolic syndrome.

Her blood pressure is above goal and would be classified as Stage 2, based on the JNC VI.

Although Mrs. Gonzalez has a normal skin exam, she has had three episodes of candidal vaginitis over the past year, which would indicate that she has had undiagnosed diabetes for some time.

Her foot exam is completely within normal limits, putting Mrs. Gonzalez at low risk for foot ulcer development or amputation at this point, although she should still be educated about proper foot care.

Practice Example

It's your turn to practice with Mr. Jones. As you recall, Mr. Jones is a 68-year-old African American man who was complaining about nocturia. Mr. Jones took the risk assessment test for diabetes and was found to have a high risk of developing diabetes. What physical assessment data would you collect on Mr. Jones? Write down what you would do. You will then be given a description of the findings for the physical assessment and be asked to interpret these findings. One limitation of a self-study format such as that used in this module is that you can only describe which physical assessment procedures you would do and how. To actually become accomplished at these procedures, you need to follow up

written instruction with experience examining patients under the supervision of a health care professional experienced in physical assessment.

You should have answered that the physical exam should include an assessment of general appearance as well as measurement of the following: respiratory rate, temperature, blood pressure, heart rate, height, weight, waist/hip ratio, BMI, and skin and foot exams.

The results of Mr. Jones' examination are as follows:

General appearance: Mr. Jones is a well-developed, overweight, African American male who appears younger than his stated age of 68 years old. He appears concerned about his health today. He is alert and oriented to person, place, and time. Patient has normal posture and gait, neat personal presentation, and normal affect and speech.

Respiratory rate: 16 breaths per minute, regular

Temperature: 98.8°F with electronic thermometer

Height: 5'8"

Weight: 240 pounds

Waist: 44"   *Hips*: 38"

Waist/Hip Ratio = 1.2

BMI = about 37

Blood pressure, right arm, seated: 152/98 mmHg

Heart rate: 84 beats per minute, regular

Blood pressure, right arm, standing: 140/90 mmHg

Heart rate: 92 beats per minute, regular

Skin exam: Skin normal color (brown) and texture. Patient shows moderate tenting and slightly dry mucous membranes. Skin appears to be generally dry. No evidence of other skin abnormalities, lesions, or edema. There are no other abnormalities located on the skin exam.

Foot screen: Patient denies any foot problems or ulcers. He denies pain on walking. On exam, his nails are longer than normal but otherwise within normal limits. No foot deformities are noted, but he does have a mild fungal foot infection in the skin fold of his little toe on the right foot. Patient also has a callus on the balls of both feet. Dorsalis pedis and posterior tibial pulses are slightly diminished on both feet and equal. Skin of both feet appears normal but dry. Patient had decreased sensation in both feet, missing two of the five areas assessed on the left foot and one area tested on the right foot.

Now interpret the findings for Mr. Jones before reading the interpretation presented below.

Based on Mr. Jones' height, he is above ideal body weight. His BMI of 37 shows he is obese. He probably has some degree of insulin resistance causing hyperglycemia. He has an "apple build," which further supports the probability that he is insulin resistant and at risk for cardiovascular dysmetabolic syndrome.

His blood pressure is above goal and would be classified as Stage 1, based on the JNC VI.

Mr. Jones' skin exam shows that he may be slightly dehydrated, as evidenced by the dry appearance of his skin and mucous membranes, poor skin turgor, and vital signs that reflect volume depletion. As you recall, Mr. Jones' initial complaint was increased urination, particularly at night. Loss of sufficient volume could account for the dry skin appearance, poor skin turgor, and vital signs.

Mr. Jones' foot exam is significant for both a foot infection and impaired sensation. The loss of protective sensation, as evidenced by his inability to feel three of the ten tests with the monofilament, puts Mr. Jones in the high-risk category. Based on this, he should have a foot exam every 3 months, be able to demonstrate preventive foot self-care, be referred to a foot care specialist, be instructed on appropriate selection of footwear, and have a "High-Risk Feet" sticker in his medical record.

Summary

Diabetes mellitus is a chronic illness with many potential acute and chronic complications. It is important to collect appropriate physical assessment data to prevent and detect these complications, as well as to monitor medication therapy. As pharmacists develop skills in this area, they are more likely to collect their own data, such as assessment of general appearance, vital signs, height and weight, and skin and foot exam.

Given the results from these assessments, pharmacists can appropriately triage patients and assess their risk for development of further complications.

References

1. American Diabetes Association. Standards of medical care for patients with diabetes mellitus. *Diabetes Care* 1999;22(*Suppl* 1):S32–41.

2. Garber AJ, Gavin JR, Goldstein BJ. Under-standing insulin resistance and syndrome X. *Patient Care* 1996;30:198–211.

3. Fagan TC, Deedwania PC. The cardiovascular dysmetabolic syndrome. *Am J Med* 1998;105(1A):77S–82S.

4. Hamaty M, Sowers JR. Antihypertensive therapy. In: Lebovitz HE, editor. *Therapy for Diabetes Mellitus and Related Disorders*. 3rd ed. Alexandria, VA: American Diabetes Association; 1998. p. 280–1.

5. The Sixth Report of the Joint National Committee on Prevention, Detection, Evaluation, and Treatment of High Blood Pressure. *Arch Int Med* 1997;157:2413–46.

6. American Diabetes Association. Diabetic retinopathy. *Diabetes Care* 1999;22(*Suppl* 1):S70–3.

7. Pickup JC, Williams G, editors. The skin in diabetes mellitus. In: *Textbook of Diabetes*. 2nd ed. Oxford, UK: Blackwell Science; 1997. p. 62.1–62.12.

8. *Dorland's Illustrated Medical Dictionary*. 26th ed. Philadelphia, PA: WB Saunders; 1981.

9. McEvoy GH, editor. *AHFS 98 Drug Information*. Bethesda, MD: American Society of Health-System Pharmacists; 1998. p. 2570–1.

10. National Institute of Diabetes and Digestive and Kidney Diseases Web site. Minor foot problems can cause amputations for people with diabetes. Available at: http:/www.niddk.nih.gov/new/releases/4-15-98.htm

11. American Diabetes Association. Foot care in patients with diabetes mellitus. *Diabetes Care* 1999;22(*Suppl* 1):S54–5.

12. National Institute of Diabetes and Digestive and Kidney Diseases (NIDDK). *Feet Can Last a Lifetime* program, 1998 edition. Bethesda, MD: NIDDK; 1998. Available at http://www.niddk.nih.gov under "Health Information." Accessed November 26, 1998.

13. Bates B. A *Guide to Physical Examination and History Taking*. 4th ed. Philadelphia, PA: JB Lippincott; 1987. p. 406–25.

Self-Study Questions

Objective

State which physical assessment procedures are routinely conducted for ambulatory patients with type 2 diabetes.

1. List the physical assessment procedures routinely conducted for patients with type 2 diabetes.

Objective

Explain the role of physical assessment information in planning for the pharmaceutical care of patients with type 2 diabetes.

2. Explain the role of height and weight assessment in planning for the pharmaceutical care of ambulatory patients with type 2 diabetes.

3. Explain the role of blood pressure assessment in planning for the pharmaceutical care of ambulatory patients with type 2 diabetes.

4. Explain the role of the foot examination in planning for the pharmaceutical care of ambulatory patients with type 2 diabetes.

Objective

Describe the correct technique for a skin exam.

5. Describe the techniques used in a skin exam.

6. What should be assessed during the skin exam?

7. What should be assessed when examining the fingertips of a patient who self-monitors for blood glucose?

Objective

Describe correct technique for a foot exam.

8. Explain the purpose and technique for visual inspection during a foot exam.

9. Explain the purpose and technique for palpating pedal pulses.

10. Explain the purpose and technique for determining sensation in the feet.

Objective

Accurately interpret the results of a physical assessment of an ambulatory patient with type 2 diabetes.

11. You obtain the following results from questioning and examining the skin of a patient with diabetes. She has had three episodes of vaginal candidiasis in the past year and has a candidal skin infection under her breasts. What is your interpretation of these results?

12. You obtain the following results of a foot exam. Patient complains of cold feet, has diminished pulses bilaterally, and shows decreased sensation using a monofilament. What is your interpretation of these results?

13. You obtain the following results of an injection site exam. Patient has areas in which the subcutaneous fat is increased where she has been injecting her insulin. What is your interpretation of these results?

Self-Study Answers

1. For the patient's initial visit, the following should be assessed: height, weight, blood pressure, and pulses. The patient should also receive a thyroid palpation and ophthalmoscopic, cardiac, foot, skin, neurological, and oral examinations.

   For continuing care visits, the following should be assessed: weight, blood pressure, and any previous abnormalities on the physical exam and foot screening. The patient should also receive a physical and dilated eye examination annually.

2. Eighty to ninety percent of patients with type 2 diabetes are obese. Patients who have a BMI >27 are considered obese, which indicates some degree of insulin resistance. This information will be useful when selecting the patient's pharmacologic and nonpharmacologic therapy.

3. The presence of high blood pressure in patients with diabetes is linked directly to morbidity and mortality. Patients with both hypertension and diabetes have an increased risk of death from cardiovascular disease, strokes, transient ischemic attacks, peripheral vascular disease, and retinopathy.

4. A very high number of patients with diabetes undergo diabetes-related lower limb amputation each year, at great expense to the health care system. A foot assessment or screening can identify patients at high risk for the development of foot ulcers that may require amputation. Part of the pharmaceutical care plan is health maintenance and interventions to reduce the risk of complications related to diabetes.

5. Physical examination techniques used to assess the skin are primarily inspection and palpation.

6. Skin color, presence of moisture or dry skin, skin temperature, texture, turgor, and lesions.

7. Observe for callus formation and signs of infection, such as inflammation, redness, and discharge.

8. It is important to inspect the patient's feet, observing for any evidence of foot deformities or peripheral vascular disease. Observe patient's nails, presence of foot deformities, skin condition including calluses, pre-ulcerative lesions, or open ulcers.

9. Palpating pedal pulses is important in assessing the presence of peripheral vascular disease. The dorsalis pedis pulse is on the dorsum of the foot, and the posterior tibial pulse is behind and below the medial malleolus. Pulses are rated normal, diminished, or absent, or graded on a four-point scale.

10. It is important to determine sensation in the feet because patients who have lost this protective sensation have an increased risk of undetected foot injury, which may lead to more serious foot complications. A 10-gram monofilament sensory testing device is used to apply force sufficient to buckle the monofilament in five distinct areas on each foot.

11. The patient's diabetes probably has not been in good control over the past year.

12. The patient is exhibiting signs and symptoms of both peripheral vascular disease and peripheral neuropathy. This puts the patient at high risk for the development of a foot ulcer.

13. The patient probably has lipohypertrophy, which occurs when repeated insulin injections at the same site cause a local lipogenic reaction. It is best treated by reviewing the patient's injection technique and recommending injection site rotation.

Creating a Patient-Specific Database
Part 2: Laboratory Data

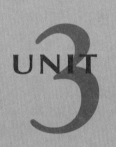
UNIT 3

In unit 2 you learned about performing physical assessments on ambulatory patients with type 2 diabetes. The remaining objective information to be included in the database is laboratory data.

Laboratory data are an essential piece of the initial and ongoing database used in the development, implementation, monitoring, and follow-up of a pharmaceutical care plan. These laboratory data are used primarily to assess the patient's degree of disease control and progression. Laboratory data may be used to assess the short-term or day-to-day control of diabetes (such as fasting or random plasma glucose) or long-term control, such as hemoglobin A_{1c}, which is a measure of blood glucose control over approximately the past 3 months. The hemoglobin A_{1c} could also be valuable information when determining a patient's adherence to his or her therapy regimen.

Other purposes for obtaining laboratory data when treating patients with type 2 diabetes include dosage calculations and assessment of patients' responses to drug therapy (both potentially toxic and therapeutic responses). Also, as the most important member of the health care team, patients need laboratory data to track their own progress in disease management.

In this unit, you will learn which laboratory data should be obtained as part of the initial patient database and which data are needed for continued monitoring. You will learn that laboratory data may be accessed from more than one source, and you will learn the reliability and meaning of each result.

Unit Objectives

After you successfully complete this unit, you will be able to:

- state laboratory tests commonly performed for ambulatory patients with type 2 diabetes,
- explain the role of laboratory data when planning for the pharmaceutical care of ambulatory patients with type 2 diabetes,
- explain unique considerations in choosing sources of laboratory data for ambulatory patients with type 2 diabetes,
- explain the unique requirements and considerations associated with conducting laboratory tests of ambulatory patients with type 2 diabetes,
- explain unique issues in appraising the reliability of laboratory tests required for ambulatory patients with type 2 diabetes, and

- accurately interpret laboratory test results for ambulatory patients with type 2 diabetes.

Unit Organization

For each laboratory test, you will learn its purpose, sources from which you may obtain this data, a description of what the data represents, and how to interpret the results. You will learn which tests the patient or pharmacist can perform versus which laboratory data will come from the physician or other sources. We will review the case of Mrs. Gonzalez and which laboratory data would be important in her care, and then you will practice by deciding which laboratory tests would be appropriate to order when developing a pharmaceutical care plan for Mr. Jones and how to interpret the results.

Commonly Performed Laboratory Tests

Before we discuss laboratory tests commonly performed for ambulatory patients with type 2 diabetes, it is appropriate to examine laboratory tests used to diagnose patients with type 2 diabetes.

You learned about the risk factors for type 2 diabetes in unit 1. Taking this a step further, the American Diabetes Association has developed criteria for testing for diabetes in asymptomatic, undiagnosed individuals who are at risk for developing type 2 diabetes.[1] These criteria include:

1. Testing for diabetes should be considered for all individuals $\geq$45 years of age and, if normal, should be repeated at 3-year intervals.
2. Testing should be considered at a younger age or be carried out more frequently among individuals who:
   - are obese ($\geq$120% desirable body weight or a body mass index [BMI] $\geq$27 kg/m^2)
   - have a first-degree relative with diabetes;
   - are members of a high-risk ethnic population (e.g., African-American, Hispanic-American, Native American, Asian-American, or Pacific Islander);
   - have delivered a baby weighing >9 lb or have been diagnosed with gestational diabetes;
   - are hypertensive ($\geq$140/90 mmHg);
   - have an HDL cholesterol level $\leq$35 mg/dl

Table 1. Diagnostic Criteria for Diabetes Mellitus

	Fasting Plasma Glucose[a]	Casual Plasma Glucose[b]	Oral Glucose Tolerance Test (OGTT)[c]
Diabetes[d,e]	≥126 mg/dl	≥200 mg/dl plus symptoms	≥200 mg/dl
Impaired Glucose Homeostasis[f]	≥110 and <126 mg/dl	N/A	≥140 and <200 mg/dl
Normal	<110 mg/dl	N/A	<140 mg/dl

[a]Fasting (as in "fasting" plasma glucose) is defined as no caloric intake for at least 8 hours. Fasting plasma glucose is the preferred diagnostic criterion.

[b]Casual (as in "casual" plasma glucose) is defined as a plasma glucose value assessed at any time of the day without regard to time since last meal.

[c]The OGTT should be performed as described by the World Health Organization, using a glucose load containing the equivalent of 75 g anhydrous glucose dissolved in water. Plasma glucose should be measured 2 hours postglucose load (2hPG). OGTT is not recommended for routine clinical use.

[d]In the absence of unequivocal hyperglycemia with acute metabolic decompensation, these criteria should be confirmed by repeat testing on a different day.

[e]If the patient is diagnosed by casual plasma glucose ≥200 mg/dl plus symptoms, be aware that classic symptoms of diabetes include polyuria, polydipsia, and unexplained weight loss.

[f]Impaired glucose homeostasis measured by fasting blood glucose is classified as impaired fasting glucose (IFG). Impaired glucose homeostasis measured by OGTT is classified as impaired glucose tolerance (IGT).

Source: data adapted from reference 1.

(0.90 mmol/L) and/or a triglyceride level ≥250 mg/dl (2.82 mmol/L); or

- on previous testing, had impaired glucose tolerance or impaired fasting glucose.

Factors leading to these recommendations include the steep rise in the incidence of diabetes after age 45, the unlikelihood of developing diabetes complications within 3 years of a negative screen, and knowledge of the well-documented risk factors for the disease.[1] The American Diabetes Association recommends using a fasting plasma glucose as the determining screen.

Some researchers have advocated the cost-effectiveness of opportunistic screening of all adults 25 years or older for type 2 diabetes.[2] If this were routinely implemented, diabetes would be diagnosed earlier and the lifetime incidence of complications might be reduced. At a minimum, we should follow the American Diabetes Association standards for diabetes screening because up to half of patients with type 2 diabetes remain undiagnosed and because many patients show signs and symptoms of diabetes complications at the time of diagnosis.[1]

Prior to June 1997, the diagnostic criteria used

for diabetes were those developed by the National Diabetes Data Group (NDDG) in 1979.[3] Under those criteria, a fasting plasma glucose of 140 mg/dl would diagnose type 2 diabetes. Using these criteria, however, 10–20% of patients had already developed complications of diabetes (e.g., retinopathy and coronary artery disease) by the time their fasting plasma glucose exceeded 140 mg/dl.[1,4]

The American Diabetes Association formed an international expert committee in May 1995 to review the diagnostic criteria and to propose new criteria if appropriate. After reviewing all the scientific data that had been accumulated since the initial guidelines were set down, in June 1997 the committee suggested new guidelines (**Table 1**), that have been accepted and endorsed by many organizations. The guidelines include diagnostic criteria for two additional classes as well: impaired fasting glucose and impaired glucose tolerance.[1]

As shown in Table 1, there are three laboratory tests that can be used to diagnose type 2 diabetes. Of the three diagnostic criteria, fasting glucose is preferred.

Let's look at an example of applying the

diagnostic criteria for diabetes. Mr. Johnson is in the medication refill clinic, complaining of symptoms of polyuria, polydipsia, and polyphagia. You recognize these as classic symptoms of hyperglycemia: an elevated blood glucose will spill into the urine at about 180 mg/dl or higher (depending on the patient's renal function). The osmotic effect of glucosuria causes polyuria, and if sufficient fluid is lost the patient experiences increased thirst. Patients who are not effectively using their glucose as an energy source (because it was eliminated via the urine instead of moving into the cells to serve as an energy substrate) may experience increased hunger. You order a plasma glucose concentration, which will be a casual plasma glucose value because Mr. Johnson had lunch 3 hours earlier. The result comes back as 238 mg/dl. Per the guidelines, this significant finding will need to be confirmed using one of the three diagnostic criteria. When the casual plasma glucose or oral glucose tolerance test (OGTT) is used as the first confirmation of diabetes, it is preferred that the fasting plasma glucose be the second confirmation. The confirmation must be on a subsequent day, so you ask Mr. Johnson to come to clinic 3 days later, first thing in the morning, so you can get a fasting plasma glucose. This value comes back as 152 mg/dl, confirming the diagnosis of type 2 diabetes.

Initial Laboratory Evaluation

Once the diagnosis of type 2 diabetes is established, there are other laboratory parameters that should be initially assessed. These values are included to help determine the degree of glycemic control and define associated complications and risk factors. The American Diabetes Association recommends the following laboratory tests[5]:

- fasting plasma glucose (or casual in undiagnosed patients);
- hemoglobin A_{1c};
- fasting lipid profile (total cholesterol, HDL cholesterol, triglycerides, and LDL cholesterol);
- serum creatinine;
- urinalysis (glucose, ketones, protein, and sediment);
- test for microalbuminuria;
- urine culture if sediment is abnormal or symptoms are present;
- thyroid function test(s) when indicated; and
- electrocardiogram in adults.

We've already discussed fasting and casual plasma glucose testing. Let's consider each of the remaining laboratory tests separately.

Hemoglobin A_{1c}

Adult hemoglobin is heterogeneous and consists of three minor protein components that may be correlated to blood glucose control: hemoglobin A_{1a}, hemoglobin A_{1b}, and hemoglobin A_{1c}. Each of these protein components are known to be elevated in patients with chronic hyperglycemia. The hemoglobin A_{1c} is the largest of the three (60–80%) and is frequently measured on its own.[6]

As with many proteins, when chronic hyperglycemia is present, glycosylation of hemoglobin takes place. In the red blood cell, glucose freely permeates from the plasma and attaches itself to the hemoglobin component in an irreversible fashion. The higher the blood glucose, the more glycosylation, and the higher the hemoglobin A values. Because the average red blood cell has a life span of 120 days, the hemoglobin A_{1c} (the hemoglobin A component used clinically) value can be considered a measure of blood glucose control during that time period. This value is a weighted average, however, with recent glycemic changes (e.g., the past 0–30 days) contributing more to the hemoglobin A_{1c} value than distant glycemic changes (e.g., 31–90 days). For example, the blood glucose level in the month preceding sampling contributes about 50% to the hemoglobin A_{1c} value, and the level of glycemic control seen 3–4 months previously only contributes about 10%.[6]

Glycosylated hemoglobin and hemoglobin A_{1c} can be measured by many different methods, including gel electrophoresis, isoelectric focusing, low-pressure and high-performance ion-exchange liquid chromatography (HPLC), immunoassay, affinity chromatography, and colorimetric procedures.[6] It is important to know whether the reported value is the total glycosylated hemoglobin or the hemoglobin A_{1c} component because there are different reference ranges for each. Another complication is the lack of standardization between assessment methods used to determine the hemoglobin A_{1c}. Efforts are underway to allow for calibration and standardization, probably at the manufacturing level. For now, it is prudent to use a single assay method, preferably from a single laboratory, to determine hemoglobin A_{1c} values in a cohort of patients. Ultimately, the goal is to have all laboratories standardize their glycosylated hemoglobin assays with those used in the Diabetes Control and Complications Trial (DCCT).[7] In this trial, the researchers were able to quantify the relationship

Table 2. Relationship Between Glycosylated Hemoglobin (HbA$_{1c}$) and Average Blood Glucose in the DCCT

%HbA$_{1c}$	Average Blood Glucose (mg/dl)
4	60
5	90
6	120
7	150
8	180
9	210
10	240
11	270
12	300
13	330

between glycosylated hemoglobin and the average blood glucose, as shown in **Table 2**.[8] Each 1% increase in hemoglobin A$_{1c}$ was related to a 30–35 mg/dl increase in average blood glucose. This type of correlation is only possible with standardized glycosylated hemoglobin assays, however.

At present, hemoglobin A$_{1c}$ is used as a long-term measure of glycemic control. The nondiabetic reference range is considered to be 4.0–6.0%; patients with uncontrolled diabetes may have a hemoglobin A$_{1c}$ reading of 15% or higher. The American Diabetes Association has stated that the goal hemoglobin A$_{1c}$ is $\leq$7.0%. This goal is mostly based on the results of the DCCT, a large clinical trial of patients with type 1 diabetes, which showed a significant reduction in diabetes-related complications among patients who achieved an average hemoglobin A$_{1c}$ of 7.2%.[7]

Some experts have suggested that hemoglobin A$_{1c}$ should be adopted as a diagnostic criteria for diabetes, or that at least it be used for patients whose fasting plasma glucose falls between 115 and 140 mg/dl.[9-11] At present, hemoglobin A$_{1c}$ is not used to diagnose diabetes, but it is obtained as a baseline and every 3–6 months thereafter.

Fasting Lipid Panel

Patients with type 2 diabetes are two- to fourfold more likely to die from coronary heart disease than patients without diabetes.[12] Hyperlipidemia is a significant risk factor in the development of coronary artery disease. It is important to obtain a baseline fasting lipid panel to assess risk status and track the efficacy of interventions. A lipid panel consists of a fasting serum cholesterol, triglyceride (TG), HDL cholesterol (HDL-C), and calculated LDL cholesterol measurements. The LDL cholesterol (LDL-C) is calculated using the following equation[13]:

$$LDL\text{-}C = Total\ Cholesterol - \left(HDL\text{-}C + \frac{TG}{5}\right)$$

Although patients do not need to fast for a total cholesterol assessment, they should be instructed to fast for 12 hours prior to having a total lipid panel drawn. Triglycerides measured without fasting for 12 hours are a reflection of triglycerides derived from endogenous sources (i.e., VLDL particles) and chylomicrons that carry fatty acids and cholesterol from exogenous sources (i.e., food). Chylomicrons are removed from blood after a 12-hour fast.

The American Diabetes Association recommends that a fasting lipid profile be performed at the initial visit for a patient with type 2 diabetes. Thereafter, adults with diabetes should have a fasting lipid profile done annually. If values fall in lower-risk levels (LDL cholesterol <100 mg/dl, HDL cholesterol >45 mg/dl, triglycerides <200 mg/dl), assessment may be repeated every 2 years. Any abnormal or borderline values should be repeated for confirmation.[14] When test results disclose abnormal values that require institution of drug therapy, the American Diabetes Association defaults to guidelines established by the National Cholesterol Education Program (NCEP) for repeat testing. The NCEP II guidelines[15] recommend the first follow-up determination should be made 6–8 weeks after initiating drug therapy (except for nicotinic acid; repeat measurements should be made 4–6 weeks after dose is stabilized, although nicotinic acid is not a first drug of choice in patients with diabetes). A second measurement should be done in another 6 weeks. After the goal LDL cholesterol has been achieved, repeat assessments should occur every 8–12 weeks for a year, and then annually (assuming the patient is still at goal and no toxicities have been noted), with interim assessment of the total cholesterol (if no hypertriglyceridemia is present).

Patients with diabetes commonly have an elevated triglyceride level and a decreased HDL cholesterol level. They may have an elevated LDL cholesterol in addition, although not necessarily

Table 3. Treatment Decisions Based on LDL Cholesterol Level in Adults with Diabetes

	Medical Nutrition Therapy		*Drug Therapy*	
	Initiation Level	LDL Cholesterol Goal	Initiation Level	LDL Cholesterol Goal
With CHD, PVD, or CVD	>100	≤100	>100	≤100
Without CHD, PVD, and CVD	>100	≤100	≥130*	≤100

Data are given in milligrams per deciliter. *For diabetic patients with CHD risk factors (low HDL [<35 mg/dl], hypertension, smoking, family history of CVD, or microalbuminuria or proteinuria), some authorities recommend initiation of drug therapy when LDL cholesterol levels are between 100 and 130 mg/dl. Caveats: 1) MNT should be attempted before starting pharmacological therapy. 2) Because diabetic men and women are considered to have equal CHD risk, age and sex are not considered risk factors. PVD, peripheral vascular disease.

Source: reprinted with permission from reference 14.

higher than nondiabetic patients. Type 2 diabetes patients may have a more atherogenic LDL cholesterol regardless of the total amount.[14]

Goals for lipid management for patients with diabetes are shown in **Table 3**.[14] The goal LDL cholesterol is ≤100 mg/dl for all patients with diabetes, with or without coronary heart disease. According to the 1999 American Diabetes Association recommendations, drug therapy should be initiated (after a trial of medical nutrition therapy) when the LDL cholesterol is >100 mg/dl in patients with a history of coronary heart disease, peripheral vascular disease, or cardiovascular disease, or ≥130 mg/dl in patients without a history of coronary heart disease, peripheral vascular disease, or cardiovascular disease. However, some experts recommend initiating drug therapy with an LDL cholesterol between 100 and 130 mg/dl, particularly in patients with multiple coronary heart disease risk factors (low HDL cholesterol [<35 mg/dl], hypertension, smoking, family history of cardiovascular disease, or microalbuminuria or proteinuria). Furthermore, the American Heart Association has noted that maximal medical nutrition therapy generally reduces LDL cholesterol by 15–25 mg/dl; therefore, patients with an LDL cholesterol that exceeds the goal by >25 mg/dl may be best treated with drug therapy at the same time behavioral therapy is implemented for high-risk patients (i.e., diabetic patients with a prior myocardial infarction and/or other coronary heart disease risk factors).[16]

Serum Creatinine

Creatinine is a byproduct of the breakdown of creatine and phosphocreatine in muscle. The amount of creatinine is fairly constant in an individual and is determined primarily by a patient's muscle mass or lean body weight. When creatinine is released into the plasma, it is excreted renally by glomerular filtration. Therefore, assessment of serum creatinine and the renal clearance of creatinine allows an approximation of a patient's glomerular filtration rate, or overall renal function. A normal serum creatinine is 0.8–1.5 mg/dl, although each laboratory will have its own reference range. As serum creatinine increases, the clearance of creatinine decreases, approximating a decline in glomerular filtration rate.

Many formulas can be used to approximate a patient's glomerular filtration rate. One popular equation is the Cockcroft and Gault formula, which correlates well with actual creatinine clearance in patients aged 18–92 with a serum creatinine <1.5 mg/dl[17]:

$$Cl_{cr} \text{ (for males) ml/min} = \frac{(140 - age)(body\ weight\ in\ kg)}{(SCr)(72\ kg)}$$

For female patients, the value calculated from this equation should be multiplied by 0.85. However, it is important to note two statements:

- This method should not be used if the last two serum creatinine values differ by >20%, and
- Lean body weight should be used in this

equation for obese patients or patients with ascites.[16] Lean or ideal body weight (IBW) can be calculated as follows[18]:

IBW in kg (males) = 50 + (2.3 × height in inches over 5 feet)

IBW in kg (females) = 45.5 + (2.3 × height in inches over 5 feet)

A normal creatinine clearance is 100–120 ml/min, and as renal function deteriorates, serum creatinine increases and creatinine clearance decreases. Nephropathy and end-stage renal disease are common complications of diabetes. Obtaining a baseline serum creatinine and calculating the creatinine clearance allows you to track the patient's degree of renal function and serves as a guide to dosage adjustment for medications that are highly renally excreted or even contraindicated for patients with impaired renal function. The patient's creatinine clearance should be calculated at the time of diagnosis. Although American Diabetes Association guidelines do not specify frequency, good clinical practice is to calculate creatinine clearance twice a year.

Urinalysis

Routine urinalysis for glucose, ketones, protein, and sediment should be performed initially and then yearly in adults. Analysis for glucosuria is useful as a screen; blood glucose monitoring is preferred for therapeutic decision-making (see the discussion on urine glucose monitoring later in this unit).

It is unlikely that a patient with type 2 diabetes would have ketonuria. Ketones of sufficient concentration to produce a positive response in testing reflect a disturbance in lipid metabolism. When a patient cannot utilize glucose as an energy source, the body uses fat as a fuel. During lipolysis, triglycerides are hydrolyzed to glycerol, which is broken down for glucose by the liver, and free fatty acids, including ketone bodies, which are waste products. The body can metabolize some ketones,

but with significantly increased ketone production the excess ketones are excreted into the urine. Patients with type 2 diabetes generally produce enough functioning insulin to prevent ketosis, but it may occur on rare occasions. Ketonuria in a patient with diabetes could represent the development of a serious complication, diabetic ketoacidosis, although this is rare among patients with type 2 diabetes.

During urinalysis the urinary sediment is centrifuged and examined for cells (desquamated urinary tract cells, epithelial cells, and white and red blood cells), casts (hyaline casts), crystals (calcium oxalate, uric acid, urate, phosphate, and carbonate), and oval fat bodies. These findings may indicate an acute complication (e.g., a urinary tract infection) or a chronic complication (e.g., renal damage). Further testing (such as a urine culture) may be indicated if white cells or urinary bacteria are detected.

Measurement of urinary protein is an important evaluation of glomerular function. With normal physiology a healthy glomerular membrane prevents most of the protein constituents of blood from entering the tubular ultrafiltrate because of the small size of the membrane filtration pores and a negative resting charge on the glomerular basement membrane. The small amount of the smaller molecular proteins that do get through may be reabsorbed by the tubules. Less than 0.1 g/24 hours is normally excreted, and this amount usually can only be detected in 24-hour samples.[19] As glomerular capillary pressure increases (because of systemic or glomerular hypertension) and the glomerular basement membrane loses negative charge, the early stages of microalbuminuria occur. With continued loss of negative charges and enlargement of the glomerular basement membrane filtration pores, albumin losses greatly increase.[20] Proteinuria is frequently quantified using a numerical scale such as that shown in **Table 4**.[19]

Table 4. Numerical Scale for Proteinuria Quantification

Protein Concentration (mg/dl)	Numerical Scale
<5	Negative
5–10	Trace
10–30	1+
40–100	2+
200–500	3+
≥500	4+

Microalbuminuria

Because of the high incidence of nephropathy among patients with diabetes, routine urinalysis should be performed yearly for adults with type 2 diabetes. If positive for protein, the amount of protein present should be quantified. If the urinalysis is negative for protein, the patient should be further tested for microalbuminuria (30–300 mg urinary albumin excreted in a 24-hour period).

Microalbuminuria may be screened using one of three methods:

- measurement of the albumin-to-creatinine ratio in a random spot collection;
- 24-hour collection with creatinine, allowing the simultaneous measurement of creatinine clearance; and
- timed (e.g., 4-hour or overnight) collection.[21]

The first method is the easiest to perform in an outpatient setting and provides accurate information.

Table 5 defines abnormalities in albumin excretion.[21] The American Diabetes Association recommends that two of three specimens should be abnormal over a 3- to 6-month period before diagnosing a patient with proteinuria. Variables that may transiently elevate urinary albumin excretion over baseline values include exercise within 24 hours, urinary tract infections, acute febrile illnesses, congestive heart failure, short-term hyperglycemia, and marked hypertension.[21]

Figure 1 illustrates the suggested process for routine urinalysis for protein and microalbuminuria.[21]

Thyroid Function Tests

Like stress, illness, and starvation, poorly controlled diabetes (both type 1 and 2) may be accompanied by alterations in the peripheral metabolism of thyroid hormones. If a patient with diabetes is exhibiting signs or symptoms consistent with hypo- or hyperthyroidism, assess the patient's thyroid function.

Electrocardiogram

Recommend an initial and annual electrocardiogram for patients with diabetes. As you have learned, cardiovascular disease is the leading complication associated with diabetes. However, many patients may have *silent ischemia*, the term used to describe ischemic changes in patients with no complaint of angina. It is important that you screen for silent ischemia prior to allowing a patient to begin an exercise program.

Follow-up Assessments

The American Diabetes Association recommends the following for laboratory evaluations during follow-up[5]:

- fasting plasma glucose (optional);
- hemoglobin A_{1c} (quarterly if treatment changes or patient is not meeting goals, and twice per year if glycemic control is stable);
- fasting lipid profile annually;
- urinalysis for protein annually; and
- microalbumin measurement annually (if urinalysis is negative for protein).

Blood Glucose

Based on the results of large studies, it is recom-

Table 5. Definitions of Abnormalities in Albumin Excretion

Category	24-hour Collection (mg/24 hour)	Timed Collection (µg/minute)	Spot Collection (µg/mg Creatinine)
Normal	<30	<20	<30
Microalbuminuria	30–300	20–200	30–300
Clinical Albuminuria	>300	>200	>300

Because of variability in urinary albumin excretion, two of three specimens collected within a 3- to 6-month period should be abnormal before considering a patient to have crossed one of these diagnostic thresholds. Exercise within 24 hours, infection, fever, congestive heart failure, marked hyperglycemia, and marked hypertension may elevate urinary albumin excretion over baseline values.

Source: reprinted with permission from reference 21.

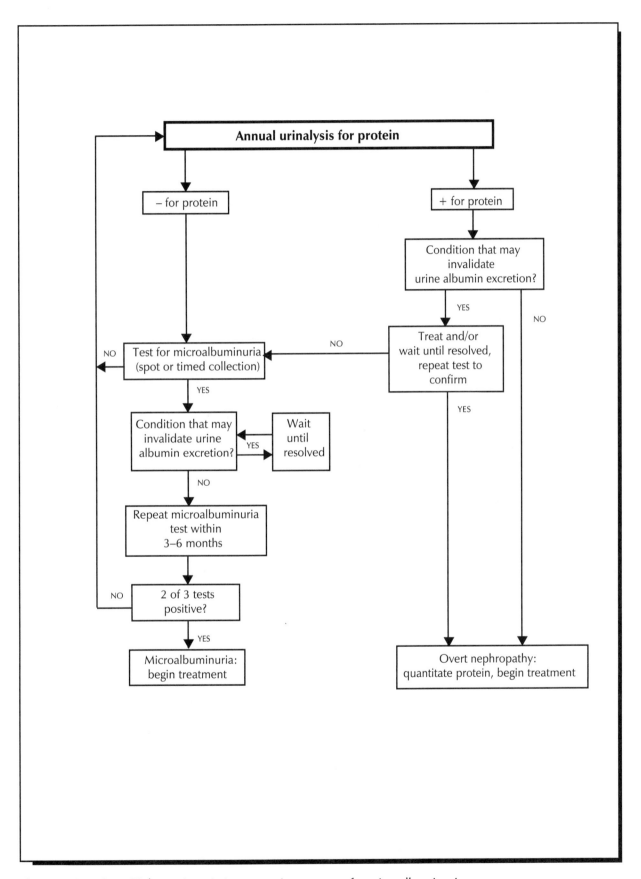

Figure 1. American Diabetes Association screening program for microalbuminuria
Source: reprinted with permission from reference 21.

mended that most patients with diabetes should attempt to achieve and maintain blood glucose levels as close to normal as is safely possible.[22] Monitoring blood glucose, in addition to other markers of glycemic status, is considered a cornerstone of diabetes care. As with all laboratory data, the results of blood glucose monitoring are used to assess patients' response to therapies and guide adjustments, as needed.

The majority of blood glucose monitoring following diagnosis is performed by the patient. Who should self-monitor blood glucose (SMBG)? The American Diabetes Association recommends that all insulin-treated patients self-monitor. Self-monitoring is also recommended for patients treated with oral agents (particularly with agents that can cause hypoglycemia [sulfonylureas and repaglinide, or combination therapy]) and for all patients not achieving glycemic goals. The number of times per day a patient should test his or her blood glucose depends on the patient's clinical situation and his or her willingness to test. The role of SMBG in the treatment of stable, diet-treated patients with type 2 diabetes is not known and may be a decision best left to the patient and the practitioner.

There are many blood glucose monitors available. **Appendix 1** lists all monitors currently on the market and their characteristics.[23] Several popular monitors are also depicted in **Figure 2**.[24]

Selecting a Blood Glucose Monitor

One of the most important considerations in selecting a blood glucose monitor is its accuracy (i.e., the extent to which the glucose values agree with the laboratory reference) and precision (i.e., the reliability of the test result or consistency of measurement).[25] The American Diabetes Association recommends strict criteria for monitoring accuracy (not to exceed 5% variance), although some consider the SMBG results acceptable and reasonable if they are within 15% of the reference method.[26] Current monitors have a high degree of accuracy if used and maintained properly. Patients and practitioners also need to know whether the monitor is calibrated to represent plasma or whole blood glucose. Concentration of plasma glucose (drawn from the patient's vein), which is assayed by the laboratory, is higher than a whole blood glucose concentration. You can calculate one value given the other using the following equation[27]:

Whole Blood Glucose (mg/dl) = Plasma Glucose (mg/dl) × 0.85

Conversely, you can determine the plasma glucose concentration by dividing the whole blood glucose concentration by 0.85.

Other features that vary between monitors include glucose testing range reported, time to complete the test, type of battery, how the monitor is calibrated, volume of blood required, size of readout display, correlation to plasma glucose, audible alarms (and ability to silence them), and data management capacity. Other deciding factors in purchasing a monitor may include availability of a voice synthesizer (One Touch II and One Touch Profile) for visually impaired patients, ability to open and manipulate the blood glucose strip container or foil wrapping, and ability to read messages in other languages (One Touch Profile has 19 language options).

Data management capabilities are present with several monitors, including the One Touch Profile, the Accu-Chek Easy, and the Precision Q.I.D. Not all patients will want or need this technology, but some patients like the feedback this data analysis provides, and improved metabolic control has clearly been shown among patients with type 1 diabetes.[28] For patients who do utilize this technology, several features in particular have been found valuable, including[29]:

- *Averages*—not only the average of all SMBG results, but averages for different times of the day (e.g., pre-lunch average).
- *Standard deviation*—how much variation there is in SMBG values. If the standard deviation is 60 mg/dl or less, this indicates blood glucose levels that are not too erratic; this would be considered good consistency. Consider two different examples: Mr. Holden has an average blood glucose of 180 mg/dl with a standard deviation of 100 mg/dl vs. Mr. Arrett, who has an average blood glucose of 260 mg/dl with a standard deviation of 40 mg/dl. Mr. Holden's high standard deviation suggests large fluctuations in caloric intake. On the other hand, Mr. Arrett's pattern of a high average with low standard deviation suggests a need for a change in his therapy regimen to better control his blood glucose.
- *Pie charts, histograms, frequency of data testing, and other features*—some patients and practitioners may find these features useful.

Another technology breakthrough that patients are eagerly awaiting is noninvasive blood glucose monitoring, which would not require a finger

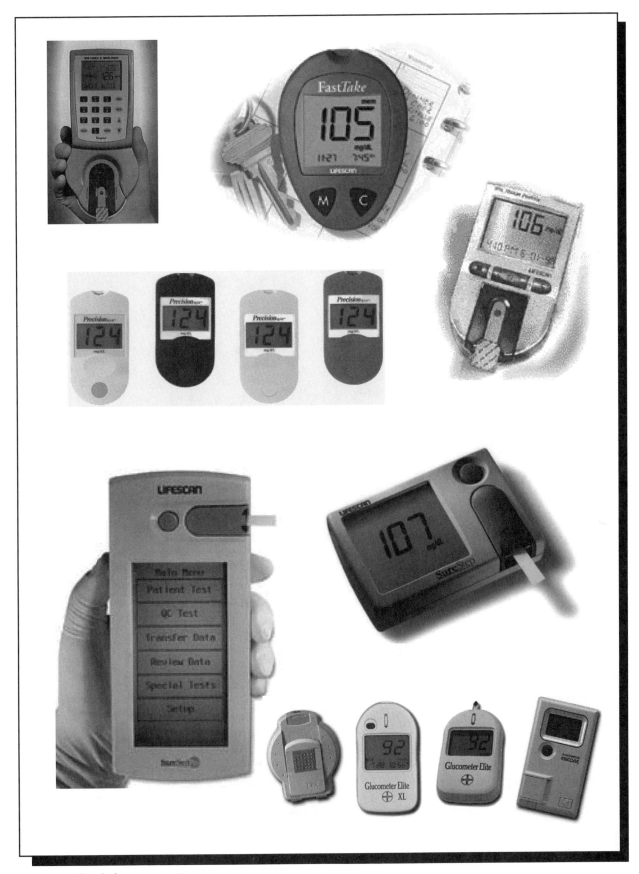

Figure 2. Blood glucose monitors

puncture. Not much has been published to date on the accuracy, reliability, and precision of the technologies under investigation. Within the next few years we may have an accurate, portable, and affordable system that does not require a finger stick, as this is one of the biggest complaints from patients.[30]

Teaching Checklist

Helping patients select the most appropriate blood glucose monitor and teaching them how to use it is a major role for pharmacists. Regardless of the type of monitor selected, we can consult a general teaching checklist with the educational aspects that should be covered for all monitors. Even if an appropriate blood glucose monitor is selected for a patient, if the patient does not use appropriate technique in maintaining and using the monitor, the results may be inaccurate. See **Figure 3** for an example blood glucose monitor teaching checklist.[24]

Fructosamine

One monitor available on the market for patient use can measure blood glucose as well as the patient's fructosamine level (Duet Glucose Control System, by LXN Corporation). Fructosamine is another example of a glycosylated protein that is a measure of blood glucose control on average over a period of time; in this case, 2–3 weeks. This frequency of measurement will enable patients to assess changes in their therapy regimen within a few weeks of implementation. The Duet monitor measures glycosylated proteins in micromoles per liter ($\mu mol/L$). **Table 6** compares average blood glucose, home fructosamine level, and hemoglobin A_{1c} level.[31] As

discussed earlier in this unit, it is important to note that these values are approximate, because home glucose meters and hemoglobin A_{1c} tests are not standardized. The manufacturer states that a reading below 310 $\mu mol/L$ is considered acceptable.[31]

Urine Glucose Testing

Although urine glucose testing strips are still available, their use is not recommended except for patients who cannot or will not perform SMBG. The information generated by urine testing is limited in its usefulness. Urine testing gives a delayed picture of blood glucose control, is not specific, is associated with poor technique, and does not permit detection of hypoglycemia.

The Pharmacist's Role in Laboratory Data Collection

Unit 5 of the *Ambulatory Care Clinical Skills Program: Core Module* includes a discussion of sources of laboratory data, including pharmacist-ordered and pharmacist-conducted laboratory tests. Laboratory tests that may be ordered by the pharmacist are more practice site specific than disease specific; any of the laboratory tests discussed in this unit may be ordered by the pharmacist in a practice setting that allows pharmacists this duty. Laboratory tests that the pharmacist can conduct related to diabetes care may include fasting or casual blood glucose assessment, hemoglobin A_{1c}, fructosamine, urine dip for gross urinalysis, urine microalbuminuria, and cholesterol. Be sure to follow the OSHA and CLIA

Table 6. Comparison of Average Blood Glucose, Home Fructosamine, and Hemoglobin A₁c (HbA₁c) Levels

Average Blood Glucose (mg/dl)	Home Fructosamine Level (μmol/liter)	HbA₁c Level (%)
300	475	12
240	400	10
180	325	8
120	250	6
60	175	4

Source: adapted with permission from reference 31.

Patient's Name:

Blood Glucose Monitor:

Quality Control	Taught	Learned
How and when to clean the monitor		
How and when to calibrate the monitor		
How and when to use the glucose control solution, and what the results mean		
How to appropriately store strips (store in original container or foil wrapping)		
Ability to manipulate/move monitor during testing process		
Meter storage		
Use of strips before expiration date		
Accuracy at high altitudes		
Finger Lancing	**Taught**	**Learned**
Wash hands well with warm soapy water to increase circulation		
Dry hands well to avoid diluting blood sample		
Do not use alcohol on fingertips (causes drying and cracking of skin)		
Dangle arm for 15–30 seconds if necessary to enhance blood flow		
Grasp finger to be used, apply pressure for 3–5 seconds in a firm stroking motion from the base of the finger toward the tip		
Keeping the hand down, prick either side of the fingertip and squeeze gently until a large, hanging drop of blood forms		
Do not milk finger vigorously; may damage blood cells		
Monitor	**Taught**	**Learned**
Review all features of the monitor (on/off, memory, calibration features, audible signal suppression, battery case, etc.)		
Describe when to turn on monitor (before or after strip insertion, or automatic)		
Describe whether blood sample should be applied before or after strip inserted into monitor		
Describe where blood sample is to be applied on the strip		
Describe size of blood sample required, and whether it needs to be placed directly on a specific area, or if wicking technology is used		
Describe how to know when the monitor has completed the assessment		
Describe where patient should record results, and what information should be recorded		
Describe whether blood glucose results are calibrated to plasma glucose readings or not		
Explain error messages, including what they mean and how to take corrective action		

Figure 3. Blood Glucose Monitoring Teaching Checklist

guidelines as described in unit 5 of the *Ambulatory Care Clinical Skills Program: Core Module*. When evaluating laboratory data, it is important to assess the information in light of the patient's other medical conditions and medication therapy.

Case Study

Now that we've discussed laboratory data necessary to follow a patient with type 2 diabetes, let's use Mrs. Gonzalez as an example. As you recall, Mrs. Gonzalez was referred by her physician because she was just diagnosed in the past few days with type 2 diabetes. In unit 2 we talked about what physical assessment procedures we should perform; now we need to decide what laboratory data would be useful in developing our pharmaceutical care plan for Mrs. Gonzalez. As we discussed earlier in this unit, the laboratory parameters that should be initially assessed for a patient with diabetes include fasting plasma glucose, hemoglobin A_{1c}, fasting lipid profile, serum creatinine, urinalysis, urine microalbuminuria, electrocardiogram, and urine culture and thyroid function tests, if indicated. Because Mrs. Gonzalez just saw her physician within the past week, and you know he did obtain some laboratory parameters, you have Mrs. Gonzalez sign a patient consent form, and you fax it to Dr. Thompson's office. You contact his secretary and determine that the following laboratory values were obtained:

February 9, 1998

Casual blood glucose	242 mg/dl
Serum creatinine	0.9 mg/dl
Total cholesterol	286 mg/dl
Electrocardiogram	within normal limits

February 18, 1998

Fasting plasma glucose	184 mg/dl
Fasting lipid panel:	
Total cholesterol	290 mg/dl
Triglycerides	280 mg/dl
HDL cholesterol	30 mg/dl
LDL cholesterol (calc.)	204 mg/dl

Our database is incomplete for the following laboratory data:
- hemoglobin A_{1c};
- urinalysis for glucose, protein, ketones, sediment; and
- urine microalbuminuria.

You are equipped with a DCA 2000+ from Bayer, which allows you to perform tests for hemoglobin A_{1c} and urine microalbuminuria in your pharmacy. You have a restroom off of your counseling room, so Mrs. Gonzalez can provide a urine specimen for both the urine microalbuminuria as well as a gross urinalysis using a dip stick.

The results you obtain that day are as follows:

February 19, 1998

Hemoglobin A_{1c}	10.2%
Urinalysis	positive for glucose, negative for ketones and protein
Urine microalbuminuria	negative

She did not complain of any symptoms suggestive of hypo- or hyperthyroidism or a urinary tract infection; therefore, further analysis in these areas was unnecessary.

Let's look at the data we now have. First, let's assess her glycemic control. Her casual plasma glucose was 242 mg/dl, and follow-up fasting plasma glucose was 184 mg/dl. Even though Mrs. Gonzalez did not come to her physician complaining of symptoms related to hyperglycemia, after you explained that increased thirst, hunger, and urination may be symptoms of diabetes, she shared with you that she had increased urination frequently in the evening, but she thought it was because she favored highly salted snacks (such as potato chips and pretzels) and drank a lot of regular soda because she was thirsty. Therefore, we agree with Dr. Thompson that the diagnosis is appropriate. Furthermore, a hemoglobin A_{1c} of 10.2% , while not a diagnostic criterion for diabetes, certainly demonstrates that she has had hyperglycemia for at least the past 3 months.

Her serum creatinine is 0.9 mg/dl, and her actual body weight is 228 pounds (103.6 kg). Using the equation for ideal body weight, we calculate 57 kg. Then, using the Cockroft and Gault equation, we can calculate that her creatinine clearance is 63.5 ml/min. Despite a normal serum creatinine, Mrs. Gonzalez is showing some decline in renal function, probably due to her age, as renal function declines after age 30.

Mrs. Gonzalez is hyperlipidemic, with an elevated total cholesterol, elevated triglycerides and LDL cholesterol, and an HDL cholesterol below goal. Goal LDL cholesterol should be <100 mg/dl, and HDL cholesterol >45 mg/dl.

Practice Example

It's your turn to practice with Mr. Jones. As you recall, on March 3, 1998, Mr. Jones was complaining about nocturia, and on evaluation of risk analysis he was found to be at high risk for diabetes. You completed your physical assessment of Mr. Jones and even checked a random whole blood glucose, which was 244 mg/dl. Mr. Jones' physician obtained a casual plasma glucose on March 18, 1998 that was 258 mg/dl and a fasting plasma glucose on March 23, 1998, of 190 mg/dl. His physician also obtained a urine culture, which was negative.

What additional laboratory data do you need for Mr. Jones?

The data you still require are hemoglobin A_{1c}, fasting lipid profile, serum creatinine, urinalysis, urine microalbuminuria, electrocardiogram, and thyroid function tests, if necessary.

Mr. Jones' physician refers the patient back to your pharmacy for monitoring. You had arranged for Mr. Jones to stop by a local laboratory on March 30 for a fasting lipid profile and serum creatinine. You also order liver function tests because of the patient's history of alcohol use. Mr. Jones is due back in his physician's office on April 1, 1998, for a physical examination and electrocardiogram. Mr. Jones does not exhibit any signs or symptoms consistent with thyroid alterations; therefore, thyroid function tests are not needed at this time. You have a DCA 2000+ Bayer machine, and on April 3, 1998, you performed a hemoglobin A_{1c} (11.6%) and urine microalbumin (35 µg/mg creatinine). You also did a gross urinalysis, which was positive for glucose and protein but negative for ketones.

Mr. Jones' laboratory work from March 30, 1998, comes back as follows:

Total cholesterol	290 mg/dl
Triglycerides	80 mg/dl
HDL cholesterol	45 mg/dl
LDL cholesterol	229 mg/dl
Serum creatinine	1.8 mg/dl
ALT	56 IU/L
AST	98 IU/L

His electrocardiogram from his physical on April 1, 1998, showed ischemic changes consistent with his history of angina and past myocardial infarction.

How would you assess Mr. Jones' laboratory data?

Mr. Jones' glycemic control clearly shows a diagnosis of diabetes based on a casual plasma glucose of 258 mg/dl with symptoms and a fasting plasma glucose of 190 mg/dl. His hemoglobin A_{1c} of 11.6% confirms that his diabetes is of at least 3 months duration (most likely longer) and is currently not controlled.

A serum creatinine of 1.8 mg/dl is above normal, and his creatinine clearance of 39 ml/min shows reduced renal function. He also has protein in his urine, a marker for continued renal decline. Mr. Jones' liver function tests are elevated above normal.

Mr. Jones has a history of angina, which is confirmed on electrocardiogram, and he has at least one significant modifiable cardiovascular risk factor, an elevated LDL cholesterol.

Summary

In this unit you have learned which laboratory data should be assessed initially for a patient with diabetes and which data should be monitored on a continuing care basis. Over the past several years, the role of pharmacists has expanded, allowing pharmacists to play more of a role in both ordering and directly performing laboratory data.

You have learned how to assess laboratory data for an ambulatory patient with diabetes and how this data affects the pharmaceutical care plan. Using the data you have collected in units 2 and 3, you are now prepared to develop a patient-specific database in unit 4.

References

1. The Expert Committee on the Diagnosis and Classification of Diabetes Mellitus. Report of the Expert Committee on the Diagnosis and Classification of Diabetes Mellitus. *Diabetes Care* 1999;22(*Suppl* 1):S5–19.
2. CDC Diabetes Cost-Effectiveness Study Group. The cost-effectiveness of screening for type 2 diabetes. JAMA 1998;280:1757–63.
3. National Diabetes Data Group. Classification and diagnosis of diabetes mellitus and other categories of glucose intolerance. *Diabetes* 1979;28:1039–57.
4. Sonnenberg GE. The new classification and diagnostic criteria for diabetes mellitus: rationale

and implications. *Wis Med J* 1998;97:27–9, 38.

5. American Diabetes Association. Standards of medical care for patients with diabetes mellitus. *Diabetes Care* 1999;22(*Suppl* 1);S32–41.

6. Pickup JC. Diabetic control and its measurement. In: Pickup JC, Williams G, editors. *Textbook of Diabetes.* 2nd ed. Oxford, UK: Blackwell Science; 1997. p. 30.1–30.15.

7. Diabetes Control and Complications Trial Research Group. The effect of intensive treatment of diabetes on the development and progression of long-term complications in insulin-dependent diabetes mellitus. *N Engl J Med* 1993;329:977–86.

8. Goldstein DE. How much do you know about glycated hemoglobin testing? *Clinical Diabetes* 1995;13:60–4.

9. Riddle MC, Karl DM. A_{1c} is our best outcome measure: let's use it. *Clinical Diabetes* 1996;14:79–82.

10. Peters AL, Davidson MB, Schriger DL, et al., for the Meta-analysis Research Group on the Diagnosis of Diabetes Using Glycated Hemoglobin Levels. A clinical approach for the diagnosis of diabetes mellitus: an analysis using glycosylated hemoglobin levels. JAMA 1996;276:1246–52.

11. Davidson MS, Schriger DL, Peters AL. An alternative approach to the diagnosis of diabetes with a review of the literature. *Diabetes Care* 1995;18:1065–71.

12. Kelley DB, editor. *Medical Management of Type 2 Diabetes.* 4th ed. Alexandria, VA: American Diabetes Association; 1998. p. 102.

13. McKenney JM. Dyslipidemias. In: Young LY, Koda-Kimble MA, editors. *Applied Therapeutics: The Clinical Use of Drugs.* 6th ed. Vancouver, WA: Applied Therapeutics, Inc; 1995. p. 9.11.

14. American Diabetes Association. Management of dyslipidemia in adults with diabetes. *Diabetes Care* 1999;22(*Suppl* 1):S56–9.

15. National Cholesterol Education Program. Second report of the expert panel on detection, evaluation, and treatment of high blood cholesterol in adults (Adult Treatment Panel II). *Circulation* 1994;89:1329–1445.

16. Grundy SM, Balady GJ, Criqui MH, et al. When to start cholesterol-lowering therapy in patients with coronary heart disease: a state-

ment for healthcare professionals from the American Heart Association task force on risk reduction. *Circulation* 1997;95:1683–5.

17. Al-Achi A, Greenwood R. Creatinine clearance: a pharmacokinetic parameter. *US Pharmacist* 1996;21:HS-2–HS-8.

18. Knoben JE, Anderson PO, editors. *Handbook of Clinical Drug Data.* 6th ed. Hamilton, IL: Drug Intelligence Publications; 1988. p. 10.

19. Treseler KM. *Clinical Laboratory Tests.* Englewood Cliffs, NJ: Prentice-Hall; 1982. p. 230–3.

20. Trevisan RM, Barnes DJ, GianCarlo V. Pathogenesis of diabetic nephropathy. In: Pickup JC, Williams G, editors. *Textbook of Diabetes.* 2nd ed. Oxford, UK: Blackwell Science; 1997. p. 52.1–.21.

21. American Diabetes Association. Diabetic nephropathy. *Diabetes Care* 1999;22(*Suppl* 1):S66–9.

22. American Diabetes Association. Tests of glycemia in diabetes. *Diabetes Care* 1999;22(*Suppl* 1):S77–9.

23. American Diabetes Association. *1999 Resource Guide.* p. 50–3.

24. Kirk JK, Rheney CC. Important features of blood glucose meters. *J Am Pharm Assoc* 1998;38:210–9.

25. Walker EA. Quality assurance for blood glucose monitoring: the balance of feasibility and standards. *Nurs Clin North Am* 1993;28:61–9.

26. Fleming DR. Accuracy of blood glucose monitoring for patients: what it is and how to achieve it. *Diabetes Educ* 1994;20:495–500.

27. Koda-Kimble MA, Carlisle BA. Diabetes mellitus. In: Young LY, Koda-Kimble MA, editors. *Applied Therapeutics: The Clinical Use of Drugs.* 6th ed. Vancouver, WA: Applied Therapeutics; 1995. p. 48–9.

28. Strowig SM, Raskin P. Improved glycemic control in intensively treated type 1 diabetic patients using blood glucose meters with storage capability and computer-assisted analyses. *Diabetes Care* 1998;21:1694–8.

29. Hirsch KB. How to use home blood glucose monitoring data most effectively. *Clin Diabetes* 1998;16:194–5.

30. Klonoff DC. Noninvasive blood glucose monitoring. *Clin Diabetes* 1998;16:43–5.

31. Dinsmoor RS. Home fructosamine test. *Diabetes Self-Management* 1998;15(3):23–5.

Self-Study Questions

Objective

State laboratory tests commonly performed for ambulatory patients with type 2 diabetes.

1. List laboratory tests commonly performed for ambulatory patients with type 2 diabetes.

Objective

Explain the role of laboratory data when planning for the pharmaceutical care of ambulatory patients with type 2 diabetes.

2. What is the role of a fasting plasma glucose when planning for the pharmaceutical care of ambulatory patients with type 2 diabetes?

3. What is the role of a serum creatinine when planning for the pharmaceutical care of ambulatory patients with type 2 diabetes?

4. What is the role of urine microalbuminuria when planning for the pharmaceutical care of patients with type 2 diabetes?

Objective

Explain unique considerations in choosing sources of laboratory data for ambulatory patients with type 2 diabetes.

5. Explain why the selection of a blood glucose monitor should be patient specific.

6. Explain why consistency in laboratory selection needs to be considered when choosing sources of laboratory data for ambulatory patients with diabetes.

7. Explain why the capacity for data management needs to be considered when choosing a home blood glucose monitor.

Objective

Explain the unique requirements and considerations associated with conducting laboratory tests of ambulatory patients with type 2 diabetes.

8. Explain why the patient's fasting status needs to be considered when obtaining a fasting lipid profile.

9. Explain why the patient's recent activities or physical presentation need to be considered when obtaining a urine protein in a patient with diabetes.

10. Explain why it is important to conduct an electrocardiogram in ambulatory patients with diabetes.

Objective

Explain unique issues in appraising the reliability of laboratory tests required for ambulatory patients with type 2 diabetes.

11. Explain the effect of patient technique when appraising the reliability of home blood glucose monitoring results performed by ambulatory patients with diabetes.

12. Explain the effect of home blood glucose monitor results being more than 15% different from plasma glucose monitoring results.

13. Explain the effect of using multiple laboratories to follow the hemoglobin A_{1c} of an ambulatory patient with type 2 diabetes and assuming hemoglobin A_{1c} correlation to average blood glucose values determined by the DCCT trial.

Objective

Accurately interpret laboratory test results for ambulatory patients with type 2 diabetes.

Consider the following patient case:

Ms. McLucas is a 70-year-old white female who had a plasma glucose drawn as part of a fasting SMA-7 at her doctor's office. The result was 142 mg/dl, and a second fasting plasma glucose a week later was 138 mg/dl. Her physician also ordered a hemoglobin A_{1c}, which was 9.4%. Her fasting lipid profile was: total cholesterol, 232 mg/dl; LDL cholesterol, 145 mg/dl; HDL cholesterol, 30 mg/dl; and triglycerides, 284 mg/dl. Serum creatinine was 0.8 mg/dl.

14. Based on Ms. McLucas' plasma glucose values, can we diagnose her with type 2 diabetes?

15. How would you interpret Ms. McLucas' hemoglobin A_{1c}?

16. How would you evaluate Ms. McLucas' lipid profile?

Self-Study Answers

1. fasting plasma glucose, casual plasma glucose, hemoglobin A_{1c}, fasting lipid profile, serum creatinine, urinalysis (glucose, ketones, protein, and sediment), urine microalbuminuria, urine culture if indicated, thyroid function tests if indicated, and electrocardiogram

2. used to diagnose diabetes initially, and to assess blood glucose control and response to therapy

3. Serum creatinine allows the pharmacist to calculate a creatinine clearance. This is an indicator of renal function, particularly glomerular filtration rate. This assists in determining the correct dosage of medications. The pharmacist can also use creatinine clearance to evaluate the appropriateness of medication dosages for those drugs that are dosed according to renal function.

4. A positive urine microalbuminuria is the first indicator of renal dysfunction in a patient. Patients with diabetes may develop nephropathy, a microvascular complication of diabetes.

5. Assuming equal accuracy among blood glucose monitors, there are several differences between monitors that may favor or discourage use by specific patients. These factors include: amount of blood sample required, ease of monitor use, size of readout display, data management capabilities, and audible alarm and voice synthesizer.

6. With the hemoglobin A_{1c} test in particular, laboratories are not as yet standardized to one reference source. Therefore, the next best thing is for a patient to consistently use one laboratory for their hemoglobin A_{1c} testing, and the laboratory will serve as its own reference.

7. Patients who are motivated to achieve tight blood glucose control and are interested in tracking and analyzing data related to their blood glucose control would benefit most from a blood glucose monitor that has these capabilities. They can track their average blood glucose values, standard deviation, pie charts, histograms, and frequency of testing.

For patients not interested in tracking data or for whom data management analysis is inappropriate, selecting a meter with these capabilities would probably not be a wise investment.

8. Chylomicrons are particles that carry fatty acids and cholesterol derived from the diet or synthesized in the intestines from the gut to the liver. These large, triglyceride-rich lipoproteins are increased after a meal, therefore the triglyceride measure would also be higher. By asking the patient to fast for 12–14 hours, the chylomicrons will have time to clear from the blood. This will allow for an accurate calculation of the LDL cholesterol.

9. Some things may elevate urinary albumin excretion over baseline values including exercise within the previous 24 hours, infection, fever, congestive heart failure, short-term hyperglycemia, and marked hypertension.

10. Patients with diabetes may have *silent ischemia*, which is ischemic changes due to damaged cardiac tissue without accompanying complaints of angina. It is particularly important that a patient have an electrocardiogram before beginning an exercise program. If a patient had silent ischemia and began an unapproved exercise program, the first manifestation of his or her cardiovascular disease might be dramatic, such as a myocardial infarction.

11. Patients who self-monitor blood glucose provide important information for their care. However, this data can be incorrect if the patient's technique in using the blood glucose monitor is incorrect. The patient must correctly calibrate, clean, and maintain the monitor to assure continued accuracy.

12. Plasma glucose values are higher than whole blood glucose concentrations. However, changes in treatment are generally not made based on one home blood glucose reading but rather observation and response to trends in readings (e.g., the glucose is generally elevated before lunch). If the blood glucose monitor is

significantly inaccurate compared to the true plasma glucose values, we are either not responding soon enough or seriously enough to blood glucose readings, or may be too aggressive. For home blood glucose monitors to provide useful information, the results must be accurate as well. Part of this is the inherent accuracy of the monitor and technology; another significant determinant of reliability is the user's skill.

13. There is no standardization between laboratories, and comparing serial hemoglobin A_{1c} values obtained from different laboratories does not give an accurate reflection of blood glucose control. At this time, laboratories are not standardized to the criteria used for hemoglobin A_{1c} determinations of patients in the DCCT; therefore, you cannot compare the hemoglobin A_{1c} drawn at one laboratory to the corresponding average blood glucose concluded from the DCCT laboratory.

14. Yes, she had two fasting plasma glucose values, on separate days, over 126 mg/dl.

15. At 9.4%, her hemoglobin A_{1c} is above the normal range of 4–6% and above the American Diabetes Association goal of 7% for patients with diabetes.

16. Ms. McLucas does not have a cardiac history, so her goal for LDL cholesterol is at least 130 mg/dl (or less). Her HDL cholesterol should be $\geq$45 mg/dl, and her triglycerides are above the goal of 200 mg/dl.

Appendix 1. Blood Glucose Monitors–
American Diabetes Association 1999 Resource Guide

Name and Manufacturer	Size (in.)	Weight (oz)	Test Strip Used[a]	Range (mg/dl)	Test Time (sec)	Battery
Accu-Chek Advantage (Roche Diagnostics)	3.6 × 2.3 × 0.6	3 with batteries	Accu-Chek Advantage or Accu-Chek Comfort Curve	10–600	40	(2) 3-volt lithium coin cell
Accu-Chek Complete (Roche Diagnostics)	4.8 × 2.8 × 1.1	4.4	Same as above	10–600	40	(2) AAA
Accu-Chek Easy (Roche Diagnostics)	4.5 × 2.5 × 0.7	3.4	Accu-Chek Easy Test Strips	20–500	15–60	Replaceable 6-volt alkaline (good for 1000 tests)
Accu-Chek Instant (Roche Diagnostics)	4.0 × 2.2 × 0.6	1.76	Accu-Chek Instant	20–500	12	(4) 1.5-volt alkaline
Assure (Chronimed)	4.8 × 2.4 × 0.9	5.3	Assure	30–550	35	1 J-cell (home change)
Checkmate Plus (Cascade Medical)	6.3 × 1.1 × 0.7	1.8 with batteries	Checkmate Plus	25–500	15–70	(2) 3-volt lithium (6–9 months, replaceable)
Diascan-S (Home Diagnostics)	3.1 × 5.2 × 0.6	4.8	Diascan	10–600	90	1 J-type (1500 tests, home change)
ExacTech (MediSense)	2.2 × 3.6 × 0.4	1.7	ExacTech	40–450	30	Permanent, no replacement required. 4000 tests
ExacTech RSG (MediSense)	3.5 × 2.1 × 0.5	1.4	ExacTech RSG	40–450	30	Permanent, no replacement required, good for a minimum of 4000 tests
Fast Take (LifeScan)	3.1 × 2.3 × 0.8	1.6	Fast Take	20–600	15	2 silver oxide #357 (1.5 volt, home change)
Glucometer DEX (Bayer Corporation Diagnostics Division)	3.2 × 2.6 × 1.0	2.8	Glucometer DEX test sensors; 10-test sensor in one cartridge	10–600	30	(2) 3-volt lithium (CR-2016)

Warranty (Years)	How Calibrated	Control Solution	Features
3	Snap-in code key	yes	No cleaning, wiping, or timing. Two steps to a result. Touchable test strips. Insufficient sample size detection; more blood can be applied if a sufficient sample isn't applied at first. 100-value memory with time and date.
3	Snap-in code key	yes	No cleaning, wiping, or timing. Large memory that collects, stores, and analyzes up to 1000 values. Records information such as blood glucose, insulin, carbohydrates, ketones, hemoglobin A_{1c}, stress, and exercise.
3	Snap-in code key	yes	Absorbent test strips with target area for easy dosing outside of the monitor. No timing or wiping of test strips. Large display; 350-value memory with time and date. 14 event codes, 7-day averaging, maximum and minimum values. Comes with carrying case and supplies, including test strips, lancet device, and control solutions.
3	Rocker button coding	yes	Uses fast-acting strip chemistry. Simple two-step procedure. No wiping or timing. Test strips provide visual backup. Nine-value memory. Temperature-warning icon marks test results outside normal operating range. Comes with carrying case and supplies, including test strips, adjustable lancet device, and control solutions.
3	Calibrator in each box of strips	yes	Data management system; biosensor technology; 180-test memory; large touch screen display.
Lifetime	Automatic calibration	yes	Display provides words for guidance. Lancing device built in. No wiping, blotting, or timing. Automatic hematocrit and temperature correction. Automatic sample volume check. Stores up to 255 results with time and date and insulin type and dosage. Average glucose reading. Clock with four alarms. Dataport allows downloading to PC. Prompts in six languages. Hands-off lancet ejection.
2	Button calibration (with safety lock) by lot of test strips	yes	Procedure requires no hanging drop of blood; extreme temperature warnings, below 41°F reads *cold* (home change) and above 98° F reads *hot*. Confidence strip supplied. Technique error notification. Automatic memory of last 10 readings. Audio signal emitted during test process can be turned off.
4	Calibrator in each box of strips	yes	Credit card size and shape; simple three-step testing procedure; biosensor technology; no cleaning, wiping, or timing; value-priced test strips; last-reading recall and calibration code.
4	Calibrator in each box of strips	yes	Better accuracy; less cost; requires no calibration or coding; simple three-step testing procedure; value-priced test strips; biosensor technology; no cleaning or maintenance required.
3	Built-in single button	yes	Smallest blood sample; fast test time; compact; 150-test memory with date and time; touchable test strip; near-monitor dosing; 14-day averaging excludes flagged control solution test; warning to check ketones from 240–600 mg/dl.
5	Automatic calibration	yes, three levels	Cartridge-based monitor eliminates strip handling. Performs 10 tests without reloading. Cartridge automatically calibrates monitor for 10 tests. Electronic functions automatically validated. Sensor actively draws just the amount of blood it needs. Advanced data management. Download memory for PC tracking. Monitor stores up to 100 results with time, date, and averages.

continued on next page

Appendix 1. Blood Glucose Monitors (cont.)
American Diabetes Association 1999 Resource Guide

Name and Manufacturer	Size (in.)	Weight (oz)	Test Strip Used[a]	Range (mg/dl)	Test Time (sec)	Battery
Glucometer Elite Diabetes Care System (Bayer Corporation, Diagnostics Division)	3.4 × 2.5 × 0.5	1.75	Glucometer Elite	20–600	30	(2) 3-volt lithium
Glucometer Encore Diabetes Care System (Bayer Corporation, Diagnostics Division)	4.3 × 2.5 × 0.7	3.6	Glucometer Encore	10–600	15	Permanent, 5-yr warranty
MediSense 2 Card (MediSense)	3.6 × 2.2 × 0.4	1.7	MediSense 2 or Precision Q.I.D.	20–600	20	Permanent, no replacement req., 4000 tests
MediSense 2 Pen (MediSense)	5.4 × 0.4	1.1	MediSense 2 or Precision Q.I.D.	20–600	20	Permanent, no replacement req., 4000 tests
One Touch Basic (LifeScan)	4.8 × 2.6 × 1.1	4.8	Genuine One Touch	0–600	45	1 J-type (6V) alkaline (home change)
One Touch Profile (LifeScan)	4.3 × 2.6 × 1.2	4.5	Genuine One Touch	0–600	45	2 AAA alkaline (home change)
PocketLab II (Clinical Diagnostics)	4.9 × 2.1 × 0.7	2.2 with batteries	PocketLab II	40–450	45	1.55 volt (silver oxide) Eveready # 357
Precision Q.I.D. (MediSense)	3.6 × 2.2 × 0.4	1.5	Precision Q.I.D.	20–600	20	Permanent, no replacement req., min. of 4000 tests
Precision Q.I.D. Pen (MediSense)	5.4 × 0.4	1.1	Precision Q.I.D.	20–600	20	Permanent, no replacement req.
Prestige (Home Diagnostics)	4.5 × 3.1 × 1.3	4.4	Prestige	25–600	10	6-volt J-cell
Select GT (Chronimed)	4.8 × 2.5 × 1.3	4.7	Select GT	30–600	50	1 J-cell (home change)
Supreme II (Chronimed)	4.8 × 2.5 × 1.3	4.7	Supreme	30–600	50	1 J-cell (home change)
SureStep (LifeScan)	3.5 × 2.4 × 0.8	3.8	SureStep	0–500	15–30	(2) AAA Alkaline (home change)

[a] These are test strips approved by the manufacturers. In some cases, manufacturers cannot guarantee results or provide assistance if any other test strips are used.

Warranty (Years)	How Calibrated	Control Solution	Features
5	Strip calibration	yes	No buttons; turned on when test strip is inserted. Blood touched to the tip of the test strip is automatically drawn into the test chamber. Twenty-test memory and a 3-minute automatic shutoff. Kit includes: blood-letting device and lancets, 10 test strips, carrying case, control solution, and log book. Videotape on request.
3	Single button calibration by lot of test strips	yes	Automatic shutoff in 3 minutes. Stores up to 10 results. Includes carrying case, control solution, 10 test strips, and lancets. Spanish instructions available.
4	Calibrator in each box of strips	yes	Provides all the same features as the MediSense 2 Pen Sensor. Credit card size; extra large display window. Uses same sensor test strips.
4	Calibrator in each box of strips	yes	Biosensor technology; automatic start with "hands-off" testing; no cleaning, no wiping, no blotting, no timing; pen size; extended memory; individually wrapped test strips.
3	Built-in single button	yes	No timing or wiping; large display; English or Spanish; detects most errors in sample application; notifies you when the monitor must be cleaned; recalls your last test result; has 30-day, money-back guarantee.
5	Built-in single button	yes	Three-step testing with no timing, wiping, or blotting; large display in English, Spanish, or 17 other languages; notifies you when the monitor must be cleaned; automatically stores last 250 results with date and time; provides a 14- and 30-day test average; insulin programming; event labeling.
Lifetime	Automatic calibration	yes	No wiping; one-button operation; large display; stores 40 results in memory. Complete starter kit available including 10 strips, a lancing device, lancets, control solution, a quickstart guide in six languages, and a log book. Monitor-only package also available.
4	Calibrator in each box of test strips	yes	Eliminates common test errors for clinical accuracy in everyday monitoring. Advanced biosensor technology; simple two-step testing; only requires 2.5 µl of blood; auto-starts when sample is detected; compact size; can apply second blood drop; not affected by many common medications; large display window; data down-loading capability; easy recall of last 10 test results.
4 yr or 4000 tests	Calibrator in each box of test strips	Precision QID high/low & norm. control solution	Identical features and benefits as the Precision Q.I.D. hand-held monitor, but in the shape of a pen for portability. Advanced biosensor technology; only requires 3.5 µl of blood. Auto-starts when sample is detected. Ability to add a second drop of blood if necessary. Not affected by common medications; data-downloading capability; recall of last 10 test results.
2	Button	yes	Non-wipe system allows user to apply the blood to test strip outside or inside the monitor; absorbable strip with sample-size verification; extreme temperature warnings; large digital display; universal symbols to guide user through test; videocassettes available in English and Spanish.
3	Built-in single button	yes	Large display; universal symbols; absorbent test strip; blood can be applied to test strip inside or outside of the monitor; 100-test memory.
3	Built-in single button	yes	Large display; universal symbols; absorbent test strip; blood can be applied to test strip inside or outside of the monitor; 100-test memory.
3	Built-in single button	yes	Large display; universal symbols; touchable, absorbent test strip allows maximum flexibility in blood application; blue confirmation dot confirms adequate blood sample; 10-test memory.

Source: reprinted with permission from American Diabetes Association. *1999 Resource Guide;* p. 50–3.

Creating a Patient-Specific Database
Part 3: Generating the Database

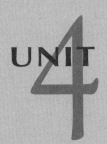

UNIT 4

You know how to establish a professional relationship with a patient and how to find and collect or generate patient-specific information. Drawing on what you learned from the *Ambulatory Care Clinical Skills Program: Core Module*, and units 1–3 of this module, you can now answer the question, "How can I generate a patient-specific database that will help me make appropriate therapy decisions?"

Unit Objective

After you successfully complete this unit, you will be able to generate a patient-specific database for a patient with type 2 diabetes.

Unit Organization

Using a diabetes patient as an example, we will focus on collecting information needed for the database in each of the following categories: demographic, administrative, medical, behavioral/lifestyle, drug therapy, social/economic/quality of life, and personal limitations/risk assessment/preventive measures. You will then practice generating a patient-specific database for an ambulatory patient with type 2 diabetes. For a complete discussion of information required in each of these categories, please refer to unit 1 of *Ambulatory Care Clinical Skills Program: Core Module*.

Case Study

Let's refer back to the first case study, Mrs. Gonzalez. When Mrs. Gonzalez presented in the pharmacy, the pharmacist asked her to complete the Pharmacist's Patient Medical History Form. Referring to this completed form in **Appendix A**, and using the techniques you learned in unit 4 of the *Ambulatory Care Clinical Skills Program: Core Module*, what information do you need to complete the Pharmacist's Patient Database Form? Let's review one category at a time.

1. What information from the demographic category do you need?

The patient's name, address, and telephone number are all important information because the pharmacist is entering into a relationship with the patient and will need to contact her occasionally. The patient's age, sex, and race or ethnic background are important information. The incidence of type 2 diabetes is higher over age 45. Also, the prevalence of type 2 diabetes is about 40% greater in women than men. There is wide variability in the risk of developing type 2 diabetes among different racial and ethnic groups. Hispanic patients have a two- or threefold higher risk of developing type 2 diabetes, even after accounting for other risk factors related to the disease.[1] Race, religion, and ethnic background can also provide useful information about a patient's dietary habits, communication style, acceptance of Western medicine, and use of alternative medicine.

Mrs. Gonzalez does not work outside her home; knowledge of the patient's occupation is valuable because it can indicate the level of physical activity (and the implications of this activity should diabetes-related complications develop) as well as the likelihood the patient will be able to adhere to a medication regimen and monitoring plan (such as checking blood glucose and injecting insulin four times daily).

2. What information from the administrative category do you need?

The pharmacist needs Mrs. Gonzalez's physician's name and telephone number to facilitate a working relationship. In this case, the pharmacist has worked with other patients of Dr. Thompson, and she is in frequent contact with him. Depending on the pharmacist's reimbursement arrangement with the third-party payer, she will require information on Mrs. Gonzalez's health insurance and her prescription plan.

3. What information from the medical category do you need?

Medical information provides important data about a patient's health status. Knowledge of Mrs. Gonzalez's current acute and chronic medical problems helps the pharmacist understand the purpose of the prescribed medications, to recommend optimal therapy, to detect drug-disease interactions, and to assess the influence of these medical problems on therapeutic decisions.

Important information from the medical category is Mrs. Gonzalez's history of hypertension (a major risk factor when combined with diabetes) and the fact that her third child, born when Mrs. Gonzalez was 35, was a large baby (10 pounds, 13.5 ounces). Mrs. Gonzalez denies having had gestational diabetes, but a large-birth-weight baby is a classic indication of uncontrolled gestational diabetes. This is important information because gestational diabetes puts a woman at greater risk for developing type 2 diabetes later in life. We've already discussed the relevance of Mrs. Gonzalez's recurrent vaginal yeast infections due to uncontrolled diabetes.

On questioning, the pharmacist learns that Mrs. Gonzalez's mother is 82 years old, has a cardiac history, and has had type 2 diabetes for 22 years. A family history of type 2 diabetes increases the likelihood a patient will develop type 2 diabetes.

The pharmacist can also review the Medical History Form that Mrs. Gonzalez completed and assess the patient's knowledge of her medical problems. For example, Mrs. Gonzalez perceived nausea secondary to codeine use as an allergy. The pharmacist questioned Mrs. Gonzalez carefully about this "allergic" reaction, probing for information such as:

- a description of the reaction,
- the dose and route of drug administration,
- when the reaction occurred,
- whether the reaction required treatment, and
- whether Mrs. Gonzalez has taken codeine since the reaction.

The pharmacist concluded that the reaction was an adverse effect of codeine, not an allergic reaction.

Mrs. Gonzalez did not realize that she had been diagnosed with hypercholesterolemia. In an interview with the patient, the pharmacist learned that Mrs. Gonzalez was asymptomatic of diabetes and had no acute complaints. In developing a care plan for Mrs. Gonzalez, the pharmacist will also need laboratory information and physical assessment results. Some of this information the pharmacist can obtain herself, and the rest she will get from Dr. Thompson. This information will help the pharmacist select and monitor the patient's drug therapy response and condition.

4. What information from the behavioral/lifestyle category do you need?

Information on diet and exercise are very important for patients with diabetes. Mrs. Gonzalez is not following a specific diet, although she has been advised to lower her salt intake because she has a history of hypertension. Mrs. Gonzalez provides details about her usual dietary intake, and how often she eats out, particularly fast food. Dietary history is important with this patient because she has diabetes, hypertension, and hypercholesterolemia.

Socially, Mrs. Gonzalez rarely drinks alcohol, and she has not smoked for 35 years. She does drink two to three regular colas a day. The colas contain caffeine and sugar, which can exacerbate her disease states.

The pharmacist determined previously that Mrs. Gonzalez does not work outside the home; she also has no regular exercise plan, performing only light housework and participating in a sewing group one night a week. This tells the pharmacist that Mrs. Gonzalez leads a basically sedentary lifestyle, which may increase her risk for insulin resistance.

5. What information from the drug therapy category do you need?

The pharmacist needs to know all medications the patient is taking to effectively evaluate her current therapy and offer recommendations. The pharmacist should ask about current prescription and nonprescription medications, herbal or natural remedies, and dietary supplements. While questioning Mrs. Gonzalez about her medications, the pharmacist can assess Mrs. Gonzalez's knowledge of drug therapy and adherence to medication regimens. Mrs. Gonzalez is fairly knowledgeable about her medications and has a good routine in place to assure adherence.

Once the pharmacist has an accurate list of Mrs. Gonzalez's medications, she can screen for drug-drug and drug-disease interactions. For example, Mrs. Gonzalez is taking HCTZ, which may increase blood glucose and LDL cholesterol.

6. What information from the social/economic/ quality of life category do you need?

Mrs. Gonzalez's living arrangement, degree of social support, and quality of life may affect adherence to medication and nondrug therapies. Diabetes is a disease that benefits from a strong support structure. Mrs. Gonzalez states that she lives with her husband and son, and that she does all meal preparation. This may be an issue with adherence to medical nutrition therapy. Mrs. Gonzalez's ethnic background has already been addressed as a risk factor for the development of type 2 diabetes.

Mrs. Gonzalez's husband has a prescription plan as part of his health benefits through his employer. Although this may decrease the financial burden on the patient, the pharmacist should assess the impact of medication costs on adherence.

The pharmacist can assess Mrs. Gonzalez's quality of life by asking if therapy is interfering with her well-being or ability to carry out daily activities. Mrs. Gonzalez confides that she found the use of Monistat 7 distasteful.

7. What information from the personal limitations/risk assessment/preventive measures category do you need?

Information on personal limitations is needed to select the most appropriate dosage forms and medication regimen as well as to help the pharmacist establish the nature of her verbal interactions with Mrs. Gonzalez. Personal limitations that are physical, cognitive, or emotional may limit a patient's ability to adhere to a therapeutic plan. The pharmacist notes that Mrs. Gonzalez speaks English fluently and does not require an interpreter. Mrs. Gonzalez is quite anxious, almost tearful, about the news that she has diabetes. This is not unusual when a patient is first diagnosed; however, the pharmacist must monitor the patient for failure to accept the diagnosis, which might require a referral to a mental health care professional. In the case of Mrs. Gonzalez, it seems that her fear stems from the unknown as well as her perceived worst possible outcomes. This will be discussed further in unit 7, when we discuss the Health Belief Model.

Pharmacists can be active in preventing disease by educating patients about screening tests and preventive health care (e.g., immunization) and by assessing patients' risk of cardiovascular disease or complications of their conditions. For example, Mrs. Gonzalez has four risk factors for cardiovascular disease: she is a female >55 years old, she has both hypertension and diabetes, and her HDL cholesterol is <35 mg/dl. This is important information because patients with type 2 diabetes are at increased risk for death from cardiovascular disease, and because three of these four risk factors can be modified, to some extent.

The information about preventive measures for Mrs. Gonzalez indicates she has not had a home fecal occult blood test, and she does not routinely get an influenza vaccine or perform monthly breast self-examinations.

Review the completed Pharmacist's Patient Database Form for Mrs. Gonzalez in **Appendix A**, which the pharmacist completed after interviewing her.

Practice Example

Now consider the case of Mr. Jones. Drawing on the information you learned in units 1, 2, and 3, the completed Pharmacist's Patient Medical History Form in **Appendix B**, and the following interview of Mr. Jones, complete the Pharmacist's Patient Database Form provided in **Appendix C**. After you have completed the Pharmacist's Patient Database Form, compare your answers to the form completed by the author shown in **Appendix D**.

Continuing the conversation with Mr. Jones on April 3, 1998, the pharmacist asks:

"Mr. Jones, I would like to get some information for my records since we'll be working together. Is that OK with you?"

MR. JONES:

"Sure, I don't have to be anywhere today. What do you want to know?"

PHARMACIST:

"First, I've reviewed the Medical History Form you completed. Let's start with some basic information. I see that you live at 321 Tydings Lane, Baltimore, Maryland. Your home telephone is 555-9876, and you are retired. Is that all correct?"

MR. JONES:

"Yes, I've lived in that same house for almost 30 years now. My wife Myrtle picked that house out, and I couldn't leave even after she died. I lived alone for years after Myrtle passed away, and my good friend Fred moved in a couple of years ago."

PHARMACIST:

"It sounds like Fred is good company for you. Do you have family in the area? Tell me about your family, including your parents."

MR. JONES:

"Both my parents have passed on, of course. Mama died when she was 72 years old, and Daddy was 60. I never thought I'd live longer than my Daddy, but I sure have."

PHARMACIST:

"What did your parents die from? Did they have any chronic diseases?"

MR. JONES:

"Mama had high blood pressure and diabetes. She died of a stroke. Daddy died when he was 60 after he had his second heart attack, probably due to his high blood pressure. He hated to take any kind of medicine. Mama always said he would come to no good, and she was right."

PHARMACIST:

"You mentioned earlier that you have three sisters with diabetes. Do your sisters have any other chronic diseases?"

MR. JONES:

"You know, I'm not sure. My sister Linnea has quite a temper, and she gets very depressed sometimes, but that's probably because her husband Norman gives her such a hard time. Renee and Elaine have high blood pressure, I think; they both take a lot of medicine, I know."

PHARMACIST:

"OK. Do you have any children Mr. Jones?"

MR. JONES:

"No children, Myrtle never could get in the family way, but I loved her anyway. We always had a couple of dogs. I would have a dog now, except Fred is allergic to dogs."

PHARMACIST:

"That's too bad, I love dogs too. Mr. Jones, you told me earlier that you don't work anymore. Where did you work before you retired?"

MR. JONES:

"At the racetrack, where I still go most days. I worked there for years and years. I used to handle all that money people would bet on the ponies. I got pretty good at picking the winners myself, and I still am!"

PHARMACIST:

"I see. Do you have health insurance or a prescription plan?"

MR. JONES:

"Oh yes. My retirement plan is great. I have Medicare, of course, and another policy to pay for whatever Medicare doesn't pay. And I have one of those cards for my medications; I only have to pay $5 or $10 every time I get my medicine."

PHARMACIST:

"That's a big help, I'm sure. Mr. Jones, you told me you go to the racetrack with your buddies most days. How does your usual day go?"

MR. JONES:

"Well, I walk to the track about 8 a.m., and stay there until around 1:00 in the afternoon. One of my buddies usually gives me a ride home. Then I watch the soap operas in the afternoon, until it's time for the news."

PHARMACIST:

"So, aside from walking to the racetrack, do you exercise routinely?"

MR. JONES:

"No, I used to walk the dogs, but now with Fred there I don't have a dog anymore. Maybe if Fred moves I'll get another dog."

PHARMACIST:

"You know, Mr. Jones, you could go for a walk even though you don't have a dog. You don't have to wait for Fred to move."

MR. JONES:

"You got me there!"

PHARMACIST:

"Mr. Jones, can you tell me a little about your medical history? Do you have any chronic diseases?"

MR. JONES:

"Well, I've had high blood pressure since 1994, and sometimes my chest hurts if I walk too fast or too far. That's been going on for about 3 years."

PHARMACIST:

"I see. Did your physician ask you to restrict your diet in any way?"

MR. JONES:

"Sure, Dr. Middleton told me to cut down on salt and fat in my diet, but it's so hard to do. For one thing, I skip meals now and then, and I don't have any set routine. I generally get up and have breakfast at 6 a.m., and if I'm in the mood I'll have lunch when I get home around 2 p.m. Then, if I'm feeling a little peckish I'll have some dinner around 6 p.m. It's too hard to plan ahead. I used to do a lot better before Myrtle passed away. And Fred is no help; he's even worse than me in the kitchen. And you know I live right across from Burger King; it's hard to say no to that!"

PHARMACIST:

"I know what you mean, it can be very hard to follow a diet. Have you ever had your cholesterol checked?"

MR. JONES:

"Oh yeah, I forgot about that. The doctor said I had high cholesterol last year. He keeps pestering me about starting to take medicine for it, but I told him I would go on a diet. Of course, I never have been too successful at dieting."

PHARMACIST:

"Mr. Jones, have you ever been in a hospital, or had any surgeries?"

MR. JONES:

"Well, I was born in a hospital, does that count? I've never had anybody cut me open, but I did have a kidney stone in '92. They put me in the hospital for that, and I had to urinate in a strainer for 3 days until it finally passed. They made me jump up and down until the little devil came out. That smarted! I still have it in a little jar at home."

PHARMACIST:

"That's something not everyone can say. Tell me about your other usual habits. Do you drink alcoholic or caffeinated beverages, or do you smoke?"

MR. JONES:

"Well, I like a cup or two of coffee a day, and I never could abide that decaffeinated nonsense. They say you can't tell the difference, but I sure can. And I'm sad to say I have smoked a pack a day of cigarettes since I was 18 years old. Myrtle used to yell at me something terrible about smoking."

PHARMACIST:

"Mr. Jones, I see on your medication profile that you use an albuterol inhaler. Why do you use that?"

MR. JONES:

"Dr. Middleton says I have asthma. He says I've had it for 5 years or so, and he says it's because I smoke."

PHARMACIST:

"Do you drink any alcoholic beverages?"

MR. JONES:

"Well, Fred and I like to have a good time. We generally have a couple of beers a night or two a week. Usually one or two on the weekend, and again on Wednesday night when we go to the 'All You Can Eat Buffet' down at the Shrimp Net."

PHARMACIST:

"I see. What other medications do you take, Mr. Jones, besides the albuterol inhaler?"

MR. JONES:

"Well, there's my fluid pill, furosemide. And I take Tylenol whenever I get a headache. Oh, and I take a multivitamin to stay healthy every day."

PHARMACIST:

"I see you have a prescription for nitroglycerin tablets to put under your tongue for chest pain. Do you carry that with you, and have you had to use it?"

MR. JONES:

"That's right, I forgot about that. Yes, I keep the little brown bottle in my pocket all the time, and I generally need it a couple of times a month."

PHARMACIST:

"Has that pattern changed? Do you ever find that you need more than a couple per month?"

MR. JONES:

"No, it's been that way for quite a while. Dr. Middleton is always asking me that too. If I walk too far or too fast, I get a little chest tightness. I sit down and take one pill under the tongue, and it goes away in a couple minutes. No problem."

PHARMACIST:

"You know you can take up to three tablets, 5 minutes apart, if the chest pain is not relieved. If you don't get relief after the three tablets, call 911. Is there anything you do not understand?"

MR. JONES:

"No, I understand."

PHARMACIST:

"Mr. Jones, I want to assess your risk for heart disease. You are at risk because you are a male over 45 years of age, you smoke, and you have high blood pressure. Also, as we've discussed, you are at high risk for diabetes, and you need to see Dr. Middleton to be evaluated for that. Next, I want to ask you about some health maintenance issues. For example, have you had a rectal and prostate exam in the past year?"

MR. JONES:

"No way! Dr. Middleton wanted to do it, but I informed him otherwise. Not in this lifetime!"

PHARMACIST:

"Why are you opposed so vehemently? I know it's not a pleasant procedure, but a prostate exam is an important part of a medical examination for men."

MR. JONES:

"I know, but I don't want any part of that nonsense. Another thing—Dr. Middleton gave me some little cards and wanted me to put my stool on them and send them back to him. You know the mailman is going to love that!"

PHARMACIST:

"Believe me, the mailman wouldn't even know it. If mailing your sample makes you uncomfortable, you could drop it off at Dr. Middleton's office. It's an important screening test for colon cancer."

MR. JONES:

"Well, I'll think about it. I just don't think it's natural."

PHARMACIST:

"Well, we can discuss it a little later. Are you careful to keep all your medical appointments with Dr. Middleton?"

MR. JONES:

"Well, most of the time. Sometimes he gets on my nerves a little by wanting to see me so often. Good grief, I have a life. If things are really hopping at the track, sometimes I just have to let an appointment slide."

PHARMACIST:

"Mr. Jones, you know it's important that you keep all your appointments with Dr. Middleton. I suggest that you discuss this with him instead of just not showing up. Do you take your medications like you're supposed to?"

MR. JONES:

"Sure. I explained about the fluid pill when I first started taking it, but that's straightened out now. I use that inhaler thing when I need to, about two or three times a week."

PHARMACIST:

"Good. I'd like you to show me how you use your inhaler before you leave today. One more question, Mr. Jones, about your vaccinations. Are you current on your tetanus/diphtheria, pneumovax, and influenza every fall?"

MR. JONES:

"Absolutely. I believe in vaccines. I grew up with too many kids who had polio. Plus, Fred gets the flu every year. He's not exactly a good patient."

PHARMACIST:

"Well, I'm glad that your immunizations are current. If it's OK with you, I'd like to check your vital signs, get your height and weight, and check your glucose. How does that sound?"

MR. JONES:

"You can do anything you want so long as it doesn't involve a rectal exam, young man!"

Summary

The system of documentation you choose to use in your practice should include the elements you observed and practiced recording in this unit. Your documentation system should allow easy access to information and facilitate efficient evaluation so recommendations can be generated. You should update the patient database continually as data becomes available. This new data will be essential for continuing care of the patient and your therapeutic decision-making process.

Reference

1. American Diabetes Association. *Diabetes 1996 Vital Statistics*. Alexandria, VA: American Diabetes Association; 1996. p. 23.

Self-Study Question

Objective

Generate a patient-specific database for an ambulatory patient with type 2 diabetes.

Refer to Case A, Ms. McLucas, as described in unit 3, and her completed Pharmacist's Patient Medical History Form in **Appendix E**. Read the following information the pharmacist obtained on interview with Ms. McLucas. Use the blank Pharmacist's Patient Database Form supplied in **Appendix F** to fill in necessary information specific for Ms. McLucas. When you are done, compare your completed forms to the ones in **Appendix G**. If you find gaps in any area of information, go back to the corresponding section in this unit, or unit 6 of the *Ambulatory Care Clinical Skills Program: Core Module*, to review the discussion.

Ms. McLucas is a Caucasian 70-year-old retired school teacher who never married and has no children. She is Lutheran (she plays the organ weekly at church) and has Medicare, but no prescription benefits. Her primary care provider is Dr. Davis. The patient has a history of hypercholesterolemia (1997), osteoarthritis (1996), hypertension (1995), gastroesophageal reflux disease, and diabetes (newly diagnosed type 2). She has seasonal allergic rhinitis, with sensitivity to both tree pollen and ragweed. She was hospitalized one time with pneumonia in 1992.

Her mother died at age 74 of myocardial infarction, and her father died at age 82 of pneumonia. She has no siblings, but her best friend was recently diagnosed with cancer.

Ms. McLucas denies alcohol, caffeine, or tobacco use. She adheres to her physician's recommendation to decrease salt but has a hard time limiting her fat intake. She is having difficulty avoiding honey-dipped donuts, which she eats for breakfast.

She serves as a volunteer at the local library every morning from 9–11 a.m., enjoys gardening, and keeps her own house. Ms. McLucas is a very matter-of-fact, practical woman and very intelligent.

She has decreased vision and wears glasses. She states that aspirin upsets her stomach. She takes naprosyn 500 mg twice daily for osteoarthritis and supplements naprosyn with nonprescription-strength ibuprofen every 4–6 hours as needed for pain. She takes Mylanta, 1 tablespoon, on occasion for indigestion. She also takes Tavist-D (one tablet, twice daily) for symptoms of allergic rhinitis. Dr. Davis prescribed cholestyramine, one scoop twice daily, in 1997, but Ms. McLucas refuses to take it.

With regard to health maintenance, Ms. McLucas is very compliant, having had a dental examination, pap smear and pelvic exam, and mammogram within the past year, as well as a fasting lipid panel, home fecal occult blood test (negative), and all immunizations. She performs monthly breast self-examinations and takes calcium supplements to prevent osteoporosis.

On physical examination on 4/23/98, the pharmacist determined Ms. McLucas' height to be 5'5"; weight 162 lb; temperature 98.6°F (oral thermometer); blood pressure 134/86 mmHg sitting, right arm; heart rate 72 beats per minute and regular; and respiratory rate 14 breaths per minute. She was alert and oriented to person, place and time, in no apparent distress, and very pleasant. She was exceptionally well groomed, and no abnormalities were noted on skin and general assessment; numerous freckles were noted. No abnormalities were noted on foot screening. Urinalysis was negative for glucose, protein, or ketones, and urine microalbuminuria was negative.

PHARMACIST'S PATIENT
MEDICAL HISTORY FORM

I. PATIENT INFORMATION

Name: __Rose Gonzalez__

Address: __344 Lombard Street Baltimore, MD 21201__

Home Phone: __555-1234__ Office Phone: __N/A__

Date of Birth: __8/12/42__ Last year of education completed: __12th grade__

Patient lives with __husband & son__

Caregiver (if applicable): __N/A__

Caregiver Phone: __N/A__

Employer: __N/A__ Job Title: __housewife__

Name of Health Insurer: __BC/BS__

Health Ins. Card #: __123-45-6789__ Social Security #: __111-22-3333__

Primary Care Physician's Name: __Dr. Thompson__ Phone: __555-CARE__

Specialist Physician's Name: __N/A__ Phone: _____

Other Health Care Practitioner: __N/A__ Phone: _____

II. MEDICAL HISTORY

Are you allergic to any prescription drugs or over-the-counter medications? _____

☑ Yes   ☐ No   If yes, please list the medications and type of allergic reaction experienced:

__codeine makes me very nauseous__

Are there any medications that you are not allergic to but cannot tolerate? _____

☐ Yes   ☑ No   If yes, please list the medications and the reaction experienced:

_____

Do you use tobacco?   __I used to smoke as a teenager, but quit during__

☐ Yes   ☑ No   If yes, what type? __my first pregnancy.__ How often? _____

Do you drink alcohol?

☐ Yes   ☑ No   If yes, what type? __whiskey sour__ How often? __~2-3x a year__

Name: __Rose Gonzalez_____

Please put a check (✔) next to those items listed below that apply to you:

HEART PROBLEMS:	✔	URINARY/REPRODUCTIVE:	✔
Chest pain (angina)		Urinary or bladder infection	
Past heart attack		Prostate problems	
Heart failure		Hysterectomy	
Irregular heartbeat		Chronic yeast infections	✓
Heart by-pass surgery		Kidney disease	
Rheumatic fever		Dialysis	
Other:		Other:	
EYES, EARS, NOSE & THROAT	✔	**MUSCLES AND BONES**	✔
Poor vision	✓	Arthritis *in my little toe-right foot*	✓
Poor hearing		Gout	
Glaucoma		Back problems	
Sinus problems		Amputation	
Balance disorder		Joint replacement	
Other: *I wear glasses*		Other:	
GASTROINTESTINAL	✔	**NEUROLOGICAL**	✔
Heartburn *once in a while*	✓	Headaches	
Ulcer		Seizures or epilepsy	
Constipation *once in a while*	✓	Parkinson's disease	
Diverticulitis		Dizziness	
Liver disease		Past stroke	
Gallbladder problems		Fainting	
Pancreatitis		Depression	
Other:		Anxiety	✓
		Other:	
DO YOU HAVE:	✔	**LUNG PROBLEMS**	✔
High blood pressure	✓	Asthma	
Low blood pressure		Emphysema	
High cholesterol		Bronchitis	
Diabetes	✓	Other:	
Cancer			
Anemia			
Bleeding disorder		**DO YOU HAVE OR USE …?**	✔
Hay fever		Glasses	✓
Sleeping problems		Hearing aid	
Other:		Other:	
DO YOU HAVE A FAMILY HISTORY OF:			
High blood pressure		Asthma	
Heart disease		Other:	
Diabetes	✓		

Name: _____ Rose Gonzalez _____

III. CURRENT PRESCRIPTION MEDICATIONS (INCLUDING ONES RECEIVED AT OTHER PHARMACIES)

Name of prescription medicine and strength (i.e., milligrams, grams, and units)	How much do you take each time?	How many times a day do you take the medicine?	Medical problem being treated	When did you start taking this medicine?	Has the medicine helped you? Yes/No	Name of doctor or specialist who prescribed the medicine
Example: Diabeta, 2.5 mg	1	2	Diabetes	1992	Yes	Dr. Harold Smith
HCTZ 25 mg.	1	1	Blood pressure	1995	yes	Dr. Thompson

IV. CURRENT NONPRESCRIPTION MEDICATIONS

EX: ANTACIDS, ANTI-DIARRHEALS, ALLERGY MEDICINES, ANTI-NAUSEA, DIET PILLS, EAR OR EYE MEDICATIONS, LAXATIVES, PAIN RELIEVERS, VITAMINS, ETC.

Name of medicine Example: Tylenol	How often do you take it? (daily, once a week, etc.)	Name of medicine	How often do you take it?
Pepcid AC	~1x a month		
Colace	~ every couple months		
Monistat	3x this year (past 12 months)		
Tylenol	~1x a month		

I certify this information is accurate and complete to the best of my knowledge. _____ Rose Gonzalez _____
                                                                                    signature/date

PHARMACIST'S PATIENT DATABASE FORM

Original Date: **2/19/98**
Date updated: _____
Date updated: _____
Date updated: _____

Demographic and Administrative Information

Name: **Mrs. Rose Gonzalez**	Social Security #: **111-22-3333**
Address: **344 Lombard Street, Baltimore, MD 21201**	
Health Care Provider's Name **Dr. Thompson**	Health Care Provider's Phone **555-CARE**
Work Phone:	Home Phone: **555-1234**	Date of Birth: **8/12/42**
Race: **Hispanic**	Gender: **F**
Religion: **Catholic**	Occupation: **housewife**
Health Insurer: **BC/BS**	Subscriber #: **123-45-6789**
Primary Card Holder: **Juan Gonzalez**	Drug Benefit: ☑ yes ☐ no copay: $ **5⁰⁰/per**

Current Symptoms   **none; diabetes picked on routine BG testing**

Past Medical History | Acute and Current Medical Problems

Past Medical History	Acute and Current Medical Problems
HTN x 4 years	1. Diabetes mellitus, type 2
no surgeries	2. Hypertension
3 children born	3. Hyperlipidemia
last child 10 lb 13 1/2 oz	4. GERD
(no dx gestational DM)	5. Constipation
	6. "Arthritis"
	7. Recurrent vag. yeast infect.
	8.

Family/Social/Economic History | Personal Limitations

Family/Social/Economic History	Personal Limitations
mother - 82-alive → MI; h/o DM x22yr.	Pt. very anxious about
father - ↓@44 2° MUA	dx DM
3 children-good health	
no siblings	
Cost of medications per month $ **40⁰⁰**	

Allergies/Intolerances | Social Drug Use

Allergies/Intolerances	Social Drug Use
☑ No known drug allergies	Alcohol **social - 2-3 drinks/yr.**
Medication Reaction	Caffeine **2-3 caffeinated colas/day**
codeine nausea	Tobacco **none x 35 yrs**
	Pregnancy/Breastfeeding Status **N/A**
	☐ Pregnant (due _____) ☐ Breastfeeding

Diet | Routine Exercise/Recreation | Daily Activities/Timing

Diet	Routine Exercise/Recreation	Daily Activities/Timing
☐ Low salt **no**	light housework	home all day
☐ Low fat **no**	otherwise ∅	sewing group 1 night/wk
☐ Diabetic **no**		
Timing of meals: **8A-12N-6P**		

Patient Name: ___Rose Gonzalez___

Physical Assessment/Laboratory Data—Initial/Follow-up

Date	2/9/98	2/18/98	2/19/98		
Height			5'5"		
Weight			228 lb		
Temp			98.6°F elec.		
BP			152/100 LA ℞		
Pulse			92 reg R/R		
Respirations			18		
Peak Flow					
FBG		184			
R. Glucose	242				
HbA$_{1c}$			10.2		
T. Chol.	286	290			
LDL		204			
HDL		30			
TG		280			
INR					
BUN					
Cr	0.9				
ALT					
AST					
Alk Phos					
EKG	WNL				
U/A			⊕glucose ⊖protein, ket.		
MicroAlb.			⊖		

Drug Serum Concentrations

Date					

Notes:

Patient Name: __Rose Gonzalez__

Current Prescription Medication Regimen

Name/Dose/Strength/Route	Schedule/Frequency of Use	Indication	Start Date (and Stop Date If Applicable)	Prescriber	Adherence Issues/Efficacy
HCTZ 25 mg po	T q AM	HTN	June 1995	Thompson	Adherent/ ?efficacy

Current Nonprescription Medication Regimen (OTC, herbal, homeopathic, nutritional, etc.)

Name/Dose/Strength/Route	Schedule/Frequency of Use	Indication	Start Date (and Stop Date If Applicable)	Prescriber	Adherence Issues/Efficacy
Docusate 100 mg po	prn	hard stool	prn x years	—	works well~ every couple months
Pepcid AC	prn (~1x q mo)	heartburn	~2 years	—	works well
Monistat-7	prn (3x last yr)	vag. yeast infection	3x in past yr	—	recurs
Acetaminophen 325 mg	prn ~1x q mo	arthritis	prn x years	—	works "OK"

Patient Name: __Rose Gonzalez__

Risk Assessment/Preventive Measures/Quality of Life

Cardiovascular Risk Assessment		
male >45 years old	1	-
female >55 years old or female <55 with history of ovarectomy not taking estrogen replacement	1	1
Definite MI or sudden death before age 55 year in father or male first-degree relative or before 65 year in mother or female first-degree relative	1	-
current cigarette smoking	1	-
hypertension	1	1
diabetes mellitus	1	1
HDL cholesterol <35 mg/dl	1	1
HDL cholesterol >60 mg/dl	-1	
Total:		**4**

Is patient at risk for complications of current conditions? ☑ Yes ☐ No

Specify: HbAlc 10.2   DM complications, both acute (vag. yeast infections)
& chronic

Preventive Measures for Adults

H = has been done   R = patient refuses   X = not applicable   Date **2/19/98**

Women						
Pap Smear/pelvic	Annually 19+	H				
Mammogram	Every 1-2Y 40-49; annually 50+	H				
Men						
Rectal/prostate	Annually 50+					
All Patients						
Total/HDL-C	Every 5Y 19+	H				
Home Fecal Occult Blood Test	Annually					
Immunizations						
Td	Every 10Y	H				
Influenza	Every fall*					
Pneumovax	Once*	H				

* if indicated

Quality of life issues

Pt. very concerned re: dx DM.

Assessment of General Appearance

Patient __Rose Gonzalez__   Date __2/19/98__

General Appearance	Observations and Comments

Level of consciousness
    alertness: alert, confused,
    delirious, stuporous, comatose,
    orientation: person, place, time
	alert & oriented to person, place & time

Signs of distress respiratory distress, pain, anxiety, etc.	somewhat anxious, near tears
Posture, motor activity, and gait *Describe*	normal posture & gait
Dress, grooming, and personal hygiene *Describe*	neat & appropriate personal appearance

Affect
    normal, inappropriate
    Describe
	normal

Speech
    normal, impaired
    Describe
	normal (accent)

Skin
    color: normal, blue, brown, red, pallor
    texture: normal, coarse, dry, oily
    turgor: good, poor
    edema
    lesions: color, type, configuration, anatomic
        distribution, consistency
	normal color, texture & turgor.
	No abnormalities, lesions or edema noted.

SCREENING FORM FOR DIABETES FOOT DISEASE

Name: **Rose Gonzalez**

Date: **2/19/98**

ID #: _____

I. Medical History

Check all that apply.

_____ Peripheral neuropathy
_____ Nephropathy
_____ Retinopathy   } denies
_____ Peripheral vascular disease
_____ Cardiovascular disease

For Sections II & III, fill in the blanks with an "R," "L," or "B" for positive findings on the right, left, or both feet.

II. Current History

1. Any change in the foot since the last evaluation?
_____ Yes _____
__✓__ No   - 1st evaluation

2. Current ulcer or history of a foot ulcer?
_____ Yes _____
__✓__ No

3. Is there pain in the calf muscles when walking that is relieved by rest?
_____ Yes _____
__✓__ No

III. Foot Exam

1. Are the nails thick, too long, ingrown, infected with fungal disease?

_____ Yes _____

__✓__ No

2. Note foot deformities

_____ Toe deformities

_____ Bunions (hallus valgus)

_____ Charcot foot   } NONE

_____ Foot drop

_____ Prominent metatarsal heads

_____ Amputation (specify date, side, and level) _____

3. Pedal Pulses *(Fill in the blanks with a "P" or an "A" to indicate present or absent.)*

Posterior tibial:

__P__ Left

__P__ Right

Dorsalis pedis: } NORMAL

__P__ Left

__P__ Right

4. Skin Condition *(Measure, draw in, and label the patient's skin condition, using the key and the foot diagram below.)*

C = Callus   PU = Pre-ulcerative lesion

U = Ulcer   F = Fissure

R = Redness   S = Swelling   } NONE Noted

W = Warmth   D = Dryness

M = Maceration

IV. Sensory Foot Exam

Label sensory level with a "+" in the five circled areas of the foot if the patient can feel the 5.07 Semmes-Weinstein (10-gram) nylon filament and "−" if the patient cannot feel the filament.

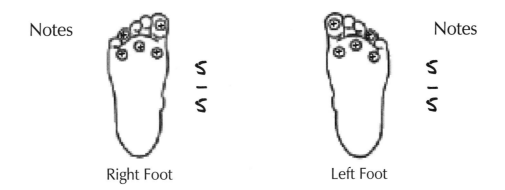

Notes   Notes

Right Foot   Left Foot

V. Risk Categorization

Check appropriate item.

✓ Low-Risk Patient
All of the following:
Intact protective sensation
Pedal pulses present
No severe deformity
No prior foot ulcer
No amputation

_____ High-Risk Patient
One or more of the following:
Loss of protective sensation
Absent pedal pulses
Severe foot deformity
History of foot ulcer
Prior amputation

VI. Footwear Assessment

Fill in the blanks.

Does the patient wear appropriate shoes?
✓ Yes   counseled pt.
_____ No

Does the patient need inserts?
_____ Yes
✓ No

Should therapeutic footwear be prescribed?
_____ Yes
✓ No

VII. Education

Fill in the blanks.

Has the patient had prior foot care education?
_____ Yes
✓ No

Can the patient demonstrate appropriate self-care?
_____ Yes   1st time seen
_____ No

VIII. Management Plan

Check all that apply.

__✓__ Provide patient education for preventive foot care.

Date: __2/20/98__

Diagnostic studies:
_____ Vascular laboratory
_____ Other: _____

Footwear recommendations:
__✓__ None
_____ Athletic shoes
_____ Accommodative inserts
_____ Custom shoes
_____ Depth shoes

Refer to:
__✓__ Primary care provider   *for scheduled follow-up*
_____ Diabetes educator
_____ Orthopedic foot surgeon
_____ RN foot specialist
_____ Orthotist
_____ Podiatrist
_____ Pedorthist
_____ Endocrinologist
_____ Rehab. specialist
_____ Vascular surgeon
_____ Other: _____
_____ Schedule follow-up visit

Date: __2/19/98__   Provider Signature: ___Jane Radcliffe, R.Ph.___

Source: http://www.niddk.nih.gov/health/diabetes/feet/feet2/screenfo.htm

PHARMACIST'S PATIENT MEDICAL HISTORY FORM

I. PATIENT INFORMATION

Name: ___George Jones___

Address: ___321 Tydings Lane Baltimore, MD 21136___

Home Phone: ___555-9876___   Office Phone: ___N/A___

Date of Birth: ___9/13/31___   Last year of education completed: ___8th grade___

Patient lives with ___friend - Fred___

Caregiver (if applicable): ___N/A___

Caregiver Phone: ___N/A___

Employer: ___N/A___   Job Title: ___N/A___

Name of Health Insurer: ___Medicare & Supplemental___

Health Ins. Card #: ___121-11-1111___   Social Security #: ___121-11-1111___

Primary Care Physician's Name: ___Dr. Middleton___   Phone: ___555-2399___

Specialist Physician's Name: ___N/A___   Phone: ___-___

Other Health Care Practitioner: ___N/A___   Phone: ___-___

II. MEDICAL HISTORY

Are you allergic to any prescription drugs or over-the-counter medications? _____

☐ Yes   ☒ No   If yes, please list the medications and type of allergic reaction experienced:

_____

Are there any medications that you are not allergic to but cannot tolerate? _____

☐ Yes   ☒ No   If yes, please list the medications and the reaction experienced:

_____

Do you use tobacco?

☒ Yes   ☐ No   If yes, what type? ___cigarettes - 1 pack a day___ How often? ___50 yrs.___

Do you drink alcohol?

☒ Yes   ☐ No   If yes, what type? ___Beer___   How often? ___3-4/week___

Name: **George Jones**

Please put a check (✔) next to those items listed below that apply to you:

HEART PROBLEMS:	✔	URINARY/REPRODUCTIVE:	✔
Chest pain (angina)	✓	Urinary or bladder infection	
Past heart attack		Prostate problems	
Heart failure		Hysterectomy	
Irregular heartbeat		Chronic yeast infections	
Heart by-pass surgery		Kidney disease	
Rheumatic fever		Dialysis	
Other:		Other: Kidney stone 1992	✓

EYES, EARS, NOSE & THROAT	✔	MUSCLES AND BONES	✔
Poor vision		Arthritis	
Poor hearing		Gout	
Glaucoma		Back problems	
Sinus problems		Amputation	
Balance disorder		Joint replacement	
Other:		Other:	

GASTROINTESTINAL	✔	NEUROLOGICAL	✔
Heartburn		Headaches	✓
Ulcer		Seizures or epilepsy	
Constipation		Parkinson's disease	
Diverticulitis		Dizziness	
Liver disease		Past stroke	
Gallbladder problems		Fainting	
Pancreatitis		Depression	
Other:		Anxiety	
		Other:	

DO YOU HAVE:	✔	LUNG PROBLEMS	✔
High blood pressure	✓	Asthma	✓
Low blood pressure		Emphysema	
High cholesterol	✓	Bronchitis	
Diabetes		Other:	
Cancer			
Anemia			
Bleeding disorder		DO YOU HAVE OR USE ...?	✔
Hay fever		Glasses	
Sleeping problems		Hearing aid	
Other:		Other:	

DO YOU HAVE A FAMILY HISTORY OF:			
High blood pressure	✓	Asthma	
Heart disease	✓	Other:	
Diabetes	✓		

Name: _George Jones_

III. CURRENT PRESCRIPTION MEDICATIONS (INCLUDING ONES RECEIVED AT OTHER PHARMACIES)

Name of prescription medicine and strength (i.e., milligrams, grams, and units)	How much do you take each time?	How many times a day do you take the medicine?	Medical problem being treated	When did you start taking this medicine?	Has the medicine helped you? Yes/No	Name of doctor or specialist who prescribed the medicine
Example: Diabeta, 2.5 mg	1	2	Diabetes	1992	Yes	Dr. Harold Smith
furosemide 20 mg	1	1	Blood pressure	2-3 yrs	yes	Middleton
Puffer	2 puffs	2-3x a month	Asthma & wheezing	years	yes	Middleton

IV. CURRENT NONPRESCRIPTION MEDICATIONS

Ex: ANTACIDS, ANTI-DIARRHEALS, ALLERGY MEDICINES, ANTI-NAUSEA, DIET PILLS, EAR OR EYE MEDICATIONS, LAXATIVES, PAIN RELIEVERS, VITAMINS, ETC.

Name of medicine Example: Tylenol	How often do you take it? (daily, once a week, etc.)	Name of medicine	How often do you take it?
Tylenol	~ once a week		
vitamin	every day		

I certify this information is accurate and complete to the best of my knowledge. _George Jones_   _3/3/98_

                                                          signature/date

Pharmacist's Patient Database Form

Original Date:_____
Date updated:_____
Date updated:_____
Date updated:_____

Demographic and Administrative Information

Name:	Social Security #:
Address:	
Health Care Provider's Name	Health Care Provider's Phone
Work Phone: Home Phone:	Date of Birth:
Race:	Gender:
Religion:	Occupation:
Health Insurer:	Subscriber #:
Primary Card Holder:	Drug Benefit: ❑ yes ❑ no copay: $_____

Current Symptoms

Past Medical History	Acute and Current Medical Problems
	1.
	2.
	3.
	4.
	5.
	6.
	7.
	8.

Family/Social/Economic History	Personal Limitations

Cost of medications per month $_____

Allergies/Intolerances	Social Drug Use
❑ No known drug allergies	Alcohol
Medication Reaction	Caffeine
	Tobacco
	Pregnancy/Breastfeeding Status
	❑ Pregnant (due _____) ❑ Breastfeeding

Diet	Routine Exercise/Recreation	Daily Activities/Timing
❑ Low salt		
❑ Low fat		
❑ Diabetic		
Timing of meals:		

Patient Name: _____

Physical Assessment/Laboratory Data—Initial/Follow-up					
Date					
Height					
Weight					
Temp					
BP					
Pulse					
Respirations					
Peak Flow					
FBG					
R. Glucose					
HbA$_{1c}$					
T. Chol.					
LDL					
HDL					
TG					
INR					
BUN					
Cr					
ALT					
AST					
Alk Phos					
Drug Serum Concentrations					
Date					
Notes:					

Patient Name: _____

Current Prescription Medication Regimen

Name/Dose/Strength/Route	Schedule/ Frequency of Use	Indication	Start Date (and Stop Date If Applicable)	Prescriber	Adherence Issues/Efficacy

Current Nonprescription Medication Regimen (OTC, herbal, homeopathic, nutritional, etc.)

Name/Dose/Strength/Route	Schedule/ Frequency of Use	Indication	Start Date (and Stop Date If Applicable)	Prescriber	Adherence Issues/Efficacy

Patient Name: _____

Risk Assessment/Preventive Measures/Quality of Life

Cardiovascular Risk Assessment		
male >45 years old	1	
female >55 years old or female <55 with history of ovarectomy not taking estrogen replacement	1	
Definite MI or sudden death before age 55 year in father or male first-degree relative or before 65 year in mother or female first-degree relative	1	
current cigarette smoking	1	
hypertension	1	
diabetes mellitus	1	
HDL cholesterol <35 mg/dl	1	
HDL cholesterol >60 mg/dl	-1	
	Total:	

Is patient at risk for complications of current conditions?   ❑ Yes   ❑ No
Specify:

Preventive Measures for Adults
H = has been done   R = patient refuses   X = not applicable   Date

Women							
Pap Smear/pelvic	Annually 19+						
Mammogram	Every 1-2Y 40-49; annually 50+						
Men							
Rectal/prostate	Annually 50+						
All Patients							
Total/HDL-C	Every 5Y 19+						
Home Fecal Occult Blood Test	Annually						
Immunizations							
Td	Every 10Y						
Influenza	Every fall*						
Pneumovax	Once*						

* if indicated

Quality of life issues

Assessment of General Appearance

Patient _____ **Date** _____

General Appearance	Observations and Comments

Level of consciousness
    alertness: alert, confused,
    delirious, stuporous, comatose,
    orientation: person, place, time	

Signs of distress respiratory distress, pain, anxiety, etc.	
Posture, motor activity, and gait _Describe_	
Dress, grooming, and personal hygiene _Describe_	

Affect
    normal, inappropriate
    Describe	

Speech
    normal, impaired
    Describe	

Skin
    color: normal, blue, brown, red, pallor
    texture: normal, coarse, dry, oily
    turgor: good, poor
    edema
    lesions: color, type, configuration, anatomic
       distribution, consistency	

SCREENING FORM FOR DIABETES FOOT DISEASE

Name: _____

Date: _____

ID #: _____

I. Medical History

Check all that apply.

_____ Peripheral neuropathy
_____ Nephropathy
_____ Retinopathy
_____ Peripheral vascular disease
_____ Cardiovascular disease

For Sections II & III, fill in the blanks with an "R," "L," or "B" for positive findings on the right, left, or both feet.

II. Current History

1. Any change in the foot since the last evaluation?
_____ Yes _____
_____ No

2. Current ulcer or history of a foot ulcer?
_____ Yes _____
_____ No

3. Is there pain in the calf muscles when walking that is relieved by rest?
_____ Yes _____
_____ No

III. Foot Exam

1. Are the nails thick, too long, ingrown, infected with fungal disease?

_____ Yes _____

_____ No

2. Note foot deformities

_____ Toe deformities

_____ Bunions (hallus valgus)

_____ Charcot foot

_____ Foot drop

_____ Prominent metatarsal heads

_____ Amputation (specify date, side, and level) _____

3. Pedal Pulses _(Fill in the blanks with a "P" or an "A" to indicate present or absent.)_

Posterior tibial:

_____ Left

_____ Right

Dorsalis pedis:

_____ Left

_____ Right

4. Skin Condition _(Measure, draw in, and label the patient's skin condition, using the key and the foot diagram below.)_

C = Callus   PU = Pre-ulcerative lesion

U = Ulcer   F = Fissure

R = Redness   S = Swelling

W = Warmth   D = Dryness

M = Maceration

IV. Sensory Foot Exam

Label sensory level with a "+" in the five circled areas of the foot if the patient can feel the 5.07 Semmes-Weinstein (10-gram) nylon filament and "–" if the patient cannot feel the filament.

Notes

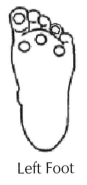

Notes

Right Foot   Left Foot

V. Risk Categorization

Check appropriate item.

_____ Low-Risk Patient
All of the following:
Intact protective sensation
Pedal pulses present
No severe deformity
No prior foot ulcer
No amputation

_____ High-Risk Patient
One or more of the following:
Loss of protective sensation
Absent pedal pulses
Severe foot deformity
History of foot ulcer
Prior amputation

VI. Footwear Assessment

Fill in the blanks.

Does the patient wear appropriate shoes?
_____ Yes
_____ No

Does the patient need inserts?
_____ Yes
_____ No

Should therapeutic footwear be prescribed?
_____ Yes
_____ No

VII. Education

Fill in the blanks.

Has the patient had prior foot care education?
_____ Yes
_____ No

Can the patient demonstrate appropriate self-care?
_____ Yes
_____ No

VIII. Management Plan

Check all that apply.

_____ Provide patient education for preventive foot care.

Date: _____

Diagnostic studies:
_____ Vascular laboratory
_____ Other: _____

Footwear recommendations:
_____ None
_____ Athletic shoes
_____ Accommodative inserts
_____ Custom shoes
_____ Depth shoes

Refer to:
_____ Primary care provider
_____ Diabetes educator
_____ Orthopedic foot surgeon
_____ RN foot specialist
_____ Orthotist
_____ Podiatrist
_____ Pedorthist
_____ Endocrinologist
_____ Rehab. specialist
_____ Vascular surgeon
_____ Other: _____
_____ Schedule follow-up visit

Date: _____   Provider Signature: _____

Source: http://www.niddk.nih.gov/health/diabetes/feet/feet2/screenfo.htm

PHARMACIST'S PATIENT DATABASE FORM

Original Date: **3/3/98**
Date updated: **4/3/98**
Date updated: _____
Date updated: _____

Demographic and Administrative Information

Name: George Jones

Social Security #: 121-11-1111

Address: 321 Tydings Lane   Baltimore, MD 21136

Health Care Provider's Name   Dr. Middleton

Health Care Provider's Phone   555-2399

Work Phone: -   Home Phone: 555-9876

Date of Birth: 9/13/31

Race: AA

Gender: M

Religion: NONE

Occupation: retired-worked at racetrack

Health Insurer: Medicare & BC/BS

Subscriber #: 121-11-1111

Primary Card Holder: pt.

Drug Benefit: ☒ yes ☐ no   copay: $ 5-10⁰⁰

Current Symptoms

c/o Nocturia (2-3 x q N) x 2-3 weeks

Past Medical History

HTN 1994

Angina 1995

Ø surgery

Hypercholesterolemia 6/97

Kidney stone 1992 → hospit.

Asthma x 5 yrs.

Acute and Current Medical Problems

1. Nocturia / Diabetes (4/3/98)
2. Hypertension
3. Angina
4. Hypercholesterolemia
5. Asthma
6. Renal dysfxn/proteinuria
7. MI (? old)
8. Insensate feet/ ↑ risk
9. fungal toe infection

Family/Social/Economic History

mother- ↓ @72 2° CVA; dxDM @50; h/o HTN

4 sisters-1 well; 3→DM & HTN

Father- ↓ @60 2° MI (MI x 2); h/o HTN

Personal Limitations

NONE

Cost of medications per month $ 15-20⁰⁰

Allergies/Intolerances

☒ No known drug allergies

Medication	Reaction

Social Drug Use

Alcohol   3-4 beers q week

Caffeine   1-2 cups coffee qd

Tobacco   50-pack year history

Pregnancy/Breastfeeding Status   N/A

☐ Pregnant (due _____)   ☐ Breastfeeding

Diet

☒ Low salt ⟩ prescribed -

☒ Low fat ⟩ not

☐ Diabetic   following

Routine Exercise/Recreation

No routine exercise

x̄ walks 1/2 mile

to race track qd

Daily Activities/Timing

Race track 8A-1P

Retires @ 10 pm

Timing of meals: 6A-2P-6P - skips meals sometimes; frequently eats fast food

Patient Name: ___George Jones___

Physical Assessment/Laboratory Data—Initial/Follow-up					
Date	3/3/98	3/18/98	3/23/98	3/30/98	4/3/98
Height	5'8"				
Weight	240 lb BMI 37				
Temp	98.8°F electron therm				
BP	152/98 ♂ 140/90 ♀				
Pulse	84 ♂ 92 ♀				
Respirations	16 reg				
Peak Flow					
FBG			190		
R. Glucose	244	258			
HbA$_{1c}$					11.6
T. Chol.				290	
LDL				229	
HDL				45	
TG				80	
INR					
BUN					
Cr				1.8	
ALT				56	
AST				98	
Alk Phos					
UCX			(−)		
EKG					4/1 ischemia c/w old MI
U/A					⊕ pro, glu ⊖ ketones
U.MicroAlb.					35 μg/mg Cr
Drug Serum Concentrations					
Date					
Notes:					

Patient Name: _____ George Jones _____

Current Prescription Medication Regimen

Name/Dose/Strength/Route	Schedule/ Frequency of Use	Indication	Start Date (and Stop Date If Applicable)	Prescriber	Adherence Issues/Efficacy
Furosemide 20 mg.	ī q AM	HTN	1994	Middleton	Adheres/eff?
NTG 0.4 mg sl prn	prn	Angina	1995	Middleton	~1/month/good
Albuterol inhaler ĪĪ puffs	prn	Asthma	1993	Middleton	~2-3 x q mo/good

Current Nonprescription Medication Regimen (OTC, herbal, homeopathic, nutritional, etc.)

Name/Dose/Strength/Route	Schedule/ Frequency of Use	Indication	Start Date (and Stop Date If Applicable)	Prescriber	Adherence Issues/Efficacy
Acetaminophen 650 mg	prn ~ weekly	headache	years	-	works well
MVI ī	QD	nutrition	years	-	perceives efficacious

Patient Name: _____George Jones_____

Risk Assessment/Preventive Measures/Quality of Life

Cardiovascular Risk Assessment		
male >45 years old	1	I
female >55 years old or female <55 with history of ovarectomy not taking estrogen replacement	1	
Definite MI or sudden death before age 55 year in father or male first-degree relative or before 65 year in mother or female first-degree relative	1	
current cigarette smoking	1	I
hypertension	1	I
diabetes mellitus	1	I
HDL cholesterol <35 mg/dl	1	
HDL cholesterol >60 mg/dl	-1	
Total:		**4**

Is patient at risk for complications of current conditions? ☒ Yes ☐ No
Specify: HbA1c 11.6%, h/o HTN & CV dz

Preventive Measures for Adults
H = has been done   R = patient refuses   X = not applicable   Date **4/3/98**

Women							
Pap Smear/pelvic	Annually 19+						
Mammogram	Every 1-2Y 40-49; annually 50+						
Men							
Rectal/prostate	Annually 50+	R					
All Patients							
Total/HDL-C	Every 5Y 19+	H					
Home Fecal Occult Blood Test	Annually	R					
Immunizations							
Td	Every 10Y	H					
Influenza	Every fall*	H					
Pneumovax	Once*	H					

* if indicated

Quality of life issues

   Nocturia is affecting his QOL

Assessment of General Appearance

Patient **George Jones**   Date **3/3/98**

General Appearance	Observations and Comments

Level of consciousness
    alertness: alert, confused,
    delirious, stuporous, comatose,
    orientation: person, place, time
	Alert & oriented to person, place & time

Signs of distress respiratory distress, pain, anxiety, etc.	Appears concerned, but not distressed
Posture, motor activity, and gait *Describe*	Normal gait & posture & motor activity
Dress, grooming, and personal hygiene *Describe*	Casual but neat personal appearance

Affect
    normal, inappropriate
    Describe
	Normal

Speech
    normal, impaired
    Describe
	Normal

Skin
    color: normal, blue, brown, red, pallor
    texture: normal, coarse, dry, oily
    turgor: good, poor
    edema
    lesions: color, type, configuration, anatomic
        distribution, consistency
	Skin normal color & texture. Turgor poor-tenting & slightly dry mucous membranes
	No other skin abnormalities, lesions or edema noted.

SCREENING FORM FOR DIABETES FOOT DISEASE

Name: _____George Jones_____

Date: _____4/3/98_____

ID #: _____

I. Medical History

Check all that apply.

_____ Peripheral neuropathy
_____ Nephropathy
_____ Retinopathy
_____ Peripheral vascular disease
__✓__ Cardiovascular disease

For Sections II & III, fill in the blanks with an "R," "L," or "B" for positive findings on the right, left, or both feet.

II. Current History

1. Any change in the foot since the last evaluation?
_____ Yes _____
_____ No   1st exam

2. Current ulcer or history of a foot ulcer?
_____ Yes _____
__✓__ No

3. Is there pain in the calf muscles when walking that is relieved by rest?
_____ Yes _____
__✓__ No

III. Foot Exam

1. Are the nails thick, too long, ingrown, infected with fungal disease?

_____ Yes _____   *A little long, but otherwise normal*

_____ No   *Also, beginnings of a fungal infection in skin crease*
                                 under toe pad of little toe on R foot

2. Note foot deformities

_____ Toe deformities

_____ Bunions (hallus valgus)   *NONE*

_____ Charcot foot

_____ Foot drop

_____ Prominent metatarsal heads   *callus on balls both feet*

_____ Amputation (specify date, side and level) _____

3. Pedal Pulses (*Fill in the blanks with a "P" or an "A" to indicate present or absent.*)

Posterior tibial:

___P___ Left

___P___ Right   *slightly*
                       diminished

Dorsalis pedis:

___P___ Left

___P___ Right

4. Skin Condition (*Measure, draw in, and label the patient's skin condition, using the key and the foot diagram below.*)

C = Callus   PU = Pre-ulcerative lesion

U = Ulcer   F = Fissure

R = Redness   S = Swelling

W = Warmth   D = Dryness

M = Maceration

IV. Sensory Foot Exam

Label sensory level with a "+" in the five circled areas of the foot if the patient can feel the 5.07 Semmes-Weinstein (10-gram) nylon filament and "−" if the patient cannot feel the filament.

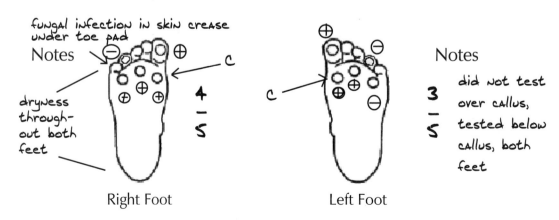

Right Foot   Left Foot

V. Risk Categorization

Check appropriate item.

_____ Low-Risk Patient
All of the following:
Intact protective sensation
Pedal pulses present
No severe deformity
No prior foot ulcer
No amputation

✓ High-Risk Patient
One or more of the following:
Loss of protective sensation ✓
Absent pedal pulses (diminished)
Severe foot deformity
History of foot ulcer
Prior amputation

VI. Footwear Assessment

Fill in the blanks.

Does the patient wear appropriate shoes?
_____ Yes
✓ No

Does the patient need inserts?
_____ Yes
✓ No

Should therapeutic footwear be prescribed?
_____ Yes **?** refer to podiatrist/primary care MD
_____ No

VII. Education

Fill in the blanks.

Has the patient had prior foot care education?
_____ Yes
✓ No

Can the patient demonstrate appropriate self-care?
_____ Yes
✓ No

VIII. Management Plan

Check all that apply.

_____√_____ Provide patient education for preventive foot care.

Date: ___*patient deferred to follow-up visit*___

Diagnostic studies:
_____ Vascular laboratory
_____ Other: _____

Footwear recommendations:
_____ None
___√___ Athletic shoes
_____ Accommodative inserts
_____ Custom shoes
_____ Depth shoes

Refer to:
___√___ Primary care provider   *possibly podiatrist*
_____ Diabetes educator
_____ Orthopedic foot surgeon
_____ RN foot specialist
_____ Orthotist
_____ Podiatrist
_____ Pedorthist
_____ Endocrinologist
_____ Rehab. specialist
_____ Vascular surgeon
_____ Other: _____
_____ Schedule follow-up visit

Date: __**4/3/98**__   Provider Signature: ___John O'Malley, PharmD.___

Source: http://www.niddk.nih.gov/health/diabetes/feet/feet2/screenfo.htm

PHARMACIST'S PATIENT
MEDICAL HISTORY FORM

I. PATIENT INFORMATION

Name: _Sarah McLucas_

Address: _4701 Stalwart Way Anywhere, USA_

Home Phone: _555-7401_   Office Phone: _-_

Date of Birth: _12/25/27_   Last year of education completed: _high school_

Patient lives with _Alone_

Caregiver (if applicable): _N/A_

Caregiver Phone: _N/A_

Employer: _N/A_   Job Title: _N/A_

Name of Health Insurer: _Medicare_

Health Ins. Card #: _111-11-1111_   Social Security #: _111-11-1111_

Primary Care Physician's Name: _Dr. Davis_   Phone: _555-1295_

Specialist Physician's Name: _N/A_   Phone: _N/A_

Other Health Care Practitioner: _N/A_   Phone: _N/A_

II. MEDICAL HISTORY

Are you allergic to any prescription drugs or over-the-counter medications? _____

☒ Yes   ☐ No   If yes, please list the medications and type of allergic reaction experienced:

aspirin ———> stomach upset

Are there any medications that you are not allergic to but cannot tolerate? _____

☐ Yes   ☒ No   If yes, please list the medications and the reaction experienced:

_____

Do you use tobacco?

☐ Yes   ☒ No   If yes, what type? _____ How often?_____

Do you drink alcohol?

☐ Yes   ☒ No   If yes, what type? _____ How often?_____

Name: **Sarah McLucas**

Please put a check (✔) next to those items listed below that apply to you:

HEART PROBLEMS:	✔	URINARY/REPRODUCTIVE:	✔
Chest pain (angina)		Urinary or bladder infection	
Past heart attack		Prostate problems	
Heart failure		Hysterectomy	
Irregular heartbeat		Chronic yeast infections	
Heart by-pass surgery		Kidney disease	
Rheumatic fever		Dialysis	
Other:		Other:	

EYES, EARS, NOSE & THROAT	✔	MUSCLES AND BONES	✔
Poor vision	✓	Arthritis	✓
Poor hearing		Gout	
Glaucoma		Back problems	
Sinus problems		Amputation	
Balance disorder		Joint replacement	
Other:		Other:	

GASTROINTESTINAL	✔	NEUROLOGICAL	✔
Heartburn	✓	Headaches (sinus)	✓
Ulcer		Seizures or epilepsy	
Constipation		Parkinson's disease	
Diverticulitis		Dizziness	
Liver disease		Past stroke	
Gallbladder problems		Fainting	
Pancreatitis		Depression	
Other:		Anxiety	
		Other:	

DO YOU HAVE:	✔	LUNG PROBLEMS	✔
High blood pressure	✓	Asthma	
Low blood pressure		Emphysema	
High cholesterol	✓	Bronchitis	
Diabetes	✓	Other:	
Cancer			
Anemia			
Bleeding disorder	✓	**DO YOU HAVE OR USE ...?**	✔
Hay fever	✓	Glasses	✓
Sleeping problems		Hearing aid	
Other:		Other:	

DO YOU HAVE A FAMILY HISTORY OF:			
High blood pressure	✓	Asthma	
Heart disease	✓	Other:	
Diabetes	✓		

Name: __Sarah McLucas__

III. Current Prescription Medications (including ones received at other pharmacies)

Name of prescription medicine and strength (i.e., milligrams, grams, and units)	How much do you take each time?	How many times a day do you take the medicine?	Medical problem being treated	When did you start taking this medicine?	Has the medicine helped you? Yes/No	Name of doctor or specialist who prescribed the medicine
Example: Diabeta, 2.5 mg	1	2	Diabetes	1992	Yes	Dr. Harold Smith
Cholestyramine	1 scoop	1 don't	cholesterol	1997	no	Davis
Naprosyn 500 mg	1	2	arthritis	1996	some	Davis
Calcium Carbonate 500 mg	1	4x/day	diet supplement	1996	yes	Davis

IV. Current Nonprescription Medications

Ex: Antacids, anti-diarrheals, allergy medicines, anti-nausea, diet pills, ear or eye medications, laxatives, pain relievers, vitamins, etc.

Name of medicine Example: Tylenol	How often do you take it? (daily, once a week, etc.)	Name of medicine	How often do you take it?
Mylanta	~ every 1-2 weeks		
Tavist-D	when needed for hay fever		
Motrin IB	3-4x a week		

I certify this information is accurate and complete to the best of my knowledge. _____

signature/date

PHARMACIST'S PATIENT DATABASE FORM

Original Date:_____
Date updated:_____
Date updated:_____
Date updated:_____

Demographic and Administrative Information

Name:	Social Security #:
Address:	
Health Care Provider's Name	Health Care Provider's Phone
Work Phone: Home Phone:	Date of Birth:
Race:	Gender:
Religion:	Occupation:
Health Insurer:	Subscriber #:
Primary Card Holder:	Drug Benefit: ❑ yes ❑ no copay: $_____

Current Symptoms

Past Medical History	Acute and Current Medical Problems
	1.
	2.
	3.
	4.
	5.
	6.
	7.
	8.

Family/Social/Economic History	Personal Limitations

Cost of medications per month $_____

Allergies/Intolerances	Social Drug Use
❑ No known drug allergies	Alcohol
Medication Reaction	Caffeine
	Tobacco
	Pregnancy/Breastfeeding Status
	❑ Pregnant (due _____) ❑ Breastfeeding

Diet	Routine Exercise/Recreation Daily Activities/Timing
❑ Low salt	
❑ Low fat	
❑ Diabetic	
Timing of meals:	

Patient Name: _____

Physical Assessment/Laboratory Data—Initial/Follow-up					
Date					
Height					
Weight					
Temp					
BP					
Pulse					
Respirations					
Peak Flow					
FBG					
R. Glucose					
HbA_{1c}					
T. Chol.					
LDL					
HDL					
TG					
INR					
BUN					
Cr					
ALT					
AST					
Alk Phos					

Drug Serum Concentrations

Date					

Notes:

Patient Name: _____

Current Prescription Medication Regimen

Name/Dose/Strength/Route	Schedule/ Frequency of Use	Indication	Start Date (and Stop Date If Applicable)	Prescriber	Adherence Issues/Efficacy

Current Nonprescription Medication Regimen (OTC, herbal, homeopathic, nutritional, etc.)

Name/Dose/Strength/Route	Schedule/ Frequency of Use	Indication	Start Date (and Stop Date If Applicable)	Prescriber	Adherence Issues/Efficacy

Patient Name: _____

Risk Assessment/Preventive Measures/Quality of Life

Cardiovascular Risk Assessment		
male >45 years old	1	
female >55 years old or female <55 with history of ovarectomy not taking estrogen replacement	1	
Definite MI or sudden death before age 55 year in father or male first-degree relative or before 65 year in mother or female first-degree relative	1	
current cigarette smoking	1	
hypertension	1	
diabetes mellitus	1	
HDL cholesterol <35 mg/dl	1	
HDL cholesterol >60 mg/dl	-1	
	Total:	

Is patient at risk for complications of current conditions? ❏ Yes ❏ No
Specify:

Preventive Measures for Adults
H = has been done   R = patient refuses   X = not applicable   Date

Women						
Pap Smear/pelvic	Annually 19+					
Mammogram	Every 1-2Y 40-49; annually 50+					
Men						
Rectal/prostate	Annually 50+					
All Patients						
Total/HDL-C	Every 5Y 19+					
Home Fecal Occult Blood Test	Annually					
Immunizations						
Td	Every 10Y					
Influenza	Every fall*					
Pneumovax	Once*					

* if indicated

Quality of life issues

Assessment of General Appearance

Patient _____   Date _____

General Appearance	Observations and Comments

Level of consciousness
    alertness: alert, confused,
    delirious, stuporous, comatose,
    orientation: person, place, time	

Signs of distress respiratory distress, pain, anxiety, etc.	
Posture, motor activity, and gait *Describe*	
Dress, grooming, and personal hygiene *Describe*	

Affect
    normal, inappropriate
    Describe	

Speech
    normal, impaired
    Describe	

Skin
    color: normal, blue, brown, red, pallor
    texture: normal, coarse, dry, oily
    turgor: good, poor
    edema
    lesions: color, type, configuration, anatomic
        distribution, consistency	

SCREENING FORM FOR DIABETES FOOT DISEASE

Name: _____

Date: _____

ID #: _____

I. Medical History

Check all that apply.

_____ Peripheral neuropathy

_____ Nephropathy

_____ Retinopathy

_____ Peripheral vascular disease

_____ Cardiovascular disease

For Sections II & III, fill in the blanks with an "R," "L," or "B" for positive findings on the right, left, or both feet.

II. Current History

1. Any change in the foot since the last evaluation?

_____ Yes _____

_____ No

2. Current ulcer or history of a foot ulcer?

_____ Yes _____

_____ No

3. Is there pain in the calf muscles when walking that is relieved by rest?

_____ Yes _____

_____ No

III. Foot Exam

1. Are the nails thick, too long, ingrown, infected with fungal disease?
_____ Yes _____
_____ No

2. Note foot deformities
_____ Toe deformities
_____ Bunions (hallus valgus)
_____ Charcot foot
_____ Foot drop
_____ Prominent metatarsal heads
_____ Amputation (specify date, side and level) _____

3. Pedal Pulses *(Fill in the blanks with a "P" or an "A" to indicate present or absent.)*
Posterior tibial:
_____ Left
_____ Right

Dorsalis pedis:
_____ Left
_____ Right

4. Skin Condition *(Measure, draw in, and label the patient's skin condition, using the key and the foot diagram below.)*

C = Callus   PU = Pre-ulcerative lesion
U = Ulcer   F = Fissure
R = Redness   S = Swelling
W = Warmth   D = Dryness
M = Maceration

IV. Sensory Foot Exam

Label sensory level with a "+" in the five circled areas of the foot if the patient can feel the 5.07 Semmes-Weinstein (10-gram) nylon filament and "−" if the patient cannot feel the filament.

Notes 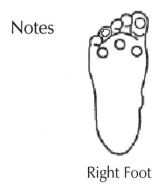 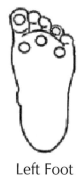 Notes

Right Foot   Left Foot

V. Risk Categorization

Check appropriate item.

_____ Low-Risk Patient
All of the following:
Intact protective sensation
Pedal pulses present
No severe deformity
No prior foot ulcer
No amputation

_____ High-Risk Patient
One or more of the following:
Loss of protective sensation
Absent pedal pulses
Severe foot deformity
History of foot ulcer
Prior amputation

VI. Footwear Assessment

Fill in the blanks.

Does the patient wear appropriate shoes?
_____ Yes
_____ No

Does the patient need inserts?
_____ Yes
_____ No

Should therapeutic footwear be prescribed?
_____ Yes
_____ No

VII. Education

Fill in the blanks.

Has the patient had prior foot care education?
_____ Yes
_____ No

Can the patient demonstrate appropriate self-care?
_____ Yes
_____ No

VIII. Management Plan

Check all that apply.

_____ Provide patient education for preventive foot care.

Date: _____

Diagnostic studies:
_____ Vascular laboratory
_____ Other: _____

Footwear recommendations:
_____ None
_____ Athletic shoes
_____ Accommodative inserts
_____ Custom shoes
_____ Depth shoes

Refer to:
_____ Primary care provider
_____ Diabetes educator
_____ Orthopedic foot surgeon
_____ RN foot specialist
_____ Orthotist
_____ Podiatrist
_____ Pedorthist
_____ Endocrinologist
_____ Rehab. specialist
_____ Vascular surgeon
_____ Other: _____
_____ Schedule follow-up visit

Date: _____   Provider Signature: _____

Source: http://www.niddk.nih.gov/health/diabetes/feet/feet2/screenfo.htm

PHARMACIST'S PATIENT DATABASE FORM

Original Date: **4/23/98**
Date updated: _____
Date updated: _____
Date updated: _____

Demographic and Administrative Information

Name: Sarah McLucas	Social Security #: 111-11-1111
Address: 4701 Stalwart Way	
Health Care Provider's Name: Dr. Davis	Health Care Provider's Phone: 555-1295
Work Phone: N/A Home Phone: 555-7401	Date of Birth: 12/25/27
Race: Caucasian	Gender: F
Religion: Lutheran	Occupation: retired school teacher
Health Insurer: Medicare	Subscriber #:
Primary Card Holder: Pt.	Drug Benefit: ❑ yes ☑ no copay: $_____

Current Symptoms
Pt. was without complaints. BG drawn on routine screen ↑; repeated →dx DM

Past Medical History	Acute and Current Medical Problems
Hypercholesterolemia-1997	1. Hypercholesterolemia
DM	2. Diabetes mellitus
OA-1996	3. Osteoarthritis
HTN-1995	4. HTN
GERD	5. GERD
Seasonal allergic rhinitis	6. Allergic rhinitis
Ø surgeries	7.
Hospitalized 1992 c̄ pneumonia	8.

Family/Social/Economic History	Personal Limitations
lives alone, never married	Decreased vision
no children	
mother ↓ @ 74; h/o HTN, CAD, DM	
father ↓ @ 82; h/o HTN, CAD, CA	
Cost of medications per month $ ~50⁰⁰	

Allergies/Intolerances	Social Drug Use	
❑ No known drug allergies	Alcohol	Ø
Medication Reaction	Caffeine	Ø
Aspirin GI upset	Tobacco	Ø

Pregnancy/Breastfeeding Status N/A
❑ Pregnant (due _____)   ❑ Breastfeeding

Diet	Routine Exercise/Recreation	Daily Activities/Timing
☑ Low salt prescribed;	Gardening	9-11 AM volunteer work
☑ Low fat ↓ salt but	light housework	
❑ Diabetic not fat		
Timing of meals:		

Patient Name: __Sarah McLucas__

Physical Assessment/Laboratory Data—Initial/Follow-up

Date	4/14/98	4/20/98	4/23/98		
Height			5'5"		
Weight			162 lb BMI 27		
Temp			98.6 °F oral		
BP			134/86 RA sitting		
Pulse			72 reg R/R		
Respirations			14		
Peak Flow					
FBG	142	138			
R. Glucose					
HbA$_{1c}$		9.4%			
T. Chol.		232			
LDL		145			
HDL		30			
TG		284			
INR					
BUN					
Cr		0.8			
ALT					
AST					
Alk Phos					
U/A			⊖ glucose		
			⊖ protein, ket		
Microalb			⊖		

Drug Serum Concentrations

Date					

Notes:

Patient Name: Sarah McLucas

Current Prescription Medication Regimen

Name/Dose/Strength/Route	Schedule/ Frequency of Use	Indication	Start Date (and Stop Date If Applicable)	Prescriber	Adherence Issues/Efficacy
Cholestyramine T scoop	BID	Hyperlipid.	1997-	Davis	not taking
Naprosyn 500	BID	OA	1996-	Davis	takes/fair
Calcium Carbonate 500 mg	QID	supplement	1996	Davis	takes/good

Current Nonprescription Medication Regimen (OTC, herbal, homeopathic, nutritional, etc.)

Name/Dose/Strength/Route	Schedule/ Frequency of Use	Indication	Start Date (and Stop Date If Applicable)	Prescriber	Adherence Issues/Efficacy
Tavist-D	T BID	allergic rhinitis	1994-	-	takes/good
Mylanta	T tablespoon	GERD	weekly 1996-	-	weekly/fair
Motrin IB	q 4-6 pm	OA	1994-	-	3-4x q wk

Patient Name: __Sarah McLucas__

Risk Assessment/Preventive Measures/Quality of Life

Cardiovascular Risk Assessment		
male >45 years old	1	
female >55 years old or female <55 with history of ovarectomy not taking estrogen replacement	1	l
Definite MI or sudden death before age 55 year in father or male first-degree relative or before 65 year in mother or female first-degree relative	1	
current cigarette smoking	1	
hypertension	1	l
diabetes mellitus	1	l
HDL cholesterol <35 mg/dl	1	l
HDL cholesterol >60 mg/dl	-1	
	Total:	**4**

Is patient at risk for complications of current conditions? ☑ Yes   ☐ No
Specify: HbAlc 9.4% above goal

Preventive Measures for Adults
H = has been done   R = patient refuses   X = not applicable   Date

Women		4/23/98				
Pap Smear/pelvic	Annually 19+	H				
Mammogram	Every 1-2Y 40-49; annually 50+	H				
Men						
Rectal/prostate	Annually 50+					
All Patients						
Total/HDL-C	Every 5Y 19+	H				
Home Fecal Occult Blood Test	Annually	H				
Immunizations						
Td	Every 10Y	H				
Influenza	Every fall*	H				
Pneumovax	Once*	H				

* if indicated

Quality of life issues

Assessment of General Appearance

Patient _____Sarah McLucas_____ Date ___4/23/98___

General Appearance	Observations and Comments

Level of consciousness
    alertness: alert, confused,
    delirious, stuporous, comatose,
    orientation: person, place, time
	alert & oriented to
	person, place & time

Signs of distress respiratory distress, pain, anxiety, etc.	no distress, very pleasant
Posture, motor activity, and gait *Describe*	normal
Dress, grooming, and personal hygiene *Describe*	exceptionally well groomed

Affect
    normal, inappropriate
    Describe
	appropriate, quiet

Speech
    normal, impaired
    Describe
	normal

Skin
    color: normal, blue, brown, red, pallor
    texture: normal, coarse, dry, oily
    turgor: good, poor
    edema
    lesions: color, type, configuration, anatomic
       distribution, consistency
	normal skin color
	(many freckles)
	good skin turgor.
	no edema or lesions

SCREENING FORM FOR DIABETES FOOT DISEASE

Name: __Sarah McLucas__

Date: __4/23/98__

ID #: _____

I. Medical History

Check all that apply.

_____ Peripheral neuropathy

_____ Nephropathy

_____ Retinopathy

_____ Peripheral vascular disease

__✓__ Cardiovascular disease   (HTN)

For Sections II & III, fill in the blanks with an "R," "L," or "B" for positive findings on the right, left, or both feet.

II. Current History

1. Any change in the foot since the last evaluation?

_____ Yes _____

_____ No   1st exam

2. Current ulcer or history of a foot ulcer?

_____ Yes _____

__✓__ No

3. Is there pain in the calf muscles when walking that is relieved by rest?

_____ Yes _____

__✓__ No

III. Foot Exam

1. Are the nails thick, too long, ingrown, infected with fungal disease?

_____ Yes _____

__✓__ No

2. Note foot deformities

_____ Toe deformities

_____ Bunions (hallus valgus)   NONE

_____ Charcot foot

_____ Foot drop

_____ Prominent metatarsal heads

_____ Amputation (specify date, side, and level) _____

3. Pedal Pulses *(Fill in the blanks with a "P" or an "A" to indicate present or absent.)*

Posterior tibial:

__P__ Left

__P__ Right

} NORMAl

Dorsalis pedis:

__P__ Left

__P__ Right

4. Skin Condition (*Measure, draw in, and label the patient's skin condition, using the key and the foot diagram below.*)

C = Callus   PU = Pre-ulcerative lesion

U = Ulcer   F = Fissure

R = Redness   S = Swelling

W = Warmth   D = Dryness

M = Maceration

IV. Sensory Foot Exam

Label sensory level with a "+" in the five circled areas of the foot if the patient can feel the 5.07 Semmes-Weinstein (10-gram) nylon filament and "−" if the patient cannot feel the filament.

Notes 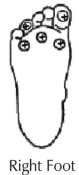 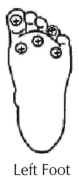 Notes

Right Foot   Left Foot

V. Risk Categorization

Check appropriate item.

___✓___ Low-Risk Patient

All of the following:

Intact protective sensation

Pedal pulses present

No severe deformity

No prior foot ulcer

No amputation

_____ High-Risk Patient

One or more of the following:

Loss of protective sensation

Absent pedal pulses

Severe foot deformity

History of foot ulcer

Prior amputation

VI. Footwear Assessment

Fill in the blanks.

Does the patient wear appropriate shoes?

___✓___ Yes

_____ No

Does the patient need inserts?

_____ Yes

___✓___ No

Should therapeutic footwear be prescribed?

_____ Yes

___✓___ No

VII. Education

Fill in the blanks.

Has the patient had prior foot care education?

_____ Yes

___✓___ No

Can the patient demonstrate appropriate self-care?

___✓___ Yes

_____ No

VIII. Management Plan

Check all that apply.

__✓__ Provide patient education for preventive foot care.

Date: **4/23/98** _____

Diagnostic studies:
_____ Vascular laboratory
_____ Other: _____

Footwear recommendations:
__✓__ None
_____ Athletic shoes
_____ Accommodative inserts
_____ Custom shoes
_____ Depth shoes

Refer to:
__✓__ Primary care provider   *for scheduled follow-up*
_____ Diabetes educator
_____ Orthopedic foot surgeon
_____ RN foot specialist
_____ Orthotist
_____ Podiatrist
_____ Pedorthist
_____ Endocrinologist
_____ Rehab. specialist
_____ Vascular surgeon
_____ Other: _____
_____ Schedule follow-up visit

Date: _____ **4/23/98** _____   Provider Signature: _**Alexa Sheffield, Pharm.D.**_____

Source: http://www.niddk.nih.gov/health/diabetes/feet/feet2/screenfo.htm

Part II

Developing an Ambulatory Pharmacist's Care Plan for Patients with Type 2 Diabetes

Assessing Current Medication and Related Therapy and Creating a Therapy Problem List

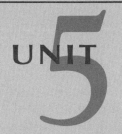

UNIT 5

As discussed in unit 7 of the *Ambulatory Care Clinical Skills Program: Core Module*, the pharmacist's care plan consists of four components:

- patient problem list and health care needs;
- pharmacotherapeutic and related health care goals;
- recommended therapy; and
- monitoring plan (parameters, endpoints, and frequency).

At this point you have followed the development of the database for several patients with type 2 diabetes. Now we need to develop the first component of the pharmacist's care plan: the therapy problem list and health care needs assessment.

It is vital the pharmacist assess the current pharmacotherapy and related health care therapy of an ambulatory patient with type 2 diabetes because assessment can identify problems and unmet needs in the patient's current therapy. This identification results in better disease management and decreased potential for the significant morbidity and mortality associated with complications of uncontrolled type 2 diabetes. You will learn more about the importance of tight blood glucose and blood pressure control and its impact on patient outcomes in unit 7.

Unit Objectives

After you successfully complete this unit, you will be able to:

- describe types of problems commonly present in the unreviewed therapy of ambulatory patients with type 2 diabetes,
- determine the presence of any of the following medication or medication-related therapy problems in the current therapy of ambulatory patients with type 2 diabetes:
  - Medication used with no therapy indication
  - Medical condition for which there is no therapy prescribed
  - Therapy prescribed inappropriately for a particular medical condition
  - Anything inappropriate in the current medication therapy regimen
  - Presence of therapeutic duplication
  - Prescription of medication to which the patient is allergic or intolerant
  - Presence or potential for adverse drug events
  - Presence or potential for clinically significant drug-drug, drug-disease, drug-nutrient, or drug–laboratory test interactions
  - Interference with medical therapy of social or cultural drug use or use of alternative therapies
  - Problems arising from financial impact of therapy on the patient
  - Patient lack of understanding of therapy
  - Patient nonadherence to therapy regimen
  - Patient at risk because of patient-specific characteristics (e.g., age and living/working environment)
  - Incomplete preventive measures
  - Adverse impact of therapy on patient's quality of life, and

- construct a therapy problem list for an ambulatory patient with type 2 diabetes.

Unit Organization

In this unit you will apply what you learned in units 7–11 of the *Ambulatory Care Clinical Skills Program: Core Module*. We will first discuss therapeutic problems commonly experienced by ambulatory patients with type 2 diabetes, with examples for each category. Then, through use of an Ambulatory Therapy Assessment Worksheet (ATAW), we will assess Mrs. Gonzalez's current therapy and prepare a Therapy Problem List (TPL) using the Ambulatory Pharmacist's Care Plan (APCP). You will then have a chance to assess the therapy and identify the pharmacotherapeutic and health care needs of Mr. Jones through a practice exercise.

Common Therapy Problems Unique to Ambulatory Patients with Type 2 Diabetes

Creation of a therapy problem list begins with an assessment of the patient's complete medical history and current therapy and includes an assessment of all drug and nondrug therapies. This assessment allows you to identify problems for setting therapeutic goals. In unit 9 of the *Ambulatory Care Clinical Skills Program: Core Module* you learned about variables such as comparative efficacy and safety, formulary issues, achievement of therapy goals, and patient-specific characteristics (such as age, gender, religion, occupation, ethnic background, pregnancy and lactation, cognitive limitations, physical limitations, social support and living arrangements, and patient preference and behavior) that guide your evaluation process. For the purposes of our discussion, we will focus on the medications that are being used to treat the patient's diabetes.

Current Medication Therapy Regimen

As described in the *Ambulatory Care Clinical Skills Program: Core Module*, one of the first steps you will take when reviewing a medication regimen is to determine a correlation between drug therapy and medical problems. This is done by matching the patient's known medical conditions with the medication list. This procedure allows you to detect the presence of medications prescribed without an indication or prescribed inappropriately as well as indications for which no medication is prescribed.

Following this, you can review the use of individual agents in the patient's therapy. Is the drug inappropriate (i.e., not the best choice for treating this patient's diabetes)? Review the dose, dosage form, schedule, duration, route of administration, method of administration, and need for adjunctive therapy.

Drug Selection

In unit 8 we will discuss how a practitioner selects and recommends the most appropriate drug therapy for an ambulatory patient with type 2 diabetes. The effectiveness of a drug is considered; for example, how well does the medication lower fasting plasma glucose, postprandial plasma glucose, and hemoglobin A_{1c}? How severe is the patient's blood glucose elevation at this time? How severe are the patient's symptoms at this time? How do the side effect profiles compare between therapeutic options? Is there a formulary consideration or other financial implications? Other considerations include patient-related variables. The following examples illustrate how patient-specific variables might affect drug selection.

Concomitant medical conditions—If a patient with type 2 diabetes also has hypercholesterolemia, metformin might be a good choice because it has a favorable effect on the lipid profile.

Physical characteristics—If a patient is obese he or she is more likely to be insulin resistant. Three medications used to enhance insulin sensitivity are metformin, rosiglitazone, and troglitazone (in combination therapy).

Allergies—If a patient has a history of allergy to sulfa products, this would be significant information when considering an oral sulfonylurea agent.

Renal and hepatic function—Patients with poor renal function should not receive metformin. Patients with impaired liver function should not receive troglitazone.

Fear of needles and injection—Some patients are afraid of giving themselves an injection. In many cases this fear can be overcome, but it should be considered a variable in drug selection.

Dose

Has the prescriber increased the dose appropriately? Many times prescribers will turn to combination drug therapy before maximizing the usefulness of a single medication.

Schedule

Most medications have recommended administration times relative to meals (**Table 1**).[1] For example, glyburide is usually administered as a single daily dose given each morning with breakfast or the first main meal of the day. However, some patients respond better to two divided daily doses, particularly patients who require >10 mg per day.

Of note are the recommendations for acarbose and repaglinide. Acarbose is an alpha-glucosidase inhibitor, which delays and decreases glucose absorption. However, it only does this if the medication precedes food into the gastrointestinal tract. Obviously, it is very important that patients take acarbose as recommended, "with the first bite of the meal," not simply "with food."

Repaglinide is an insulin secretagogue chemically unrelated to the oral sulfonylurea agents. Repaglinide's mechanism of action is to stimulate the release of insulin from the pancreas. The drug is rapidly and completely absorbed after oral administration, reaching peak effect within 1 hour. Repaglinide should be administered 15 minutes before a meal. If the patient skips a meal, skip the repaglinide dose. If a meal is added, they should take an additional dose.

Need for Combination Therapy

If the patient was on the correct medication and the dose was optimized but the patient still has not achieved his or her glycemic goal, you would consider using combination therapy. There are many possible combinations of two or perhaps even three diabetes medications. Combination therapy will be discussed in greater detail in unit 8.

Method of Administration

Is the therapy being administered correctly? For example, insulin is administered subcutaneously. Incorrect administration technique (in the example of insulin, intramuscular administration) may alter the pharmacokinetics. Another insulin administration issue is the actual injection site. The absorption rate varies between the abdomen, thigh, upper arm, and flank. Many diabetes treatment centers are now recommending use of the abdomen exclusively to standardize and optimize insulin's absorption.

Presence or Potential for Adverse Drug Events

Therapy assessment should evaluate each drug's real or potential ability to cause the patient's symptoms or medical conditions. For example, a common adverse drug effect associated with diabetes therapy is drug-induced hypoglycemia, which occurs with

Table 1. Recommended Oral Antidiabetic Medication Administration Times with Respect to Meals

Agent	Recommendation
Acarbose	Administered at the beginning (with the first bite) of each main meal
Acetohexamide	Administered once or twice a day before the morning (and evening) meal(s)
Chlorpropamide	Administered in the morning with breakfast
Glimepiride	Administered once daily each morning with breakfast or the first main meal
Glipizide	Administered once a day approximately 30 minutes before a meal
Glyburide	Administered once a day with breakfast or the first main meal
Repaglinide	Administered 15 minutes before each meal
Metformin	Administered two to three times daily with food
Miglitol	Administered at the beginning (with the first bite) of each main meal
Rosiglitazone	Administered once or twice a day without respect to meals
Tolazamide	Administered once or twice a day with food
Tolbutamide	Administered once or twice a day after meals
Troglitazone	Administered as a single daily dose given each morning with breakfast or the first main meal

several agents. Oral sulfonylurea agents, repaglinide, and insulin are the only drugs used to treat diabetes that are commonly associated with hypoglycemia. Metformin, troglitazone, miglitol, and acarbose rarely cause hypoglycemia, unless used in combination with one of the agents listed above. Therefore, any patient on an oral sulfonylurea, repaglinide, or insulin, as monotherapy or in combination therapy, has the potential to develop hypoglycemia.

Troglitazone has been associated with several deaths from liver failure. Therefore, if a patient had elevated liver function tests, this would be a significant adverse event.

As described in the *Ambulatory Care Clinical Skills Program: Core Module*, you should ask yourself several questions when evaluating a potential drug-induced adverse event:

- Did the adverse effect occur after the patient started using the medication?
- Did the adverse effect cease when the medication was discontinued?
- Did the adverse effect return when the medication was re-initiated?
- Is the symptom a known adverse effect associated with the medication?
- What is the incidence of the adverse effect?
- Does the patient have risk factors for adverse effects (e.g., advanced age, impaired renal function, impaired liver function, etc.)?

If you suspect the adverse event is drug-related and it is not a very common adverse effect, you are obliged to report it to the FDA.

Table 2 lists some of the more commonly experienced adverse drug events associated with diabetes therapies.[1-5]

Presence or Potential for Clinically Significant Drug Interactions

The current therapy regimen should be assessed for potential or actual drug-drug, drug-disease, drug-nutrient, or drug–laboratory test interactions. Consider the case of Mrs. Webster, an 82-year-old woman in a long-term care facility. She has a long history of type 2 diabetes and hypertension. Her medication regimen is as follows: glyburide 10 mg every morning and propanolol extended release capsules 160 mg every morning.

Mrs. Webster doesn't like the food in the long-term care facility, so her family continually brings food in "to make Mama and us feel better." However, the week the family went on vacation, Mrs. Webster was found unconscious, with a blood glucose of 38 mg/dl. What happened? Why didn't

Mrs. Webster complain of symptoms of hypoglycemia? When the family went on vacation, she wasn't getting all the food she normally ate, so her blood glucose dropped. She didn't complain of hypoglycemia because her nonselective beta-adrenergic blocking agent, propranolol, masked all symptoms of hypoglycemia except sweating.

There are many medications that can interact with the medications used to treat diabetes, or worsen blood glucose control (drug-disease interaction). With the case of Mrs. Webster, it would be important to recognize the potential for this drug-disease interaction before it occurs. **Tables 3 through 6** list some common drug interactions experienced by patients with diabetes.[6]

Problems Arising from Financial Impact of Therapy

We are very fortunate to have so many therapeutic options available to treat type 2 diabetes today. However, they range in price from <$4 per month to almost $100 per month, at starting doses. When we use combination therapy at maximum doses, the costs for patients who do not have a prescription benefit can be prohibitive.

You also need to consider the total cost of therapy with a specific agent. Associated costs include laboratory tests, follow-up visits, and dosing aids. For example, patients taking troglitazone must also have regular liver function tests assessed to make sure they are not experiencing adverse effects. Considering all variables will help you answer the question, Is this medication regimen and its ancillary expenses cost-effective? Even if you determine it is cost-effective and the best possible treatment for the patient, if the answer to the question, Does the cost of therapy represent a financial hardship for the patient? is yes, then the patient may not get the prescription filled at all.

Table 7 shows the average wholesale price (AWP) comparison of oral antidiabetic agents.[7]

Patient Lack of Understanding of Medication Therapy

This drug-related problem can overlap with several of the others discussed above. A patient's failure to take his or her acarbose with the first bite of a meal is a scheduling problem, but it may be caused by the patient's lack of understanding. Patients may also experience an adverse drug reaction and not realize it is due to their diabetes medication. As discussed in the *Ambulatory Care Clinical Skills Program: Core Module*, use your time wisely when interviewing your

Table 2. Adverse Effects Experienced with Diabetes Therapies

Agent	*Adverse Effects*
Acarbose	• Hypoglycemia, when used in combination treatment with insulin or oral sulfonylurea agents • Increased liver enzymes • Gastrointestinal distress: abdominal pain, diarrhea, and flatulence • Slight decrease in hematocrit
Insulin	• Hypoglycemia • Weight gain • Dermatologic reactions: pruritus, erythema, swelling, and stinging at injection site • Lipohypertrophy/lipoatrophy
Metformin	• Hypoglycemia, when used in combination treatment with insulin or oral sulfonylurea agent • Gastrointestinal distress: diarrhea, nausea, vomiting, abdominal bloating, flatulence, anorexia, and metallic taste • Reduced vitamin B_{12} levels (asymptomatic cases) • Lactic acidosis (rare; occurred in cases where drug was contraindicated). Symptoms include: malaise, myalgias, respiratory distress, increased somnolence, and abdominal distress.
Miglitol	• Hypoglycemia, when used in combination treatment with insulin or oral sulfonylurea agent • Gastrointestinal distress: abdominal pain, diarrhea, and flatulence
Repaglinide	• Hypoglycemia • Upper respiratory infection • Sinusitis/rhinitis/bronchitis • Gastrointestinal distress: nausea, vomiting, diarrhea, constipation, and dyspepsia • Arthralgia/back pain • Headache
Rosiglitazone	• Weight gain • Adversely affects lipid profile
Sulfonylureas	• Hypoglycemia • Gastrointestinal distress: nausea, fullness, and heartburn • Dermatologic reactions: pruritus and rash • Weight gain • Blood dyscrasias (rare) • Alcohol intolerance (mostly with chlorpropamide) • Hepatotoxicity (rare) • Syndrome of Inappropriate Antidiuretic Hormone (SIADH) (mostly with chlorpropamide)
Troglitazone	• Hypoglycemia, when used in combination treatment with insulin or oral sulfonylurea agents • Increased liver enzymes; idiosyncratic hepatocellular injury (rare). Hepatic failure and death have been reported. Symptoms of hepatic injury include nausea, vomiting, abdominal pain, fatigue, anorexia, dark urine, and increased liver enzymes.

Table 3. Effects of Drugs of Abuse on Diabetes Management

Drug of Abuse	Effect
Alcohol	Hypoglycemia; impairs judgment, possibly leading to failure to self-manage therapy appropriately; alters insulin response when taken with carbohydrate sources; alters glycogen manufacture, release, and storage
Caffeine (large amounts)	Increases blood glucose levels
Central nervous system stimulants	Increases blood glucose levels; causes hyperglycemia by increasing liver glycogen breakdown; may cause anorexia, resulting in increased blood glucose levels; alters time perception, possibly leading to failure to self-manage therapy appropriately
Marijuana	Stimulates increased food intake; alters time perception, possibly leading to failure to self-manage therapy appropriately; impairs glucose tolerance in large doses
Nicotine	Alters oral and intravenous glucose tolerance tests; risk factor for development of diabetic nephropathy; may decrease subcutaneous absorption of insulin; may increase insulin requirements by 15–20%
Opiates	Causes euphoria, possibly leading to failure to self-manage therapy appropriately
Sedatives and hypnotics	Impaired thought, possibly leading to failure to self-manage therapy appropriately

patient to assess the patient's knowledge of his or her medications. If nonadherence or lack of understanding is found to be a problem, the patient may benefit from medication counseling and patient education tools (e.g., written information, audio or videotaped information, and wallet cards) or adherence aids. This need should be noted on your problem list.

Patient Not Adhering to Medication Regimen

As described in the *Ambulatory Care Clinical Skills Program: Core Module*, nonadherence can represent several behaviors. These may include:

- failure to fill the prescription,
- taking the incorrect dose,
- taking the medication at the wrong time,
- omission of one or more doses,
- stopping the medication too soon, or
- administering medication with incorrect procedure or technique.

Consider the case of Mr. Simpson, who is on insulin (NPH and regular twice daily) for treatment of his type 2 diabetes. Mr. Simpson considers himself to be very well educated about his disease and insulin therapy. Whenever Mr. Simpson wants to deviate from his meal plan (which is frequently), he self-adjusts his insulin therapy. Unfortunately, Mr. Simpson doesn't have a clear understanding of which insulin to adjust or how much to adjust it. Consequently, his blood glucose control is very erratic. Mr. Simpson should be referred to a dietician so he can learn to plan his meals better, or learn to carbohydrate count and adjust his insulin therapy appropriately.

Incorrect administration procedure or technique is commonly seen with patients who inject insulin. Patients are often fearful of injecting themselves, their technique may get sloppy over time, or they may take shortcuts. This is an educational intervention that must be revisited occasionally to assure continued competence.

Patient at Risk Due to Patient-Specific Characteristics

Patient-specific characteristics that place the patient at risk for drug therapy problems should also be assessed. Characteristics that may increase therapy risk in patients with type 2 diabetes include young or old age, pregnancy, and occupation.

Age

Suppose you are the parent of a not quite 2-year-old child recently diagnosed with diabetes. Of course, she is treated with insulin (type 1 diabetics are insulin-requiring) and has had several frightening episodes of hypoglycemia. At her age, the child cannot adequately describe symptoms of developing hypoglycemia, so you must be acutely alert to signs of hypoglycemia. The six S's of hypoglycemia in young children include: feeling shaky, sweaty (but cool to touch), sleepy, staring (will happily eat their least favorite foods), stubborn, and spacey.[8] Other physical clues include pallor, change in activity

Table 4. Medications That Cause or Exacerbate Peripheral Neuropathies

amitriptyline
amphetamines
amphotericin B
carbamazepine
chlorambucil
cimetidine
clofibrate
colchicine
colistin
cytarabine
disopyramide
ergotamine
ethambutol
gold compounds
hydralazine
indomethacin
isoniazid
methysergide
metronidazole
nitrofurantoin
penicillamine
phenytoin
procarbazine
streptomycin
vincristine

Table 5. Medications That May Induce Diabetic Nephropathy

cephaloridine
cyclophosphamide
gentamicin
gold compounds
heroin
kanamycin
methotrexate
methylsergide
neomycin
nonsteroidal analgesics (large doses)
penicillamine
rifampin
tobramycin

level, rubbing the head, and looking for food. It is important not to establish unrealistic goals of euglycemia with children; their central nervous system is still developing, and episodes of hypoglycemia may not be recognized. Other issues with pediatrics include the goal to maintain a normal growth rate (uncontrolled diabetes delays growth) and the wide glucose fluctuations that accompany acute illnesses. Children often seem to have a cold in the winter, and it is important to monitor blood glucose closely to avoid hypoglycemia and diabetic ketoacidosis. When children are ill they are also very susceptible to dehydration.[8]

On the other end of the age spectrum are geriatric patients. Diabetes is not only more common but also more serious in older patients. Older adults with diabetes have a higher incidence of hospitalization and long-term care institution admission rates than older adults who do not have diabetes. There are several challenges in caring for older adults with diabetes, such as an asymptomatic or atypical presentation (e.g., blurred vision may be the only complaint, or the development of a long-term complication may be the first clinical sign of diabetes). Older adults typically have more than one chronic disease, which when coupled with pharmacokinetic and pharmacodynamic changes that accompany aging may result in a complicated

Table 6. Medications That Alter Blood Glucose Levels

Hyperglycemia

acetazolamide	alcohol (chronic use)	amiodarone
asparginase	beta-adrenergic agonists	caffeine
calcium channel blockers	chlorpromazine	chlorthalidone
corticosteroids	cyclosporine	diazoxide
encainide	estrogens	ethacrynic acid
fentanyl	furosemide	indapamide
interferon alpha	lactulose	nalidixic acid
niacin	nicotinic acid	oral contraceptives
pentamidine	phenytoin	probenecid
rifampin	sulfasalazine	sympathomimetic amines
thiazide diuretics	thyroid preparations	tricyclic antidepressants

Hypoglycemia

acetaminophen	alcohol (acute use)	amitriptyline
anabolic steroids	beta-adrenergic blockers	biguanides
chloroquine	clofibrate	disopyramide
fluphenazine	guanethidine	haloperidol
imipramine	insulin	lithium
MAO inhibitors	norfloxacin	pentamidine
perphenazine	phenobarbital	prazosin
propoxyphene	quinine	salicylates (large doses)
sulfonamide antibiotics	sulfonylureas	

medication regimen. A diagnosis of diabetes may necessitate learning a variety of new skills, such as medication management (e.g., insulin administration), blood glucose monitoring, meal planning, regular foot and skin care, exercise, management of blood glucose excursions, smoking cessation, achievement and maintenance of acceptable body weight, and management of concurrent illnesses. An older adult may be unable or unwilling to accept these responsibilities.[9]

Pregnancy

Women who develop glucose intolerance during pregnancy are diagnosed with gestational diabetes. Women in this diagnostic category, as well as women with diabetes who elect to become pregnant, must achieve as near to euglycemic control as possible. Uncontrolled diabetes during pregnancy is associated with adverse outcomes for both mother and child. An in-depth discussion on the treatment of diabetes during pregnancy is beyond the scope of this unit, but general principles of treatment include the use of nonpharmacologic treatment (medical nutrition therapy and exercise), if sufficient. If these are not sufficient, insulin is used. Oral antidiabetes therapies are not indicated during pregnancy and may be teratogenic.

For more information on the management of diabetes in pediatrics, geriatrics, and during pregnancy, refer to **Table 8** for a resource list.

Occupation

Many patients must contend with the prevailing circumstances at their place of work. Some occupational-related diabetes management issues include privacy for blood glucose monitoring and insulin injection as well as the hours involved in swing shift work. Suppose you are meeting with a patient, Ms. Walker, who works as a security guard on the 3–11 p.m. shift. Ms. Walker is on combination therapy, metformin plus insulin (regular and NPH twice daily).

PHARMACIST:

"Ms. Walker, I can tell from your blood glucose log that you are injecting your regular insulin immediately before you eat. This affects your blood glucose readings after dinner such that your blood glucose rises before the insulin is effective. I think it's important that you inject 30 minutes before you eat."

MS. WALKER:

"I know, but I only have 40 minutes for dinner. What else can I do?"

PHARMACIST:

"Well, I'm sure there must be options. Is there any way you can think of that you could check your glucose and give your injection half an hour before your dinner break?"

MS. WALKER:

"I go to dinner every night at 6 p.m. I guess I could ask the guard on rounds to stop by every day at 5:30 p.m. so I can go to the ladies room for 5 minutes and give myself the injection. That way I could do as you suggest."

PHARMACIST:

"That sounds like a good suggestion. Do you think it's feasible?"

MS. WALKER:

"Sure, the guard on foot comes by my station once an hour anyway, I'll just ask him to make sure he comes at 5:30 p.m."

Therapy is Adversely Impacting Patient's Quality of Life

While managing a patient's diabetes, it is important to consider the impact therapy, monitoring, and follow-up have on the patient's quality of life. Some experts argue that excellent glycemic control comes with too high a price tag for many patients. Patients complain, "I can go on vacation, but I can never take a vacation from my diabetes." This is a disease that requires constant attention to diet, exercise, medications, monitoring, and health maintenance. You should evaluate the patient's quality of life (as described in the *Ambulatory Care Clinical Skills Program: Core Module*) as well as his or her satisfaction with treatment.

Consider the example of Mrs. Hammond, a 62-year-old woman recently diagnosed with type 2 diabetes. Her predominant abnormality is postprandial hyperglycemia. In response to this pattern, her physician prescribed acarbose 25 mg three times daily before each meal.

Mrs. Hammond calls you a week after starting

Table 7. Acquisition Cost Comparison of Oral Antidiabetic Agents

Oral Agent	Usual Starting Dose	Cost per Month
Acarbose	25 mg tid	$41.05
Acetohexamide	250 mg/day	$ 8.40
Chlorpropamide	250 mg/day	$ 4.22
Glimepiride	1 mg/day	$ 6.78
Glipizide	5 mg/day	$ 9.55
Glipizide XL	5 mg/day	$10.07
Glyburide	2.5 mg/day	$ 8.99
Glyburide micronized	1.5 mg/day	$10.62
Metformin	500 mg bid	$32.26
Miglitol	25 mg tid	$35.10
Repaglinide	1 mg tid	$66.96
Rosiglitizone	4 mg/day	$60.00
Tolazamide	100 mg/day	$ 3.72
Tolbutamide	500 mg bid	$ 3.72
Troglitazone	200 mg/day	$89.28

Note: generic prices vary among manufacturers.

Table 8. Diabetes in Pediatrics, Geriatrics, and Pregnancy Resources

Pediatrics

1. Daneman D. Childhood, adolescence, and diabetes: a delicate developmental balance. *Diabetes Spectrum* 1989;2:225–43.

2. Lorenz R, Wysocki T. The family and childhood diabetes. *Diabetes Spectrum* 1991;4:261-92.

3. Vandagriff J, Marrero D, Ingersoll GM, Fineberg NS. Parents of children with diabetes: what are they worried about? *Diabetes Educator* 1992;18:299–302.

4. American Diabetes Association. Care of children with diabetes in the school and day care setting. *Diabetes Care* 1999;22(*Suppl* 1):S94–7.

Geriatrics

1. Bohannon NJ, Jack DB. Type II diabetes: tips for managing your older patients. *Geriatrics* 1996;51(3):28–35.

2. Lardinois CK. Type 2 diabetes: glycemic targets and oral therapies for older patients. *Geriatrics* 1998;53(11):22–3, 27–8, 33–4.

3. Samos LF, Roos BA. Diabetes mellitus in older persons. *Medical Clinics of North America* 1998;82:791–803.

Pregnancy

1. American Diabetes Association. *Medical Management of Pregnancy Complicated by Diabetes*, 2nd ed. Alexandria, VA: American Diabetes Association; 1995.

2. Carr DB, Gabbe S. Gestational diabetes: detection, management and implications. *Clinical Diabetes* 1998;16:4–11.

3. Sullivan BA, Henderson ST, Davis JM. Gestational diabetes. *J Am Pharm Assoc* 1998;38:364–71.

4. American Diabetes Association. Preconception care of women with diabetes. *Diabetes Care* 1999;22(*Suppl* 1):S62–5.

5. American Diabetes Association. Gestational diabetes mellitus. *Diabetes Care* 1999;22(*Suppl* 1):S74–6.

therapy to complain:

"I can't stand it any more. The side effects are unacceptable. Can you think of something else I can take, or do I even need anything at all?"

PHARMACIST:

"Which side effect are you referring to, Mrs. Hammond?"

MRS. HAMMOND:

"Well, it's very embarrassing, but it's flatulence. My stomach hurts, and the rumbling is awful. Then I have these embarrassing episodes of flatulence. I'm virtually house-bound. I refuse to keep taking this medication. What should I do?"

PHARMACIST:

"Let me speak with your physician, Mrs. Hammond. Many patients do better starting at a lower dose and then gradually increasing. I'll get right back to you. Is that OK?"

MRS. HAMMOND:

"Yes, thank you."

Obviously, this adverse drug effect is impacting Mrs. Hammond's quality of life, because she won't even leave her house.

Case Study

You will now learn how to determine the presence of therapy problems in a patient with type 2 diabetes. If you wish to review, refer to unit 9 of the *Ambulatory Care Clinical Skills Program: Core Module*.

Refer to Mrs. Gonzalez. Her Pharmacist's Patient Database Form, completed Ambulatory Therapy Assessment Worksheet (ATAW), and TPL are found in **Appendix A**. Let's work through her case and identify her drug-related problems, using the ATAW.

Correlation Between Drug Therapy and Medical Problems

We can match up each of Mrs. Gonzalez's medications with a medical condition as follows:

Hydrochlorothiazide—hypertension
Docusate—constipation
Pepcid AC—GERD
Monistat-7—vaginal yeast infections
Acetaminophen—arthritis pain

She is not receiving any unidentified medications at this time. She is not receiving any medications for her new diagnoses of type 2 diabetes mellitus or hyperlipidemia. Pharmacist Radcliffe needs to determine whether either or both of these conditions require drug therapy at this time, but the first step is medical nutrition therapy and adherence to an exercise plan.

The American Diabetes Association recommends that an aspirin a day (81–325 mg/day) be taken as secondary prevention by all patients with diabetes and cardiovascular risk factors (e.g., history of myocardial infarction, vascular bypass procedure, CVA or TIA, peripheral vascular disease, or claudication and/or angina), as well as primary prevention in patients with[10]:

- a family history of coronary heart disease,
- a practice of cigarette smoking,
- hypertension,
- obesity (>120% desirable body weight); BMI >28 in women, >27.3 in men
- albuminuria (micro- or macro-), or
- lipids:
  - cholesterol >200 mg/dl
  - LDL cholesterol >130 mg/dl
  - HDL cholesterol <40 mg/dl
  - Triglycerides >250 mg/dl

Mrs. Gonzalez is postmenopausal and is not receiving hormone replacement therapy. She also has several identifiable risk factors for osteoporosis, including her gender, sedentary lifestyle, and increased age. Calcium therapy is indicated for Mrs. Gonzalez.

Appropriate Therapy

One potential problem in a patient with diabetes is the use of hydrochlorothiazide, as it may increase the blood glucose and adversely effect the lipid profile. Furthermore, ACE inhibitors have been shown to be beneficial in patients with diabetes, reducing the risk of nephropathy.

The pharmacist has noted the recommendation for medical nutrition therapy and an exercise plan, because diabetes and hyperlipidemia were just diagnosed.

Drug Regimen

No problems noted.

Therapeutic Duplication

No problems noted.

Drug Allergy or Intolerance

Mrs. Gonzalez claimed an allergy to codeine. On closer questioning, she stated the nature of the allergy was nausea. Nausea is an adverse effect of codeine, which occurs at a higher incidence than with other opioids. This is an important distinction because if Mrs. Gonzalez had a true codeine allergy (e.g., hives, rash, difficulty breathing) she would not be able to take any morphine-like opioids, because cross-sensitivity is high. However, the pharmacist has noted the intolerance to codeine.

Adverse Drug Events

No problems noted.

Interactions: Drug-Drug, Drug-Disease, Drug-Nutrient, and Drug–Laboratory Test

As noted previously, hydrochlorothiazide can worsen blood glucose control and hyperlipidemia.

Social or Recreational Drug Use

Mrs. Gonzalez states that she drinks two or three 16-oz regular colas per day. The carbohydrate content in a regular cola is probably too high to be consistent with the diet she should be following, and the caffeine may exacerbate her hypertension.

Financial Impact

No problem noted. Mrs. Gonzalez has no difficulty with her co-pay at this time.

Patient Knowledge of Therapy

No problem noted.

Adherence

No problem noted.

Self-Monitoring

Mrs. Gonzalez requested a blood glucose monitor when she initially met with the pharmacist, per her physician's order. She will need to learn to use the monitor selected. She also needs to learn blood pressure measurement.

Risks and Quality of Life Impacts

Mrs. Gonzalez scored 4 on the Cardiovascular Risk Assessment. Also, she has never done a home fecal occult blood test. She has never had an influenza vaccine, which was noted to serve as a reminder for fall 1998. Mrs. Gonzalez should also be instructed to begin monthly breast self-examinations. It was also noted that she is very anxious about being diagnosed with type 2 diabetes.

Now that we have completed an ATAW for Mrs. Gonzalez, we can transfer all identified therapy problems to the Ambulatory Pharmacist's Care Plan (APCP). Review the APCP to see how each problem we identified for Mrs. Gonzalez has been entered in the "problem" column of the APCP. We will discuss completion and implementation of the APCP in subsequent units.

Practice Example

Now that you have followed through our assessment of Mrs. Gonzalez's problems, it's your turn to practice with Mr. Jones. Turn to **Appendix B** and assess his problems based on the information you had as of 3/3/98 using the blank ATAW form. How would your assessment change once you have the information available as of 4/3/98? Prepare an ATAW for Mr. Jones. Then, based on your assessment, create a TPL using the blank APCP found in **Appendix B**. When you are finished, compare your completed forms to the ones found in **Appendix C**. If you find gaps in any area of information, go back to the corresponding section in this unit or to the *Ambulatory Care Clinical Skills Program: Core Module*.

Correlation Between Drug Therapy and Medical Problems

We can match Mr. Jones' medications and medical problems as follows:

> Furosemide—hypertension
> Nitroglycerin sublingual tablets—angina/coronary artery disease
> Albuterol—asthma
> Acetaminophen, as needed—headaches
> MVI—dietary supplementation

No treatment has been noted for hyperlipidemia (diagnosed in June 1997), the nocturia for which he is currently complaining, possible dehydration, insensate feet, or fungal skin infection on the large toe detected on physical examination.

When he saw the patient again on April 3, 1998, the pharmacist could add newly diagnosed type 2 diabetes mellitus as an untreated indication. Mr. Jones' fasting lipid profile from March 30, 1998, enables the pharmacist to add hyperlipidemia, which is currently not controlled. The foot screen performed by the pharmacist on April 3, 1998, allows addition of insensate feet and detection of a skin fungal infection to the ATAW. In addition, Mr. Jones should be on daily aspirin therapy.

Appropriate Therapy

The pharmacist questioned the use of furosemide as an antihypertensive agent. Generally, thiazide diuretics are preferred to treat hypertension (although his creatinine clearance is close to the point at which thiazide diuretics begin to lose effectiveness); furosemide is more commonly used in patients who have consistent hypervolemic states, such as congestive heart failure. Also, on March 3, 1998, the pharmacist obtained a casual whole blood glucose reading of 244 mg/dl. Although Mr. Jones was not officially diagnosed with type 2 diabetes that day, it can be noted that furosemide may increase the blood glucose (which was measured when a diagnosis of type 2 diabetes was confirmed) as well as worsen the lipid values.

The pharmacist noted that Mr. Jones has not been adhering to his prescribed diet of restricted salt and fat intake.

Drug Regimen

No problems were noted, but the pharmacist did note several potentially problematic points. The patient had stated initially that even though he knew his furosemide should have been taken first thing in the morning, it interfered with his social activities. He only returned to the appropriate administration time when he realized the consequences of taking it in the evening led to even less desirable consequences. Mr. Jones correctly described the use of his sublingual nitroglycerin tablets, which he takes about once a month with good results (this is a stable pattern for him). He also had his albuterol inhaler with him, and he demonstrated good technique to the pharmacist.

Therapeutic Duplication

No problems noted.

Drug Allergy or Intolerance

No problems noted.

Adverse Drug Events

The pharmacist circled "no problem exists" but carefully evaluated furosemide as the cause of Mr. Jones' nocturia. The pharmacist concluded that it was unlikely, because the furosemide was administered at approximately 6 a.m., and Mr. Jones retires around 11 p.m.

Interactions: Drug-Drug, Drug-Disease, Drug-Nutrient, and Drug–Laboratory Test

The pharmacist again noted that furosemide may worsen blood glucose control and hyperlipidemia.

Social or Recreational Drug Use

The patient has a 50-pack-year history of smoking, and he drinks three to four beers a week. Even before the pharmacist knew Mr. Jones was diagnosed with type 2 diabetes, drinking three to four beers a week contributes to his caloric intake and may worsen his obesity. The smoking is a significant cardiovascular risk factor, and should be discouraged.

Financial Impact

No problems noted.

Patient Knowledge of Therapy

No problem was noted regarding knowledge of therapy, but the pharmacist did indicate that while Mr. Jones understood the importance of dietary modification, he did not wish to comply with the recommendation.

Adherence

A problem exists with adherence to therapy. Mr. Jones had a history of changing his medication administration time to suit his personal schedule (regardless of what was best for him), and he does not comply with recommended follow-up appointments. It took a month for Mr. Jones to be diagnosed with diabetes and return to the pharmacist for follow-up, instead of a week or less. Also, he does not adhere to his prescribed diet and exercise program.

Self-Monitoring

Patient stated that he used his albuterol inhaler about two or three times a month when he felt "wheezy," with good results. He had never heard of a peak flow meter but was interested in obtaining one and learning to use it, to better guide him when to use his albuterol. The pharmacist also explained that Mr. Jones should track how often he needs to use the albuterol; if his use increases, his therapy may need to be amended.

On April 3, the pharmacist added that the patient does not self-monitor blood glucose, because the diabetes was just diagnosed.

Risks and Quality of Life Impacts

Mr. Jones scored a 4 on the cardiovascular risk assessment, which is significant particularly because he has active coronary artery disease. He has refused a rectal or prostate examination by his physician, and he has never performed a home fecal occult blood test. Mr. Jones is not distressed about the nocturia but is concerned, which is impacting his quality of life.

Summary

Drug therapy evaluation using the ATAW enables you to identify the problems that will need to be addressed when setting pharmacotherapeutic goals and designing therapy for the patients you follow with type 2 diabetes.

This assessment tool provides a list of factors for you to consider in evaluating current therapy; the series of evaluative questions ensure that you will do a complete, thorough assessment of the patient's therapy problems. As stated in the *Ambulatory Care Clinical Skills Program: Core Module*, you must also have a feel for the relative importance of these influencing factors, with relative efficacy and safety being the primary concern.

References

1. McEvoy GK. *AHFS 98 Drug Information*. Bethesda, MD: American Society of Health-System Pharmacists; 1998. p. 2567–2618.

2. Prandin package insert, Novo Nordisk Pharmaceuticals, Inc., December 1997.

3. Glucophage package insert, Bristol-Myers Squibb Co., January 1998.

4. Rezulin package insert, Parke-Davis, July 1998.

5. Precose package insert, Baker, October 1997.

6. Steil CF, Campbell RK, White JR. Diabetes Care Products and Monitoring Devices. In: Covington TR, ed. *Handbook of Nonprescription Drugs*, 11th ed. Washington, DC: American Pharmaceutical Association; 1996. p. 326–7.

7. *Redbook 1998*. Montvale, NJ: Medical Economics Co.

8. Pontious SL. Diabetes mellitus and the preschool child. In: Haire-Joshe D, editor. *Management of Diabetes Mellitus: Perspectives of Care Across the Life Span*, 2nd ed. St Louis, MO: Mosby; 1996. p. 579–634.

9. Funnell MM, Herritt JH. Diabetes mellitus and the older adult. In: Haire-Joshe D, editor. *Management of Diabetes Mellitus: Perspectives of Care Across the Life Span*, 2nd ed. St Louis, MO: Mosby; 1996. p. 755–833.

10. American Diabetes Association. Aspirin therapy in diabetes. *Diabetes Care* 1999;22 (*Suppl* 1):S60–1.

Self-Study Questions

Objective

Describe types of problems commonly present in the unreviewed therapy of ambulatory patients with type 2 diabetes.

1. Name and describe problems commonly present in the unreviewed therapy of ambulatory patients with type 2 diabetes.

Objective

Determine the presence of any of the following medication or medication-related therapy problems in the current therapy of ambulatory patients with diabetes:

*   *medication used with no therapy indication*
*   *medical condition for which there is no therapy prescribed*
*   *therapy prescribed inappropriately for a particular medical condition*
*   *anything inappropriate in the current medication therapy regimen*
*   *presence of therapeutic duplication*
*   *prescription of medication to which the patient is allergic or intolerant*
*   *presence or potential for adverse drug events*
*   *presence or potential for clinically significant drug-drug, drug-disease, drug-nutrient, or drug–laboratory test interactions*
*   *interference with medical therapy of social or cultural drug use or use of alternative therapies*
*   *problems arising from financial impact of therapy on the patient*
*   *patient lack of understanding of therapy*
*   *patient nonadherence to therapy regimen*
*   *patient at risk because of patient-specific characteristics (e.g., age and living/working environment)*
*   *incomplete preventive measures*
*   *adverse impact of therapy on patient's quality of life*

2. Refer to Ms. McLucas' Pharmacist's Patient Database Form in **Appendix D**. Using the blank ATAW form, evaluate her current therapy to determine the presence of any medication or medication-related therapy problems.

Objective

Construct a therapy problem list for an ambulatory patient with type 2 diabetes.

3. Create a TPL for Ms. McLucas, using the blank APCP in **Appendix D**.

Self-Study Answers

1. There are many problems commonly present in the unreviewed therapy of ambulatory patients with type 2 diabetes, including undiagnosed, untreated, and undertreated diabetes (poor blood glucose control); actual or potential drug interactions or adverse drug events; and patient lack of knowledge and poor adherence to therapy (pharmacologic and nonpharmacologic).

2. Refer to the completed ATAW for Ms. McLucas (**Appendix E.**)

3. Refer to the APCP for Ms. McLucas (**Appendix E**)

PHARMACIST'S PATIENT DATABASE FORM

Original Date: **2/19/98**
Date updated: _____
Date updated: _____
Date updated: _____

Demographic and Administrative Information

Name: **Mrs. Rose Gonzalez**

Social Security #: **111-22-3333**

Address: **344 Lombard Street, Baltimore, MD 21201**

Health Care Provider's Name **Dr. Thompson**

Health Care Provider's Phone **555-CARE**

Work Phone: Home Phone: **555-1234**

Date of Birth: **8/12/42**

Race: **Hispanic**

Gender: **F**

Religion: **Catholic**

Occupation: **housewife**

Health Insurer: **BC/BS**

Subscriber #: **123-45-6789**

Primary Card Holder: **Juan Gonzalez**

Drug Benefit: ☑ yes ☐ no   copay: $ **5⁰⁰/per**

Current Symptoms   **none; diabetes picked on routine BG testing**

Past Medical History	Acute and Current Medical Problems
HTN x 4 years	1. Diabetes mellitus, type 2
no surgeries	2. Hypertension
3 children born	3. Hyperlipidemia
last child 10 lb 13 1/2 oz	4. GERD
(no dx gestational DM)	5. Constipation
	6. "Arthritis"
	7. Recurrent vag. yeast infect.
	8.

Family/Social/Economic History	Personal Limitations
mother – 82-alive → MI; h/o DM x22yr.	Pt. very anxious about
father – ↓@44 2° MUA	dx DM
3 children-good health	
no siblings	
Cost of medications per month $ **40⁰⁰**	

Allergies/Intolerances	Social Drug Use
☑ No known drug allergies	Alcohol **social – 2-3 drinks/yr.**
Medication Reaction	Caffeine **2-3 caffeinated colas/day**
codeine nausea	Tobacco **none x 35 yrs**
	Pregnancy/Breastfeeding Status **n/a**
	☐ Pregnant (due _____) ☐ Breastfeeding

Diet	Routine Exercise/Recreation	Daily Activities/Timing
☐ Low salt **no**	light housework	home all day
☐ Low fat **no**	otherwise ∅	sewing group 1 night/wk
☐ Diabetic **no**		
Timing of meals: **8A-12N-6P**		

Patient Name: _____Rose Gonzalez_____

Physical Assessment/Laboratory Data—Initial/Follow-up

Date	2/9/98	2/18/98	2/19/98		
Height			5'5"		
Weight			228 lb		
Temp			98.6°F elec.		
BP			152/100 LA sitting		
Pulse			92 reg R/R		
Respirations			18		
Peak Flow					
FBG		184			
R. Glucose	242				
HbA$_{1c}$			10.2		
T. Chol.	286	290			
LDL		204			
HDL		30			
TG		280			
INR					
BUN					
Cr	0.9				
ALT					
AST					
Alk Phos					
EKG	WNL				
U/A			⊕glucose ⊖protein, ket.		
MicroAlb.			⊖		

Drug Serum Concentrations

Date					

Notes:

Patient Name: __Rose Gonzalez__

Current Prescription Medication Regimen

Name/Dose/Strength/Route	Schedule/Frequency of Use	Indication	Start Date (and Stop Date If Applicable)	Prescriber	Adherence Issues/Efficacy
HCTZ 25 mg po	T ḡ AM	HTN	June 1995	Thompson	Adherent/ ?efficacy

Current Nonprescription Medication Regimen (OTC, herbal, homeopathic, nutritional, etc.)

Name/Dose/Strength/Route	Schedule/Frequency of Use	Indication	Start Date (and Stop Date If Applicable)	Prescriber	Adherence Issues/Efficacy
Docusate 100 mg po	prn	hard stool	prn x years	–	works well~ every couple months
Pepcid AC	prn ("1x ḡ mo)	heartburn	~2 years	–	works well
Monistat-7	prn (3x last yr)	vag. yeast infection	3x in past yr	–	recurs
Acetaminophen 325 mg	prn "1x ḡ mo	arthritis	prn x years	–	works "OK"

Patient Name: __Rose Gonzalez__

Risk Assessment/Preventive Measures/Quality of Life

Cardiovascular Risk Assessment		
male >45 years old	1	-
female >55 years old or female <55 with history of ovarectomy not taking estrogen replacement	1	I
Definite MI or sudden death before age 55 year in father or male first-degree relative or before 65 year in mother or female first-degree relative	1	-
current cigarette smoking	1	-
hypertension	1	I
diabetes mellitus	1	I
HDL cholesterol <35 mg/dl	1	I
HDL cholesterol >60 mg/dl	-1	
	Total:	4

Is patient at risk for complications of current conditions? ☑ Yes   ☐ No
Specify: HbA1c 10.2   DM complications, both acute (vag. yeast infections)
                  & chronic

Preventive Measures for Adults
H = has been done   R = patient refuses   X = not applicable   Date **2/19/98**

Women						
Pap Smear/pelvic	Annually 19+	H				
Mammogram	Every 1-2Y 40-49; annually 50+	H				
Men						
Rectal/prostate	Annually 50+					
All Patients						
Total/HDL-C	Every 5Y 19+	H				
Home Fecal Occult Blood Test	Annually					
Immunizations						
Td	Every 10Y	H				
Influenza	Every fall*					
Pneumovax	Once*	H				

* if indicated

Quality of life issues

Pt. very concerned re: dx DM.

Assessment of General Appearance

Patient **Rose Gonzalez** _____ Date **2/19/98**

General Appearance	Observations and Comments

Level of consciousness
  alertness: alert, confused,
  delirious, stuporous, comatose,
  orientation: person, place, time
	Alert & oriented to person, place & time

Signs of distress respiratory distress, pain, anxiety, etc.	somewhat anxious, near tears
Posture, motor activity, and gait _Describe_	normal posture & gait
Dress, grooming, and personal hygiene _Describe_	neat & appropriate personal appearance

Affect
  normal, inappropriate
  Describe
	normal

Speech
  normal, impaired
  Describe
	normal (accent)

Skin
  color: normal, blue, brown, red, pallor
  texture: normal, coarse, dry, oily
  turgor: good, poor
  edema
  lesions: color, type, configuration, anatomic
    distribution, consistency
	normal color, texture & turgor. No abnormalities, lesions or edema noted.

SCREENING FORM FOR DIABETES FOOT DISEASE

Name: **Rose Gonzalez**

Date: **2/19/98**

ID #: _____

I. Medical History

Check all that apply.

_____ Peripheral neuropathy
_____ Nephropathy
_____ Retinopathy   > denies
_____ Peripheral vascular disease
_____ Cardiovascular disease

For Sections II & III, fill in the blanks with an "R," "L," or "B" for positive findings on the right, left, or both feet.

II. Current History

1. Any change in the foot since the last evaluation?

_____ Yes _____
✓ No - 1ˢᵗ evaluation

2. Current ulcer or history of a foot ulcer?

_____ Yes _____
✓ No

3. Is there pain in the calf muscles when walking that is relieved by rest?

_____ Yes _____
✓ No

III. Foot Exam

1. Are the nails thick, too long, ingrown, infected with fungal disease?

_____ Yes _____

__✓__ No

2. Note foot deformities

_____ Toe deformities

_____ Bunions (hallus valgus)

_____ Charcot foot   } NONE

_____ Foot drop

_____ Prominent metatarsal heads

_____ Amputation (specify date, side, and level) _____

3. Pedal Pulses *(Fill in the blanks with a "P" or an "A" to indicate present or absent.)*

Posterior tibial:

__P__ Left

__P__ Right
                          } NORMAL
Dorsalis pedis:

__P__ Left

__P__ Right

4. Skin Condition *(Measure, draw in, and label the patient's skin condition, using the key and the foot diagram below.)*

C = Callus   PU = Pre-ulcerative lesion

U = Ulcer   F = Fissure

R = Redness   S = Swelling   ) NONE Noted

W = Warmth   D = Dryness

M = Maceration

IV. Sensory Foot Exam

Label sensory level with a "+" in the five circled areas of the foot if the patient can feel the 5.07 Semmes-Weinstein (10-gram) nylon filament and "−" if the patient cannot feel the filament.

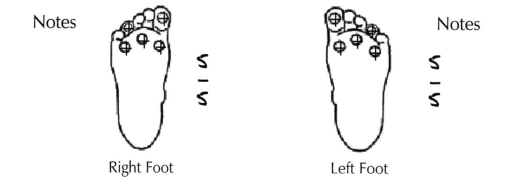

Notes   Notes

Right Foot   Left Foot

V. Risk Categorization

Check appropriate item.

✓ Low-Risk Patient
All of the following:
Intact protective sensation
Pedal pulses present
No severe deformity
No prior foot ulcer
No amputation

_____ High-Risk Patient
One or more of the following:
Loss of protective sensation
Absent pedal pulses
Severe foot deformity
History of foot ulcer
Prior amputation

VI. Footwear Assessment

Fill in the blanks.

Does the patient wear appropriate shoes?
✓ Yes   counseled pt.
_____ No

Does the patient need inserts?
_____ Yes
✓ No

Should therapeutic footwear be prescribed?
_____ Yes
✓ No

VII. Education

Fill in the blanks.

Has the patient had prior foot care education?
_____ Yes
✓ No

Can the patient demonstrate appropriate self-care?
_____ Yes   1st time seen
_____ No

VIII. Management Plan

Check all that apply.

___✓___ Provide patient education for preventive foot care.

Date: **2/20/98**

Diagnostic studies:
_____ Vascular laboratory
_____ Other: _____

Footwear recommendations:
___✓___ None
_____ Athletic shoes
_____ Accommodative inserts
_____ Custom shoes
_____ Depth shoes

Refer to:
___✓___ Primary care provider   **for scheduled follow-up**
_____ Diabetes educator
_____ Orthopedic foot surgeon
_____ RN foot specialist
_____ Orthotist
_____ Podiatrist
_____ Pedorthist
_____ Endocrinologist
_____ Rehab. specialist
_____ Vascular surgeon
_____ Other: _____
_____ Schedule follow-up visit

Date: **2/19/98**   Provider Signature: ___**Jane Radcliffe, R.Ph.**___

Source: http://www.niddk.nih.gov/health/diabetes/feet/feet2/screenfo.htm

AMBULATORY THERAPY ASSESSMENT WORKSHEET (ATAW)

Patient **Rose Gonzalez**

Pharmacist **Jane Radcliffe, R.Ph.**

Date **2/19/98**

Correlation Between Drug Therapy and Medical Problems

ASSESSMENT	PRESENCE OF PROBLEM*	COMMENTS/NOTES
Any drugs without a medical indication? Any unidentified medications? Any untreated medical conditions? Do they require drug therapy?	(1.) A problem exists. 2. More information is needed for determination. 3. No problem exists or an intervention is not needed.	- DM & hypercholesterolemia just dx, requires nonpharmacologic tx - should be on an ASA qd. - postmenopausal & no HRT - no calcium tx to prevent osteoarthritis

Appropriate Therapy

ASSESSMENT	PRESENCE OF PROBLEM*	COMMENTS/NOTES
Comparative efficacy of chosen medication(s)? Relative safety of chosen medication(s)? Is medication on formulary? Is nondrug therapy appropriately used (e.g., diet and exercise)? Is therapy achieving desired goals or outcomes? Is therapy tailored to this patient (e.g., age, comorbid conditions, and living/working environment)?	(1.) A problem exists. 2. More information is needed for determination. 3. No problem exists or an intervention is not needed.	- reconsider use of HCTZ due to possible adverse effects on BG & lipids - recommend MNT & exercise for DM, HTN, hyperchol.

Drug Regimen

ASSESSMENT	PRESENCE OF PROBLEM*	COMMENTS/NOTES
Are dose and dosing regimen appropriate and/or within usual therapeutic range and/or modified for patient factors? Appropriateness of PRN medications (prescribed or taken that way) Is route/dosage form/mode of administration appropriate, length or course of therapy considering efficacy, safety, convenience, patient limitations, length or course of therapy, and cost?	1. A problem exists. 2. More information is needed for determination. (3.) No problem exists or an intervention is not needed.	

*Problem denotes any pharmacotherapeutic or related health care problem.

MNT = medical nutrition tx

Therapeutic Duplication

ASSESSMENT	PRESENCE OF PROBLEM*	COMMENTS/NOTES
Any therapeutic duplications?	1. A problem exists. 2. More information is needed for determination. (3.) No problem exists or an intervention is not needed.	

Drug Allergy or Intolerance

ASSESSMENT	PRESENCE OF PROBLEM*	COMMENTS/NOTES
Allergy or intolerance to any medications (or chemically related medications) currently being taken? Is patient using a method to alert health care providers of the allergy/intolerance or serious health problem?	1. A problem exists. 2. More information is needed for determination. (3.) No problem exists or an intervention is not needed.	intolerance to codeine noted

Adverse Drug Events

ASSESSMENT	PRESENCE OF PROBLEM*	COMMENTS/NOTES
Are symptoms or medical problems drug induced? What is the likelihood the problem is drug related?	1. A problem exists. 2. More information is needed for determination. (3.) No problem exists or an intervention is not needed.	

Interactions: Drug-Drug, Drug-Disease, Drug-Nutrient, Drug–Laboratory Test

ASSESSMENT	PRESENCE OF PROBLEM*	COMMENTS/NOTES
Any drug-drug interactions? Clinical significance? Any relative or absolute contraindications given patient characteristics and current/past disease states? Any drug-nutrient interactions? Clinical significance? Any drug-laboratory test interactions? Clinical significance?	(1.) A problem exists. 2. More information is needed for determination. 3. No problem exists or an intervention is not needed.	HCTZ can worsen BG control & hypercholesterolemia.

*Problem denotes any pharmacotherapeutic or related health care problem.

Social or Recreational Drug Use

ASSESSMENT	PRESENCE OF PROBLEM*	COMMENTS/NOTES
Is current use of social drugs problematic? Are symptoms related to sudden withdrawal or discontinuation of social drugs?	(1) A problem exists. 2. More information is needed for determination. 3. No problem exists or an intervention is not needed.	*Drinks 2-3 16-oz. Regular colas per day. Caffeine may ↑BP; sugar may ↑BG*

Financial Impact

ASSESSMENT	PRESENCE OF PROBLEM*	COMMENTS/NOTES
Is therapy cost-effective? Does cost of therapy represent a financial hardship for the patient?	1. A problem exists. 2. More information is needed for determination. (3.) No problem exists or an intervention is not needed.	

Patient Knowledge of Therapy

ASSESSMENT	PRESENCE OF PROBLEM*	COMMENTS/NOTES
Does patient understand the role of his/her medication(s), how to take it, and potential side effects? Would patient benefit from education tools (e.g., written patient education sheets, wallet cards, or reminder package?) Does the patient understand the role of nondrug therapy?	1. A problem exists. 2. More information is needed for determination. (3.) No problem exists or an intervention is not needed.	

Adherence

ASSESSMENT	PRESENCE OF PROBLEM*	COMMENTS/NOTES
Is there a problem with nonadherence to drug or nondrug therapy (e.g., diet and exercise)? Are there barriers to adherence or factors hindering the achievement of therapeutic efficacy?	1. A problem exists. 2. More information is needed for determination. (3.) No problem exists or an intervention is not needed.	

*Problem denotes any pharmacotherapeutic or related health care problem.

Self-Monitoring

ASSESSMENT	PRESENCE OF PROBLEM*	COMMENTS/NOTES
Does patient perform appropriate self-monitoring? (e.g., peak flow and blood glucose) Is correct technique employed? Is self-monitoring performed consistently, at appropriate times, and with appropriate frequency?	(1.) A problem exists. 2. More information is needed for determination. 3. No problem exists or an intervention is not needed.	*Needs to learn SMBG* *Needs to learn blood pressure monitoring*

Risks and Quality of Life Impacts

ASSESSMENT	PRESENCE OF PROBLEM*	COMMENTS/NOTES
Is patient at risk for complications with an existing disease state (i.e., risk factor assessment)? Is patient on track for preventive measures (e.g., immunizations, mammograms, prostate exams, eye exams)? Is therapy adversely impacting patient's quality of life? How so?	(1.) A problem exists. 2. More information is needed for determination. 3. No problem exists or an intervention is not needed.	- *multiple CV risk factors* - *Has not done home fecal occult blood test* - *needs influenza vaccine Fall 98* - *needs ophthalmologic exam* - *initiate monthly breast self-examination* - *anxious about dx of diabetes*

*Problem denotes any pharmacotherapeutic or related health care problem.

AMBULATORY PHARMACIST'S CARE PLAN

Patient _____ Rose Gonzalez _____   Pharmacist _____ Jane Radcliffe _____   Date _ 2/20/98

DATE IDENTIFIED	PROBLEM (TPL)	PHARMACOTHERAPEUTIC AND RELATED HEALTH CARE GOAL	RECOMMENDATIONS FOR THERAPY	MONITORING PARAMETER(S)	DESIRED ENDPOINT(S)	MONITORING FREQUENCY
2/20/98	poor control of diabetes					
"	poor control of HTN					
"	poor control of cholest.					
"	not on daily ASA tx					
"	post menopausal s̄ HRT					
"	not receiving calcium tx					
"	Potential of HCTZ to affect DM & chol.					
"	no exercise plan					

Ambulatory Pharmacist's Care Plan

Patient _Rose Gonzalez_   Pharmacist _Jane Radcliffe_   Date _2/20/98_

DATE IDENTIFIED	PROBLEM (TPL)	PHARMACOTHERAPEUTIC AND RELATED HEALTH CARE GOAL	RECOMMENDATIONS FOR THERAPY	MONITORING PARAMETER(S)	DESIRED ENDPOINT(S)	MONITORING FREQUENCY
2/20/98	no MNT plan					
'	no home BG monitoring					
'	no home BP monitoring					
''	no home fecal test					
''	no influenza vaccine					
''	no monthly breast self-exam					

PHARMACIST'S PATIENT DATABASE FORM

Original Date: **3/3/98**
Date updated: **4/3/98**
Date updated: _____
Date updated: _____

Demographic and Administrative Information

Name: George Jones	Social Security #: 121-11-1111

Address: **321 Tydings Lane   Baltimore, MD 21136**

Health Care Provider's Name Dr. Middleton	Health Care Provider's Phone 555-2399
Work Phone: - Home Phone: 555-9876	Date of Birth: 9/13/31
Race: AA	Gender: M
Religion: None	Occupation: retired-worked at racetrack
Health Insurer: Medicare & BC/BS	Subscriber #: 121-11-1111
Primary Card Holder: pt.	Drug Benefit: ☒ yes ☐ no copay: $ 5-10⁰⁰

Current Symptoms   c/o Nocturia (2-3 x q N) x 2-3 weeks

Past Medical History

HTN 1994

Angina 1995

∅ surgery

Hypercholesterolemia 6/97

Kidney stone 1992 → hospit.

Asthma x 5 yrs.

Acute and Current Medical Problems

1. Nocturia / Diabetes (4/3/98)
2. Hypertension
3. Angina
4. Hypercholesterolemia
5. Asthma
6. Renal dysfxn/proteinuria
7. MI (? old)
8. Insensate feet/ ↑ risk

Family/Social/Economic History

mother- ↓ @72 2° CVA; dxDM @50; h/o HTN

4 sisters-1 well; 3 → DM & HTN

Father- ↓ @60 2° MI (MI x 2); h/o HTN

Personal Limitations 9. fungal toe infection

None

Cost of medications per month $ 15-20⁰⁰

Allergies/Intolerances

☒ No known drug allergies

Medication	Reaction

Social Drug Use

Alcohol	3-4 beers q week
Caffeine	1-2 cups coffee qd
Tobacco	50-pack year history

Pregnancy/Breastfeeding Status   N/A

☐ Pregnant (due _____)   ☐ Breastfeeding

Diet

☒ Low salt ⟩ prescribed -

☒ Low fat ⟩ not

☐ Diabetic   following

Timing of meals: 6A-2P-6P - skips meals sometimes; frequently eats fast food

Routine Exercise/Recreation

no routine exercise

x̄ walks 1/2 mile

to race track qd

Daily Activities/Timing

Race track 8A-1P

Retires @ 10 pm

Patient Name: ___George Jones___

Physical Assessment/Laboratory Data—Initial/Follow-up

Date	3/3/98	3/18/98	3/23/98	3/30/98	4/3/98
Height	5'8"				
Weight	240 lb BMI 37				
Temp	98.8F electron therm				
BP	152/98 ↑ 140/90 ↓				
Pulse	84 ↑ 92 ↓				
Respirations	16 reg				
Peak Flow					
FBG			190		
R. Glucose	244	258			
HbA$_{1c}$					11.6
T. Chol.				290	
LDL				229	
HDL				45	
TG				80	
INR					
BUN					
Cr				1.8	
ALT				56	
AST				98	
Alk Phos					
UCX			⊖		
EKG					4/) ischemia c/w old MI
U/A					⊕ pro, glu ⊖ ketones
U.MicroAlb.					35 µg/mg Cr

Drug Serum Concentrations

Date					

Notes:

Patient Name: ___George Jones___

Current Prescription Medication Regimen

Name/Dose/Strength/Route	Schedule/ Frequency of Use	Indication	Start Date (and Stop Date If Applicable)	Prescriber	Adherence Issues/Efficacy
Furosemide 20 mg.	T q AM	HTN	1994	Middleton	Adheres/eff?
NTG 0.4 mg sl prn	prn	Angina	1995	Middleton	~1/month/good
Albuterol inhaler TT puffs	prn	Asthma	1993	Middleton	"2-3 x q mo/good

Current Nonprescription Medication Regimen (OTC, herbal, homeopathic, nutritional, etc.)

Name/Dose/Strength/Route	Schedule/ Frequency of Use	Indication	Start Date (and Stop Date If Applicable)	Prescriber	Adherence Issues/Efficacy
Acetaminophen 650 mg	prn ~ weekly	headache	years	—	works well
MVI T	QD	nutrition	years	—	perceives efficacious

Patient Name: _____ George Jones _____

Risk Assessment/Preventive Measures/Quality of Life

Cardiovascular Risk Assessment		
male >45 years old	1	ı
female >55 years old or female <55 with history of ovarectomy not taking estrogen replacement	1	
Definite MI or sudden death before age 55 year in father or male first-degree relative or before 65 year in mother or female first-degree relative	1	
current cigarette smoking	1	ı
hypertension	1	ı
diabetes mellitus	1	ı
HDL cholesterol <35 mg/dl	1	
HDL cholesterol >60 mg/dl	-1	
	Total:	**4**

Is patient at risk for complications of current conditions? ☒ Yes   ☐ No
Specify: HbA1c 11.6%, h/o HTN & CV dz

Preventive Measures for Adults
H = has been done   R = patient refuses   X = not applicable   Date   4/3/98

Women					
Pap Smear/pelvic	Annually 19+				
Mammogram	Every 1-2Y 40-49; annually 50+				
Men					
Rectal/prostate	Annually 50+	R			
All Patients					
Total/HDL-C	Every 5Y 19+	H			
Home Fecal Occult Blood Test	Annually	R			
Immunizations					
Td	Every 10Y	H			
Influenza	Every fall*	H			
Pneumovax	Once*	H			

* if indicated

Quality of life issues
Nocturia is affecting his QOL

Assessment of General Appearance

Patient   George Jones   Date   3/3/98

General Appearance	Observations and Comments

Level of consciousness
    alertness: alert, confused,
    delirious, stuporous, comatose,
    orientation: person, place, time
	Alert & oriented to person, place & time

Signs of distress respiratory distress, pain, anxiety, etc.	Appears concerned, but not distressed
Posture, motor activity, and gait *Describe*	Normal gait & posture & motor activity
Dress, grooming, and personal hygiene *Describe*	Casual but neat personal appearance

Affect
    normal, inappropriate
    Describe
	Normal

Speech
    normal, impaired
    Describe
	Normal

Skin
    color: normal, blue, brown, red, pallor
    texture: normal, coarse, dry, oily
    turgor: good, poor
    edema
    lesions: color, type, configuration, anatomic
       distribution, consistency
	Skin normal color & texture. Turgor poor-tenting & slightly dry mucous membranes
	No other skin abnormalities, lesions or edema noted.

SCREENING FORM FOR DIABETES FOOT DISEASE

Name: _____George Jones_____

Date: _____4/3/98_____

ID #: _____

I. Medical History

Check all that apply.

_____ Peripheral neuropathy
_____ Nephropathy
_____ Retinopathy
_____ Peripheral vascular disease
__✓__ Cardiovascular disease

For Sections II & III, fill in the blanks with an "R," "L," or "B" for positive findings on the right, left, or both feet.

II. Current History

1. Any change in the foot since the last evaluation?
_____ Yes _____
_____ No   **1st EXAM**

2. Current ulcer or history of a foot ulcer?
_____ Yes _____
__✓__ No

3. Is there pain in the calf muscles when walking that is relieved by rest?
_____ Yes _____
__✓__ No

III. Foot Exam

1. Are the nails thick, too long, ingrown, infected with fungal disease?

_____ Yes _____   *A little long, but otherwise normal*

_____ No   *Also, beginnings of a fungal infection in skin crease*

under toe pad of little toe on R foot

2. Note foot deformities

_____ Toe deformities

_____ Bunions (hallus valgus)   *NONE*

_____ Charcot foot

_____ Foot drop

_____ Prominent metatarsal heads   *callus on balls both feet*

_____ Amputation (specify date, side, and level) _____

3. Pedal Pulses *(Fill in the blanks with a "P" or an "A" to indicate present or absent.)*

Posterior tibial:

___P__ Left

___P__ Right   *slightly*
                    diminished

Dorsalis pedis:

___P__ Left

___P__ Right

4. Skin Condition *(Measure, draw in, and label the patient's skin condition, using the key and the foot diagram below.)*

C = Callus   PU = Pre-ulcerative lesion

U = Ulcer   F = Fissure

R = Redness   S = Swelling

W = Warmth   D = Dryness

M = Maceration

IV. Sensory Foot Exam

Label sensory level with a "+" in the five circled areas of the foot if the patient can feel the 5.07 Semmes-Weinstein (10-gram) nylon filament and "−" if the patient cannot feel the filament.

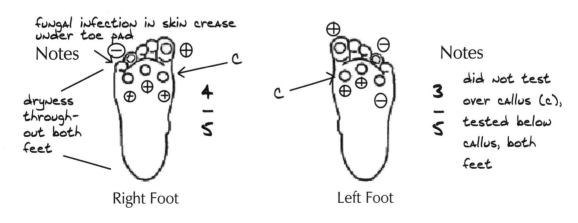

Right Foot   Left Foot

V. Risk Categorization

Check appropriate item.

_____ Low-Risk Patient	✓ High-Risk Patient
All of the following:	*One or more of the following:*
Intact protective sensation	Loss of protective sensation ✓
Pedal pulses present	Absent pedal pulses (diminished)
No severe deformity	Severe foot deformity
No prior foot ulcer	History of foot ulcer
No amputation	Prior amputation

VI. Footwear Assessment

Fill in the blanks.

Does the patient wear appropriate shoes?
_____ Yes
✓ No

Does the patient need inserts?
_____ Yes
✓ No

Should therapeutic footwear be prescribed?
_____ Yes **?** refer to podiatrist/primary care MD
_____ No

VII. Education

Fill in the blanks.

Has the patient had prior foot care education?
_____ Yes
✓ No

Can the patient demonstrate appropriate self-care?
_____ Yes
✓ No

VIII. Management Plan

Check all that apply.

√ Provide patient education for preventive foot care.

Date: _patient deferred to follow-up visit_

Diagnostic studies:
_____ Vascular laboratory
_____ Other: _____

Footwear recommendations:
_____ None
√ Athletic shoes
_____ Accommodative inserts
_____ Custom shoes
_____ Depth shoes

Refer to:
√ Primary care provider   *possibly podiatrist*
_____ Diabetes educator
_____ Orthopedic foot surgeon
_____ RN foot specialist
_____ Orthotist
_____ Podiatrist
_____ Pedorthist
_____ Endocrinologist
_____ Rehab. specialist
_____ Vascular surgeon
_____ Other: _____
_____ Schedule follow-up visit.

Date: **4/3/98**   Provider Signature: _John O'Malley, PharmD._

Source: http://www.niddk.nih.gov/health/diabetes/feet/feet2/screenfo.htm

AMBULATORY THERAPY ASSESSMENT WORKSHEET (ATAW)

Patient _____

Pharmacist _____

Date _____

Correlation Between Drug Therapy and Medical Problems

ASSESSMENT	PRESENCE OF PROBLEM*	COMMENTS/NOTES
Any drugs without a medical indication? Any unidentified medications? Any untreated medical conditions? Do they require drug therapy?	1. A problem exists. 2. More information is needed for determination. 3. No problem exists or an intervention is not needed.	

Appropriate Therapy

ASSESSMENT	PRESENCE OF PROBLEM*	COMMENTS/NOTES
Comparative efficacy of chosen medication(s)? Relative safety of chosen medication(s)? Is medication on formulary? Is nondrug therapy appropriately used (e.g., diet and exercise)? Is therapy achieving desired goals or outcomes? Is therapy tailored to this patient (e.g., age, comorbid conditions, and living/working environment)?	1. A problem exists. 2. More information is needed for determination. 3. No problem exists or an intervention is not needed.	

Drug Regimen

ASSESSMENT	PRESENCE OF PROBLEM*	COMMENTS/NOTES
Are dose and dosing regimen appropriate and/or within usual therapeutic range and/or modified for patient factors? Appropriateness of PRN medications (prescribed or taken that way) Is route/dosage form/mode of administration appropriate, length or course of therapy considering efficacy, safety, convenience, patient limitations, length or course of therapy, and cost?	1. A problem exists. 2. More information is needed for determination. 3. No problem exists or an intervention is not needed.	

*Problem denotes any pharmacotherapeutic or related health care problem.

Therapeutic Duplication

ASSESSMENT	PRESENCE OF PROBLEM*	COMMENTS/NOTES
Any therapeutic duplications?	1. A problem exists. 2. More information is needed for determination. 3. No problem exists or an intervention is not needed.	

Drug Allergy or Intolerance

ASSESSMENT	PRESENCE OF PROBLEM*	COMMENTS/NOTES
Allergy or intolerance to any medications (or chemically related medications) currently being taken? Is patient using a method to alert health care providers of the allergy/intolerance or serious health problem?	1. A problem exists. 2. More information is needed for determination. 3. No problem exists or an intervention is not needed.	

Adverse Drug Events

ASSESSMENT	PRESENCE OF PROBLEM*	COMMENTS/NOTES
Are symptoms or medical problems drug induced? What is the likelihood the problem is drug related?	1. A problem exists. 2. More information is needed for determination. 3. No problem exists or an intervention is not needed.	

Interactions: Drug-Drug, Drug-Disease, Drug-Nutrient, Drug–Laboratory Test

ASSESSMENT	PRESENCE OF PROBLEM*	COMMENTS/NOTES
Any drug-drug interactions? Clinical significance? Any relative or absolute contraindications given patient characteristics and current/past disease states? Any drug-nutrient interactions? Clinical significance? Any drug-laboratory test interactions? Clinical significance?	1. A problem exists. 2. More information is needed for determination. 3. No problem exists or an intervention is not needed.	

*Problem denotes any pharmacotherapeutic or related health care problem.

Social or Recreational Drug Use

ASSESSMENT	PRESENCE OF PROBLEM*	COMMENTS/NOTES
Is current use of social drugs problematic? Are symptoms related to sudden withdrawal or discontinuation of social drugs?	1. A problem exists. 2. More information is needed for determination. 3. No problem exists or an intervention is not needed.	

Financial Impact

ASSESSMENT	PRESENCE OF PROBLEM*	COMMENTS/NOTES
Is therapy cost-effective? Does cost of therapy represent a financial hardship for the patient?	1. A problem exists. 2. More information is needed for determination. 3. No problem exists or an intervention is not needed.	

Patient Knowledge of Therapy

ASSESSMENT	PRESENCE OF PROBLEM*	COMMENTS/NOTES
Does patient understand the role of his/her medication(s), how to take it, and potential side effects? Would patient benefit from education tools (e.g., written patient education sheets, wallet cards, or reminder package?) Does the patient understand the role of nondrug therapy?	1. A problem exists. 2. More information is needed for determination. 3. No problem exists or an intervention is not needed.	

Adherence

ASSESSMENT	PRESENCE OF PROBLEM*	COMMENTS/NOTES
Is there a problem with nonadherence to drug or nondrug therapy (e.g., diet and exercise)? Are there barriers to adherence or factors hindering the achievement of therapeutic efficacy?	1. A problem exists. 2. More information is needed for determination. 3. No problem exists or an intervention is not needed.	

*Problem denotes any pharmacotherapeutic or related health care problem.

Self-Monitoring

ASSESSMENT	PRESENCE OF PROBLEM*	COMMENTS/NOTES
Does patient perform appropriate self-monitoring? (e.g., peak flow and blood glucose) Is correct technique employed? Is self-monitoring performed consistently, at appropriate times, and with appropriate frequency?	1. A problem exists. 2. More information is needed for determination. 3. No problem exists or an intervention is not needed.	

Risks and Quality of Life Impacts

ASSESSMENT	PRESENCE OF PROBLEM*	COMMENTS/NOTES
Is patient at risk for complications with an existing disease state (i.e., risk factor assessment)? Is patient on track for preventive measures (e.g., immunizations, mammograms, prostate exams, eye exams)? Is therapy adversely impacting patient's quality of life? How so?	1. A problem exists. 2. More information is needed for determination. 3. No problem exists or an intervention is not needed.	

*Problem denotes any pharmacotherapeutic or related health care problem.

AMBULATORY PHARMACIST'S CARE PLAN

Patient _____   Pharmacist _____   Date _____

DATE IDENTIFIED	PROBLEM (TPL)	PHARMACOTHERAPEUTIC AND RELATED HEALTH CARE GOAL	RECOMMENDATIONS FOR THERAPY	MONITORING PARAMETER(S)	DESIRED ENDPOINT(S)	MONITORING FREQUENCY

AMBULATORY PHARMACIST'S CARE PLAN

Patient _____   Pharmacist _____   Date _____

DATE IDENTIFIED	PROBLEM (TPL)	PHARMACOTHERAPEUTIC AND RELATED HEALTH CARE GOAL	RECOMMENDATIONS FOR THERAPY	MONITORING PARAMETER(S)	DESIRED ENDPOINT(S)	MONITORING FREQUENCY

AMBULATORY PHARMACIST'S CARE PLAN

Patient _____   Pharmacist _____   Date _____

DATE IDENTIFIED	PROBLEM (TPL)	PHARMACOTHERAPEUTIC AND RELATED HEALTH CARE GOAL	RECOMMENDATIONS FOR THERAPY	MONITORING PARAMETER(S)	DESIRED ENDPOINT(S)	MONITORING FREQUENCY

AMBULATORY THERAPY ASSESSMENT WORKSHEET (ATAW)

Patient   George Jones

Pharmacist   John O'Malley

Date   3/3/98; updated 4/3

Correlation Between Drug Therapy and Medical Problems

ASSESSMENT	PRESENCE OF PROBLEM*	COMMENTS/NOTES
Any drugs without a medical indication? Any unidentified medications? Any untreated medical conditions? Do they require drug therapy?	(1.) A problem exists. 2. More information is needed for determination. 3. No problem exists or an intervention is not needed.	New c/o nocturia, poor skin turgor 4/3/98—DM dx; no tx - fungal toe infection - insensate feet/high risk - should be on daily ASA— No tx for hypercholesterolemia

Appropriate Therapy

ASSESSMENT	PRESENCE OF PROBLEM*	COMMENTS/NOTES
Comparative efficacy of chosen medication(s)? Relative safety of chosen medication(s)? Is medication on formulary? Is nondrug therapy appropriately used (e.g., diet and exercise)? Is therapy achieving desired goals or outcomes? Is therapy tailored to this patient (e.g., age, comorbid conditions, and living/working environment)?	(1.) A problem exists. 2. More information is needed for determination. 3. No problem exists or an intervention is not needed.	Question use of furosemide as best anti-HTN agent Pt not following diet 4/3/98- Hypercholesterolemia not controlled DM dx - needs exercise and MNT tx Furosemide may worsen glucose and cholesterol.

Drug Regimen

ASSESSMENT	PRESENCE OF PROBLEM*	COMMENTS/NOTES
Are dose and dosing regimen appropriate and/or within usual therapeutic range and/or modified for patient factors? Appropriateness of PRN medications (prescribed or taken that way) Is route/dosage form/mode of administration appropriate, length or course of therapy considering efficacy, safety, convenience, patient limitations, length or course of therapy, and cost?	1. A problem exists. 2. More information is needed for determination. (3.) No problem exists or an intervention is not needed.	Pt. confirmed he is taking furosemide in AM. Pt. correctly describes use of SL NTG. Pt. correctly demonstrated use of albuterol inhaler

*Problem denotes any pharmacotherapeutic or related health care problem.

Therapeutic Duplication

ASSESSMENT	PRESENCE OF PROBLEM*	COMMENTS/NOTES
Any therapeutic duplications?	1. A problem exists. 2. More information is needed for determination. (3.) No problem exists or an intervention is not needed.	

Drug Allergy or Intolerance

ASSESSMENT	PRESENCE OF PROBLEM*	COMMENTS/NOTES
Allergy or intolerance to any medications (or chemically related medications) currently being taken? Is patient using a method to alert health care providers of the allergy/intolerance or serious health problem?	1. A problem exists. 2. More information is needed for determination. (3.) No problem exists or an intervention is not needed.	

Adverse Drug Events

ASSESSMENT	PRESENCE OF PROBLEM*	COMMENTS/NOTES
Are symptoms or medical problems drug induced? What is the likelihood the problem is drug related?	1. A problem exists. 2. More information is needed for determination. (3.) No problem exists or an intervention is not needed.	Furosemide-induced nocturia unlikely.

Interactions: Drug-Drug, Drug-Disease, Drug-Nutrient, Drug–Laboratory Test

ASSESSMENT	PRESENCE OF PROBLEM*	COMMENTS/NOTES
Any drug-drug interactions? Clinical significance? Any relative or absolute contraindications given patient characteristics and current/past disease states? Any drug-nutrient interactions? Clinical significance? Any drug-laboratory test interactions? Clinical significance?	(1.) A problem exists. 2. More information is needed for determination. 3. No problem exists or an intervention is not needed.	Furosemide may worsen hypercholesterol-emia. 4\3\98 – Furo-semide may increase BG

*Problem denotes any pharmacotherapeutic or related health care problem.

Social or Recreational Drug Use

ASSESSMENT	PRESENCE OF PROBLEM*	COMMENTS/NOTES
Is current use of social drugs problematic? Are symptoms related to sudden withdrawal or discontinuation of social drugs?	(1.) A problem exists. 2. More information is needed for determination. 3. No problem exists or an intervention is not needed.	Pt. has 50-pack yr. smoking history. Pt. drinks 3-4 beers/wk.

Financial Impact

ASSESSMENT	PRESENCE OF PROBLEM*	COMMENTS/NOTES
Is therapy cost-effective? Does cost of therapy represent a financial hardship for the patient?	1. A problem exists. 2. More information is needed for determination. (3.) No problem exists or an intervention is not needed.	

Patient Knowledge of Therapy

ASSESSMENT	PRESENCE OF PROBLEM*	COMMENTS/NOTES
Does patient understand the role of his/her medication(s), how to take it, and potential side effects? Would patient benefit from education tools (e.g., written patient education sheets, wallet cards, or reminder package?) Does the patient understand the role of nondrug therapy?	1. A problem exists. 2. More information is needed for determination. (3.) No problem exists or an intervention is not needed.	Pt. understands importance of dietary modifications but doesn't want to do it.

Adherence

ASSESSMENT	PRESENCE OF PROBLEM*	COMMENTS/NOTES
Is there a problem with nonadherence to drug or nondrug therapy (e.g., diet and exercise)? Are there barriers to adherence or factors hindering the achievement of therapeutic efficacy?	(1.) A problem exists. 2. More information is needed for determination. 3. No problem exists or an intervention is not needed.	Pt. has history of changing medication administration time to suit his schedule. Pt. not always adherent to flu appointments Pt. does not adhere to dietary and exercise recommendations.

*Problem denotes any pharmacotherapeutic or related health care problem.

Self-Monitoring

ASSESSMENT	PRESENCE OF PROBLEM*	COMMENTS/NOTES
Does patient perform appropriate self-monitoring? (e.g., peak flow and blood glucose) Is correct technique employed? Is self-monitoring performed consistently, at appropriate times, and with appropriate frequency?	(1.) A problem exists. 2. More information is needed for determination. 3. No problem exists or an intervention is not needed.	Pt. does not have a peak flow meter. 4/3/98 Pt. does not SMBG.

Risks and Quality of Life Impacts

ASSESSMENT	PRESENCE OF PROBLEM*	COMMENTS/NOTES
Is patient at risk for complications with an existing disease state (i.e., risk factor assessment)? Is patient on track for preventive measures (e.g., immunizations, mammograms, prostate exams, eye exams)? Is therapy adversely impacting patient's quality of life? How so?	(1.) A problem exists. 2. More information is needed for determination. 3. No problem exists or an intervention is not needed.	Pt. refuses rectal and prostate exam and home fecal occult blood test. Nocturia ↓QOL Multiple CV risk factors Renal impairment Hepatic impairment

*Problem denotes any pharmacotherapeutic or related health care problem.

AMBULATORY PHARMACIST'S CARE PLAN

Patient George Jones   Pharmacist John O'Malley   Date 3-3-98

Page 1 of 3

DATE IDENTIFIED	PROBLEM (TPL)	PHARMACOTHERAPEUTIC AND RELATED HEALTH CARE GOAL	RECOMMENDATIONS FOR THERAPY	MONITORING PARAMETER(S)	DESIRED ENDPOINT(S)	MONITORING FREQUENCY
3/3/98	SX and BG suggestive of DM. High risk status					
	poor control of hypertension					
	nonadherence to diet					
	h/o med schedule nonadherence					
	Furosemide may worsen lipids					
	smoking history					
	Alcohol use history					

AMBULATORY PHARMACIST'S CARE PLAN

Patient ___George Jones___   Pharmacist ___John O'Malley___   Date ___3-3-98___

Page 2 of 3

DATE IDENTIFIED	PROBLEM (TPL)	PHARMACOTHERAPEUTIC AND RELATED HEALTH CARE GOAL	RECOMMENDATIONS FOR THERAPY	MONITORING PARAMETER(S)	DESIRED ENDPOINT(S)	MONITORING FREQUENCY
3/3/98	h/o non-adherence to flu appts					
	nonadherence to exercise					
	Not doing peak flow monitoring					
	No rectal/ prostate exam					
	no home fecal test					
4/3/98	poor control of diabetes					
	Furosemide may ↑ BG					
	Fungal skin infection on toe					

AMBULATORY PHARMACIST'S CARE PLAN

Patient __George Jones__   Pharmacist __John O'Malley__   Date __3-3-98__

Page 3 of 3

DATE IDENTIFIED	PROBLEM (TPL)	PHARMACOTHERAPEUTIC AND RELATED HEALTH CARE GOAL	RECOMMENDATIONS FOR THERAPY	MONITORING PARAMETER(S)	DESIRED ENDPOINT(S)	MONITORING FREQUENCY
4/3	Insensate feet					
	Not on daily ASA tx					
	Poor control of cholesterol					
	Not doing SMBG					
	No dilated retinal exam					
	No recent dental exam					
	liver dysfunction					

Original Date: **4/23/98**
Date updated:_____
Date updated:_____
Date updated:_____

PHARMACIST'S PATIENT DATABASE FORM

Demographic and Administrative Information

Name: Sarah McLucas	Social Security #: 111-11-1111
Address: 4701 Stalwart Way	
Health Care Provider's Name: Dr. Davis	Health Care Provider's Phone: 555-1295
Work Phone: N/A Home Phone: 555-7401	Date of Birth: 12/25/27
Race: Caucasian	Gender: F
Religion: Lutheran	Occupation: retired school teacher
Health Insurer: Medicare	Subscriber #:
Primary Card Holder: Pt.	Drug Benefit: ☐ yes ☒ no copay: $_____

Current Symptoms
Pt. was without complaints. BG drawn on routine screen ↑; repeated → dx DM

Past Medical History	Acute and Current Medical Problems
Hypercholesterolemia-1997	1. Hypercholesterolemia
DM	2. Diabetes mellitus
OA-1996	3. Osteoarthritis
HTN-1995	4. HTN
GERD	5. GERD
Seasonal allergic rhinitis	6. Allergic rhinitis
Ø surgeries	7.
Hospitalized 1992 c̄ pneumonia	8.

Family/Social/Economic History	Personal Limitations
lives alone, never married	Decreased vision
no children	
mother ↓ @ 74; h/o HTN, CAD, DM	
father ↓ @ 82; h/o HTN, CAD, CA	
Cost of medications per month $ ~50⁰⁰	

Allergies/Intolerances	Social Drug Use	
☐ No known drug allergies	Alcohol	Ø
Medication Reaction	Caffeine	Ø
aspirin GI upset	Tobacco	Ø
	Pregnancy/Breastfeeding Status N/A	
	☐ Pregnant (due _____) ☐ Breastfeeding	

Diet	Routine Exercise/Recreation	Daily Activities/Timing
☒ Low salt prescribed;	Gardening	9-11 AM volunteer work
☒ Low fat ↓ salt but	light housework	
☐ Diabetic not fat		
Timing of meals:		

Patient Name: **Sarah McLucas**

Physical Assessment/Laboratory Data—Initial/Follow-up

Date	4/14/98	4/20/98	4/23/98		
Height			5'5"		
Weight			162 lb BMI 27		
Temp			98.6 oral		
BP			134/86 RA sitting		
Pulse			72 reg R/R		
Respirations			14		
Peak Flow					
FBG	142	138			
R. Glucose					
HbA$_{1c}$		9.4%			
T. Chol.		232			
LDL		145			
HDL		30			
TG		284			
INR					
BUN					
Cr		0.8			
ALT					
AST					
Alk Phos					
U/A		⊖ glucose ⊖ protein, ket			
U. Microalb.		⊖			

Drug Serum Concentrations

Date					

Notes:

Patient Name: __Sarah McLucas__

Current Prescription Medication Regimen

Name/Dose/Strength/Route	Schedule/ Frequency of Use	Indication	Start Date (and Stop Date If Applicable)	Prescriber	Adherence Issues/Efficacy
Cholestyramine T̄ scoop	BID	Hyperlipid.	1997-	Davis	not taking
Naprosyn 500	BID	OA	1996-	Davis	takes/fair
Calcium Carbonate 500 mg	QID	supplement	1996	Davis	takes/good

Current Nonprescription Medication Regimen (OTC, herbal, homeopathic, nutritional, etc.)

Name/Dose/Strength/Route	Schedule/ Frequency of Use	Indication	Start Date (and Stop Date If Applicable)	Prescriber	Adherence Issues/Efficacy
Tavist-D	T̄ BID	allergic rhinitis	1994-	-	takes/good
Mylanta	T̄ tablespoon	GERD	weekly 1996-	-	weekly/fair
Motrin IB	q 4-6 pm	OA	1994-	-	3-4x q wk

Patient Name: **Sarah McLucas**

Risk Assessment/Preventive Measures/Quality of Life

Cardiovascular Risk Assessment		
male >45 years old	1	
female >55 years old or female <55 with history of ovarectomy not taking estrogen replacement	1	l
Definite MI or sudden death before age 55 year in father or male first-degree relative or before 65 year in mother or female first-degree relative	1	
current cigarette smoking	1	
hypertension	1	l
diabetes mellitus	1	l
HDL cholesterol <35 mg/dl	1	l
HDL cholesterol >60 mg/dl	-1	
	Total:	**4**

Is patient at risk for complications of current conditions? ☑ Yes   ☐ No

Specify: HbA1c 9.4% above goal

Preventive Measures for Adults

H = has been done   R = patient refuses   X = not applicable   Date

Women		4/23/98				
Pap Smear/pelvic	Annually 19+	H				
Mammogram	Every 1-2Y 40-49; annually 50+	H				
Men						
Rectal/prostate	Annually 50+					
All Patients						
Total/HDL-C	Every 5Y 19+	H				
Home Fecal Occult Blood Test	Annually	H				
Immunizations						
Td	Every 10Y	H				
Influenza	Every fall*	H				
Pneumovax	Once*	H				

* if indicated

Quality of life issues

Assessment of General Appearance

Patient _____Sarah McLucas_____   Date ____4/23/98____

General Appearance	Observations and Comments

Level of consciousness
   alertness: alert, confused,
   delirious, stuporous, comatose,
   orientation: person, place, time
	alert & oriented to person, place & time

Signs of distress respiratory distress, pain, anxiety, etc.	No distress, very pleasant
Posture, motor activity, and gait *Describe*	Normal
Dress, grooming, and personal hygiene *Describe*	exceptionally well groomed

Affect
   normal, inappropriate
   Describe
	Appropriate, quiet

Speech
   normal, impaired
   Describe
	Normal

Skin
   color: normal, blue, brown, red, pallor
   texture: normal, coarse, dry, oily
   turgor: good, poor
   edema
   lesions: color, type, configuration, anatomic
     distribution, consistency
	Normal skin color (many freckles) good skin turgor. No edema or lesions

SCREENING FORM FOR DIABETES FOOT DISEASE

Name: __Sarah McLucas__

Date: __4/23/98__

ID #: _____

I. Medical History

Check all that apply.

_____ Peripheral neuropathy
_____ Nephropathy
_____ Retinopathy
_____ Peripheral vascular disease
__✓__ Cardiovascular disease **(HTN)**

For Sections II & III, fill in the blanks with an "R," "L," or "B" for positive findings on the right, left, or both feet.

II. Current History

1. Any change in the foot since the last evaluation?
_____ Yes _____ **1st exam**
_____ No

2. Current ulcer or history of a foot ulcer?
_____ Yes _____
__✓__ No

3. Is there pain in the calf muscles when walking that is relieved by rest?
_____ Yes _____
__✓__ No

III. Foot Exam

1. Are the nails thick, too long, ingrown, infected with fungal disease?

_____ Yes _____

☑ No

2. Note foot deformities

_____ Toe deformities

_____ Bunions (hallus valgus)   NONE

_____ Charcot foot

_____ Foot drop

_____ Prominent metatarsal heads

_____ Amputation (specify date, side, and level) _____

3. Pedal Pulses *(Fill in the blanks with a "P" or an "A" to indicate present or absent.)*

Posterior tibial:

___P_ Left

___P_ Right   } NORMAl

Dorsalis pedis:

___P_ Left

___P_ Right

4. Skin Condition *(Measure, draw in, and label the patient's skin condition, using the key and the foot diagram below.)*

C = Callus	PU = Pre-ulcerative lesion
U = Ulcer	F = Fissure
R = Redness	S = Swelling
W = Warmth	D = Dryness
M = Maceration	

IV. Sensory Foot Exam

Label sensory level with a "+" in the five circled areas of the foot if the patient can feel the 5.07 Semmes-Weinstein (10-gram) nylon filament and "−" if the patient cannot feel the filament.

Notes 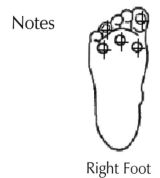   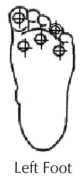 Notes

Right Foot   Left Foot

V. Risk Categorization

Check appropriate item.

____✓____ Low-Risk Patient
All of the following:
Intact protective sensation
Pedal pulses present
No severe deformity
No prior foot ulcer
No amputation

_____ High-Risk Patient
One or more of the following:
Loss of protective sensation
Absent pedal pulses
Severe foot deformity
History of foot ulcer
Prior amputation

VI. Footwear Assessment

Fill in the blanks.

Does the patient wear appropriate shoes?
____✓____ Yes
_____ No

Does the patient need inserts?
_____ Yes
____✓____ No

Should therapeutic footwear be prescribed?
_____ Yes
____✓____ No

VII. Education

Fill in the blanks.

Has the patient had prior foot care education?
_____ Yes
____✓____ No

Can the patient demonstrate appropriate self-care?
____✓____ Yes
_____ No

VIII. Management Plan

Check all that apply.

✓ Provide patient education for preventive foot care.

Date: **4/23/98**

Diagnostic studies:
_____ Vascular laboratory
_____ Other: _____

Footwear recommendations:
✓ None
_____ Athletic shoes
_____ Accommodative inserts
_____ Custom shoes
_____ Depth shoes

Refer to:
✓ Primary care provider   **for scheduled follow-up**
_____ Diabetes educator
_____ Orthopedic foot surgeon
_____ RN foot specialist
_____ Orthotist
_____ Podiatrist
_____ Pedorthist
_____ Endocrinologist
_____ Rehab. specialist
_____ Vascular surgeon
_____ Other: _____
_____ Schedule follow-up visit

Date: _____**4/23/98**_____ Provider Signature: _____*Alexa Sheffield, Pharm.D.*_____

Source: http://www.niddk.nih.gov/health/diabetes/feet/feet2/screenfo.htm

AMBULATORY THERAPY ASSESSMENT WORKSHEET (ATAW)

Patient _____

Pharmacist _____

Date _____

Correlation Between Drug Therapy and Medical Problems

ASSESSMENT	PRESENCE OF PROBLEM*	COMMENTS/NOTES
Any drugs without a medical indication? Any unidentified medications? Any untreated medical conditions? Do they require drug therapy?	1. A problem exists. 2. More information is needed for determination. 3. No problem exists or an intervention is not needed.	

Appropriate Therapy

ASSESSMENT	PRESENCE OF PROBLEM*	COMMENTS/NOTES
Comparative efficacy of chosen medication(s)? Relative safety of chosen medication(s)? Is medication on formulary? Is nondrug therapy appropriately used (e.g., diet and exercise)? Is therapy achieving desired goals or outcomes? Is therapy tailored to this patient (e.g., age, comorbid conditions, and living/working environment)?	1. A problem exists. 2. More information is needed for determination. 3. No problem exists or an intervention is not needed.	

Drug Regimen

ASSESSMENT	PRESENCE OF PROBLEM*	COMMENTS/NOTES
Are dose and dosing regimen appropriate and/or within usual therapeutic range and/or modified for patient factors? Appropriateness of PRN medications (prescribed or taken that way) Is route/dosage form/mode of administration appropriate, length or course of therapy considering efficacy, safety, convenience, patient limitations, length or course of therapy, and cost?	1. A problem exists. 2. More information is needed for determination. 3. No problem exists or an intervention is not needed.	

*Problem denotes any pharmacotherapeutic or related health care problem.

Therapeutic Duplication

ASSESSMENT	PRESENCE OF PROBLEM*	COMMENTS/NOTES
Any therapeutic duplications?	1. A problem exists. 2. More information is needed for determination. 3. No problem exists or an intervention is not needed.	

Drug Allergy or Intolerance

ASSESSMENT	PRESENCE OF PROBLEM*	COMMENTS/NOTES
Allergy or intolerance to any medications (or chemically related medications) currently being taken? Is patient using a method to alert health care providers of the allergy/intolerance or serious health problem?	1. A problem exists. 2. More information is needed for determination. 3. No problem exists or an intervention is not needed.	

Adverse Drug Events

ASSESSMENT	PRESENCE OF PROBLEM*	COMMENTS/NOTES
Are symptoms or medical problems drug induced? What is the likelihood the problem is drug related?	1. A problem exists. 2. More information is needed for determination. 3. No problem exists or an intervention is not needed.	

Interactions: Drug-Drug, Drug-Disease, Drug-Nutrient, Drug–Laboratory Test

ASSESSMENT	PRESENCE OF PROBLEM*	COMMENTS/NOTES
Any drug-drug interactions? Clinical significance? Any relative or absolute contraindications given patient characteristics and current/past disease states? Any drug-nutrient interactions? Clinical significance? Any drug-laboratory test interactions? Clinical significance?	1. A problem exists. 2. More information is needed for determination. 3. No problem exists or an intervention is not needed.	

*Problem denotes any pharmacotherapeutic or related health care problem.

Social or Recreational Drug Use

ASSESSMENT	PRESENCE OF PROBLEM*	COMMENTS/NOTES
Is current use of social drugs problematic? Are symptoms related to sudden withdrawal or discontinuation of social drugs?	1. A problem exists. 2. More information is needed for determination. 3. No problem exists or an intervention is not needed.	

Financial Impact

ASSESSMENT	PRESENCE OF PROBLEM*	COMMENTS/NOTES
Is therapy cost-effective? Does cost of therapy represent a financial hardship for the patient?	1. A problem exists. 2. More information is needed for determination. 3. No problem exists or an intervention is not needed.	

Patient Knowledge of Therapy

ASSESSMENT	PRESENCE OF PROBLEM*	COMMENTS/NOTES
Does patient understand the role of his/her medication(s), how to take it, and potential side effects? Would patient benefit from education tools (e.g., written patient education sheets, wallet cards, or reminder package?) Does the patient understand the role of nondrug therapy?	1. A problem exists. 2. More information is needed for determination. 3. No problem exists or an intervention is not needed.	

Adherence

ASSESSMENT	PRESENCE OF PROBLEM*	COMMENTS/NOTES
Is there a problem with nonadherence to drug or nondrug therapy (e.g., diet and exercise)? Are there barriers to adherence or factors hindering the achievement of therapeutic efficacy?	1. A problem exists. 2. More information is needed for determination. 3. No problem exists or an intervention is not needed.	

*Problem denotes any pharmacotherapeutic or related health care problem.

Self-Monitoring

ASSESSMENT	PRESENCE OF PROBLEM*	COMMENTS/NOTES
Does patient perform appropriate self-monitoring? (e.g., peak flow and blood glucose) Is correct technique employed? Is self-monitoring performed consistently, at appropriate times, and with appropriate frequency?	1. A problem exists. 2. More information is needed for determination. 3. No problem exists or an intervention is not needed.	

Risks and Quality of Life Impacts

ASSESSMENT	PRESENCE OF PROBLEM*	COMMENTS/NOTES
Is patient at risk for complications with an existing disease state (i.e., risk factor assessment)? Is patient on track for preventive measures (e.g., immunizations, mammograms, prostate exams, eye exams)? Is therapy adversely impacting patient's quality of life? How so?	1. A problem exists. 2. More information is needed for determination. 3. No problem exists or an intervention is not needed.	

*Problem denotes any pharmacotherapeutic or related health care problem.

AMBULATORY PHARMACIST'S CARE PLAN

Patient _____

Pharmacist _____ Date _____

DATE IDENTIFIED	PROBLEM (TPL)	PHARMACOTHERAPEUTIC AND RELATED HEALTH CARE GOAL	RECOMMENDATIONS FOR THERAPY	MONITORING PARAMETER(S)	DESIRED ENDPOINT(S)	MONITORING FREQUENCY

AMBULATORY PHARMACIST'S CARE PLAN

Patient _____   Pharmacist _____   Date _____

DATE IDENTIFIED	PROBLEM (TPL)	PHARMACOTHERAPEUTIC AND RELATED HEALTH CARE GOAL	RECOMMENDATIONS FOR THERAPY	MONITORING PARAMETER(S)	DESIRED ENDPOINT(S)	MONITORING FREQUENCY

AMBULATORY THERAPY ASSESSMENT WORKSHEET (ATAW)

Patient __Sarah McLucas__

Pharmacist __Alexa Sheffield, Pharm.D.__

Date __4-23-98__

Correlation Between Drug Therapy and Medical Problems

ASSESSMENT	PRESENCE OF PROBLEM*	COMMENTS/NOTES
Any drugs without a medical indication? Any unidentified medications? Any untreated medical conditions? Do they require drug therapy?	(1.) A problem exists. 2. More information is needed for determination. 3. No problem exists or an intervention is not needed.	-HTN not treated -Postmenopausal -no HRT -DM just diagnosed; no tx yet -should be on daily ASA tx

Appropriate Therapy

ASSESSMENT	PRESENCE OF PROBLEM*	COMMENTS/NOTES
Comparative efficacy of chosen medication(s)? Relative safety of chosen medication(s)? Is medication on formulary? Is nondrug therapy appropriately used (e.g., diet and exercise)? Is therapy achieving desired goals or outcomes? Is therapy tailored to this patient (e.g., age, comorbid conditions, and living/working environment)?	(1.) A problem exists. 2. More information is needed for determination. 3. No problem exists or an intervention is not needed.	-Diabetes not controlled -BP not at goal; need tx -Hypercholesterolemia not controlled -Pt. ↓ salt, but not fat in diet

Drug Regimen

ASSESSMENT	PRESENCE OF PROBLEM*	COMMENTS/NOTES
Are dose and dosing regimen appropriate and/or within usual therapeutic range and/or modified for patient factors? Appropriateness of PRN medications (prescribed or taken that way) Is route/dosage form/mode of administration appropriate, length or course of therapy considering efficacy, safety, convenience, patient limitations, length or course of therapy, and cost?	(1.) A problem exists. 2. More information is needed for determination. 3. No problem exists or an intervention is not needed.	-Pt. taking Tavist-D year-round -prn ibuprofen use in addition to naprosyn RX.

*Problem denotes any pharmacotherapeutic or related health care problem.

Therapeutic Duplication

ASSESSMENT	PRESENCE OF PROBLEM*	COMMENTS/NOTES
Any therapeutic duplications?	(1.) A problem exists. 2. More information is needed for determination. 3. No problem exists or an intervention is not needed.	−Naprosyn and nonprescription ibuprofen use

Drug Allergy or Intolerance

ASSESSMENT	PRESENCE OF PROBLEM*	COMMENTS/NOTES
Allergy or intolerance to any medications (or chemically related medications) currently being taken? Is patient using a method to alert health care providers of the allergy/intolerance or serious health problem?	1. A problem exists. 2. More information is needed for determination. (3.) No problem exists or an intervention is not needed.	Pt. c/o GI upset c̄ ASA but denies c̄ Naprosyn and ibuprofen (c/o GERD however)

Adverse Drug Events

ASSESSMENT	PRESENCE OF PROBLEM*	COMMENTS/NOTES
Are symptoms or medical problems drug induced? What is the likelihood the problem is drug related?	1. A problem exists. 2. More information is needed for determination. (3.) No problem exists or an intervention is not needed.	

Interactions: Drug-Drug, Drug-Disease, Drug-Nutrient, Drug–Laboratory Test

ASSESSMENT	PRESENCE OF PROBLEM*	COMMENTS/NOTES
Any drug-drug interactions? Clinical significance? Any relative or absolute contraindications given patient characteristics and current/past disease states? Any drug-nutrient interactions? Clinical significance? Any drug-laboratory test interactions? Clinical significance?	(1.) A problem exists. 2. More information is needed for determination. 3. No problem exists or an intervention is not needed.	−PPA in Tavist-D may ↑ BP and BG −NSAID may ↑ BP −Possible NSAID-induced GERD

*Problem denotes any pharmacotherapeutic or related health care problem.

Social or Recreational Drug Use

ASSESSMENT	PRESENCE OF PROBLEM*	COMMENTS/NOTES
Is current use of social drugs problematic? Are symptoms related to sudden withdrawal or discontinuation of social drugs?	1. A problem exists. 2. More information is needed for determination. (3.) No problem exists or an intervention is not needed.	

Financial Impact

ASSESSMENT	PRESENCE OF PROBLEM*	COMMENTS/NOTES
Is therapy cost-effective? Does cost of therapy represent a financial hardship for the patient?	1. A problem exists. 2. More information is needed for determination. (3.) No problem exists or an intervention is not needed.	Pt. denies financial hardship despite lack of RX benefit

Patient Knowledge of Therapy

ASSESSMENT	PRESENCE OF PROBLEM*	COMMENTS/NOTES
Does patient understand the role of his/her medication(s), how to take it, and potential side effects? Would patient benefit from education tools (e.g., written patient education sheets, wallet cards, or reminder package?) Does the patient understand the role of nondrug therapy?	(1.) A problem exists. 2. More information is needed for determination. 3. No problem exists or an intervention is not needed.	-Did not realize naprosyn and ibuprofen were both NSAIDs. -Did not know allergy med should be used prn.

Adherence

ASSESSMENT	PRESENCE OF PROBLEM*	COMMENTS/NOTES
Is there a problem with nonadherence to drug or nondrug therapy (e.g., diet and exercise)? Are there barriers to adherence or factors hindering the achievement of therapeutic efficacy?	(1.) A problem exists. 2. More information is needed for determination. 3. No problem exists or an intervention is not needed.	-Pt. refuses to take cholestyramine -Pt. will not ↓ fat in diet

*Problem denotes any pharmacotherapeutic or related health care problem.

Self-Monitoring

ASSESSMENT	PRESENCE OF PROBLEM*	COMMENTS/NOTES
Does patient perform appropriate self-monitoring? (e.g., peak flow and blood glucose) Is correct technique employed? Is self-monitoring performed consistently, at appropriate times, and with appropriate frequency?	(1.) A problem exists. 2. More information is needed for determination. 3. No problem exists or an intervention is not needed.	*Needs to learn SMBG*

Risks and Quality of Life Impacts

ASSESSMENT	PRESENCE OF PROBLEM*	COMMENTS/NOTES
Is patient at risk for complications with an existing disease state (i.e., risk factor assessment)? Is patient on track for preventive measures (e.g., immunizations, mammograms, prostate exams, eye exams)? Is therapy adversely impacting patient's quality of life? How so?	(1.) A problem exists. 2. More information is needed for determination. 3. No problem exists or an intervention is not needed.	*Current on health maintenance, but has multiple CV risk factors.*

*Problem denotes any pharmacotherapeutic or related health care problem.

AMBULATORY PHARMACIST'S CARE PLAN

Patient __Sarah McLucas__   Pharmacist __Alexa Sheffield__   Date __4-23-98__

DATE IDENTIFIED	PROBLEM (TPL)	PHARMACOTHERAPEUTIC AND RELATED HEALTH CARE GOAL	RECOMMENDATIONS FOR THERAPY	MONITORING PARAMETER(S)	DESIRED ENDPOINT(S)	MONITORING FREQUENCY
4/23/98	Poor control of diabetes					
"	Poor control of HTN					
"	Poor control of lipids					
"	Postmenopausal w/o HRT					
"	Not on ASA GPD tx					
"	PPA in Tavist-D may worsen BP & BG					
"	Nonadherence to diet					
"	NSAID may ↑ BP					

AMBULATORY PHARMACIST'S CARE PLAN

Patient __Sarah McLucas__   Pharmacist __Alexa Sheffield__   Date __4-23-98__

Page 2

DATE IDENTIFIED	PROBLEM (TPL)	PHARMACOTHERAPEUTIC AND RELATED HEALTH CARE GOAL	RECOMMENDATIONS FOR THERAPY	MONITORING PARAMETER(S)	DESIRED ENDPOINT(S)	MONITORING FREQUENCY
4/23/98	Taking Tavist-D year-round					
"	Taking Naprosyn and ibuprofen					
"	Poor control of OA pain					
"	NSAID may ↑ Sxs of GERD					
"	Nonadherence to cholestyramine					
"	No SMBG					
"	No exercise plan					

Considering the Big Picture: Health Care Needs, Triage, and Referral

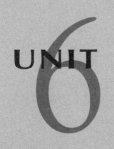

UNIT

6

Pharmacists are widely recognized as drug experts; however, pharmaceutical care emphasizes dealing with the patient as a whole person rather than just treating drug-related problems. Even though the *Ambulatory Care Clinical Skills Program: Type 2 Diabetes Mellitus Management Module* is specifically about type 2 diabetes, you are still obliged to consider all the patient's health care needs, not just the diabetes.

Patients with type 2 diabetes benefit most from a team approach; the patient carries the ball, but receives input from all the other members of the team. It is important for us as pharmacists to know which other members of the health care team should be involved in diabetes care and when those referrals should be made. The pharmacist's relationship with other health care providers should be *inter*disciplinary (integrated care), not just *multi*disciplinary (independent, parallel care). In working collaboratively with the patient and other health care professionals, the pharmacist will help ensure the patient's overall treatment and successful drug therapy outcomes.

Unit Objectives

After you successfully complete this unit, you will be able to:
- define the health care needs of an ambulatory patient with type 2 diabetes,
- explain portions of the pharmacist's care plan for an ambulatory patient with type 2 diabetes that should be managed by health care professionals other than the pharmacist, and
- explain situations unique to the treatment of ambulatory patients with type 2 diabetes that require immediate attention.

Unit Organization

This unit begins by reviewing the concept of patient health care needs and illustrates how to determine a diabetes patient's overall health care needs, using Mrs. Gonzalez as an example. Next, you will learn what routine and unanticipated health care needs of the ambulatory patient with type 2 diabetes necessitate triage and referral to other health care providers. We will review the case of Mrs. Gonzalez to determine her referral needs. Finally, you will practice determining health care and referral needs

for a patient with type 2 diabetes with the case of Mr. Jones.

Health Care Needs of Ambulatory Patients with Type 2 Diabetes

In unit 11 of the *Ambulatory Care Clinical Skills Program: Core Module*, you learned that health care providers have three basic goals when caring for a patient:
- identifying all actual or potential health care problems,
- alleviating actual problems, and
- avoiding potential problems.

These goals illustrate that a patient's health care needs are elements of care required to improve or prevent deterioration of health and well-being.

Diabetes is a complex, chronic disease with many possible complications. Health care needs for the ambulatory patient with type 2 diabetes include adequate control of the diabetes as well as common comorbid conditions, such as hypertension and hypercholesterolemia. The term *adequate control* refers to the control of markers of the disease, such as hemoglobin A_{1c}, blood pressure, and LDL cholesterol.

An important aspect of these common conditions is their propensity to lead to chronic complications. For example, diabetes may cause macrovascular disease (cardiovascular, cerebrovascular, and peripheral vascular disease), microvascular disease (nephropathy and retinopathy), neuropathy (peripheral and autonomic neuropathy), and complications caused by a hybrid of these (e.g., foot and leg ulcers caused by vascular disease and peripheral neuropathy). Poorly controlled hypertension causes target organ damage, including retinopathy and nephropathy, and cardiovascular, cerebrovascular, and peripheral vascular disease. Hypercholesterolemia is a major risk factor for cardiovascular disease. An important health care need of a patient with diabetes, hypertension, and hypercholesterolemia is to prevent the long-term complications associated with each, or to slow their progression should they occur.

Another health care need closely related to the complications of these comorbid conditions is to decrease modifiable risk factors for the development of each. For example, risk factors for cardiovascular disease include smoking, obesity, and hypercholesterolemia. Some risk factors cannot be modified, such as sex and age. Preventive care, particularly prevention of the complications of diabetes, is the best defense and an important health care goal.

Type 2 diabetes and associated conditions are managed with both nonpharmacologic and pharmacologic interventions. Important health care needs are to improve adherence to both drug and nondrug therapies, to prevent medication-related adverse effects, and to optimize therapy to avoid drug-disease interactions.

A final health care need to consider is a patient's self-care. Because a patient is responsible for the majority of the care in type 2 diabetes and other related conditions, education and self-monitoring are very important. Initiation and adherence to home blood glucose or blood pressure monitoring is another health care need.

As you learned in the *Ambulatory Care Clinical Skills Program: Core Module*, the pharmacist's care plan is a dynamic tool; you need to continually reassess the patient and his or her health care needs as the patient's health status changes. Although you will not record the patient's health care needs on the APCP, you should observe relationships between information on the patient's database and items listed on the therapy problem list (TPL) and identify health care needs.

Case Study

Let's look at the case of Mrs. Gonzalez. Her APCP is **Appendix A**. What are her health care needs?

Mrs. Gonzalez has just been diagnosed with type 2 diabetes and hypercholesterolemia, and she has had hypertension for 4 years. Based on this information, we can identify these health care needs:

- adequate control of type 2 diabetes
- adequate control of hypertension
- adequate control of hypercholesterolemia
- prevention of long-term complications of type 2 diabetes, hypertension, and hypercholesterolemia

Mrs. Gonzalez has several modifiable risk factors for cardiovascular disease: She is not receiving an aspirin daily, she has high cholesterol, and she is postmenopausal but is not having hormone replacement therapy. Therefore, we can add another health care need to Mrs. Gonzalez's list:

- decrease modifiable cardiovascular risk factors

Mrs. Gonzalez has never been prescribed a meal or exercise plan, so we can list these health care needs as follows:

- improve knowledge of diabetes medical nutrition therapy
- improve knowledge of exercise options
- ensure adherence to nonpharmacologic therapeutic interventions

Additional health care needs for Mrs. Gonzalez follow:

- improve knowledge of drug therapy and monitoring
- ensure adherence to pharmacologic therapeutic interventions
- prevent adverse effects from drug therapy
- optimize therapy and reduce risk of drug-disease interactions
- avoid interactions of medications with other diseases
- initiate home blood glucose monitoring
- initiate home blood pressure monitoring

Mrs. Gonzalez is also missing several health maintenance interventions, such as an annual home fecal occult blood test, annual influenza vaccine, calcium therapy to prevent osteoporosis, and monthly breast self-examinations. We can add one last health care need:

- screen for and minimize the risk for developing significant comorbid conditions

Although Mrs. Gonzalez's health care needs are not recorded, you should observe relationships between information on her database and items listed on the TPL and identify health care needs.

Triage and Referral of Ambulatory Patients with Type 2 Diabetes

Portions of the APCP Requiring Services of Other Health Care Professionals

In unit 12 of the *Ambulatory Care Clinical Skills Program: Core Module*, you learned there are three factors to consider in deciding when to refer a patient to another health care provider: the nature of the problem, its urgency, and the patient's preference.

There are several clear examples of type 2 diabetes management issues that are outside the usual scope of practice for a pharmacist. These include services provided by a dietitian, exercise physiologist, podiatrist, ophthalmologist, and dentist, as well as the patient's primary care provider.

The urgency of a problem also affects your triage decision. If a patient states that she has trouble cutting her toenails, you might recommend that she make an appointment with her podiatrist, to be seen within the next week or so. If the same patient states that the toenail on her great toe turned black a few days ago, and it looks as if it's going to fall off, this is a podiatric emergency requiring immediate attention.

As we have discussed, patients will do what they think is in their own best interest, so it is prudent to prospectively solicit the patient's preference. If the patient expresses no interest in seeing the dietitian, attempting to make the referral may be futile. It would be more appropriate to explore with the patient why she didn't want to see the dietitian and formulate a plan *with* the patient instead of *for* the patient. Let's examine each of the potential referrals that arise while caring for ambulatory patients with type 2 diabetes.

Medical Nutrition Therapy

The term *medical nutrition therapy* (MNT) was introduced in 1994 by the American Dietetic Association largely because of legislative efforts to promote reimbursement. It is defined as the use of specific nutrition services to treat an illness, injury, or condition and involves two phases:

- assessment of the nutrition status of the patient, and
- treatment, which includes diet therapy, counseling, and the use of specialized nutrition supplements.[1]

Diabetes MNT encompasses four distinct functions:

- assessment of the patient's metabolic, nutrition, and lifestyle parameters;
- identification and negotiation of nutrition goals;
- intervention designed to achieve the individualized goals; and
- evaluation of outcomes.[2]

The evolution from diet counseling to diabetes medical nutrition therapy occurred under the influence of several factors. First, the Diabetes Control and Complications Trial (DCCT) results highlighted the use of contemporary meal-planning approaches and teaching techniques.[3] Second, the American Diabetes Association published the "1994 Diabetes Nutrition Recommendations," which emphasized the need for individualizing diabetes

MNT.[4] Last, practice guidelines for professionals who work in dietetics have delineated roles and responsibilities within diabetes MNT.[6-8] The importance of diet in the management of type 2 diabetes clearly exceeds the need for simple counseling. Dietary and behavioral modification is a therapeutic intervention. Dietitians, particularly Registered Dietitians (RDs) and Certified Diabetes Educators (CDEs) are specifically trained to perform the four functions of MNT described previously.

The most recent Clinical Practice Recommendations published by the American Diabetes Association include the position statement, "Nutrition Recommendations and Principles for People with Diabetes Mellitus."[9] The goals of MNT for patients with diabetes per this position statement include:

- maintenance of as near-normal blood glucose levels as possible by balancing food intake with medications and physical activity;
- achievement of optimal serum lipid levels;
- provision of adequate calories for maintaining or attaining reasonable weights for adults, normal growth and development rates in children and adolescents, and to meet the increased metabolic needs during pregnancy and lactation or recovery from catabolic illness;
- prevention and treatment of acute and long-term complications of diabetes; and
- improvement of overall health through optimal nutrition.

Goals specific for patients with type 2 diabetes include achievement and maintenance of glucose, lipid, and blood pressure goals. Because the majority of patients with type 2 diabetes are obese, a hypocaloric diet aimed to achieve slow, steady weight loss will probably be prescribed.

The distribution of calories between carbohydrates, protein, and fat should be individualized for each patient. For example, 10–20% of daily calories should be from protein sources. Patients with overt nephropathy would likely be restricted to the 10% protein allowance.

The daily total fat allowance is also customized based on any identified lipid problems the patient has and treatment goals for glucose, lipids, and weight. The American Diabetes Association recommends that patients of healthy body weight with no lipid abnormalities follow the recommendations of the National Cholesterol Education Program (NCEP), which are that all individuals >2 years of age limit fat intake to <30% of total calories, with saturated fat restricted to <10% of total calories, polyunsaturated fat intake <10% of calories, and monounsaturated fat 10–15% of calories.[8] For patients who have lipid abnormalities or are obese, the fat allowance would be redistributed between saturated, polyunsaturated, and monounsaturated fats and/or the fat content would be reduced altogether.

The remaining calories are from carbohydrate sources.

Patients diagnosed with type 2 diabetes generally have many questions about their meal plan. Pharmacists should at least be familiar with the basic principles of meal planning, such as the Food Guide Pyramid, produced by the United States Department of Agriculture (USDA).[10] The Food Guide Pyramid is shown in **Figure 1**; a copy of the complete brochure can be viewed at the Web site of the USDA (www.usda.gov). To order multiple copies of the brochure you should contact the Government Printing Office.

Patients with type 2 diabetes should be referred to a dietitian at the time of diagnosis, and whenever the patient feels the need, or when the health care team feels the patient could benefit from a dietary consult. You can find dietitians at your local hospital or clinic, or you can contact your state chapter or the national office of the American Association of Diabetes Educators (1-800-338-3633) to get a listing of dietitians providing diabetes MNT in your area.

Exercise

Exercise is a therapeutic tool in the management of ambulatory patients with type 2 diabetes. Research has shown a consistent beneficial effect of regular exercise training on carbohydrate metabolism and insulin sensitivity, with long-lasting effects.[11] Exercise has been shown to reduce the risk of cardiovascular disease, triglyceride levels, blood pressure, and weight in patients with type 2 diabetes.

As discussed in previous units, it is essential that patients be evaluated by their physician prior to beginning an exercise program. The patient should be screened for macrovascular and microvascular complications that may be worsened by an exercise program. Specifically, a pre-exercise evaluation may consist of a graded exercise test, an evaluation of peripheral arterial disease, an eye examination for retinopathy, and screening for nephropathy and neuropathy (both peripheral and autonomic). Based on the findings of this assessment, appropriate exercises may be offered as options to the patient. Patients with preexisting complications may not participate in selected exercise activities. For example, a patient with insensate feet cannot participate in repetitive, weight-bearing activities and should select activities such as swimming, bicycling, rowing, chair and arm exercise, or another

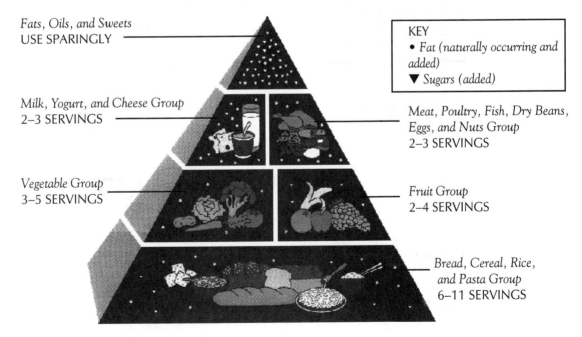

Figure 1. The Food Guide Pyramid
Source: U.S. Department of Agriculture Web site (www.usda.gov).

non-weight-bearing exercise.[11] The pharmacist should get clearance from the patient's physician prior to recommending an exercise program, including regular walking.

After screening, the patient may benefit from a referral to an exercise physiologist. The exercise physiologist will work with the patient to select appropriate exercise activities and develop the four components of an exercise program: frequency, intensity, time, and type of exercise.[12] An exercise physiologist can also be identified from your state chapter or the national office of the American Association of Diabetes Educators.

Podiatry

Foot ulcers and related problems are a major cause of morbidity, mortality, and disability for patients with diabetes. The American Diabetes Association recommends a comprehensive screening including vascular, neurological, musculoskeletal, and skin and soft tissue evaluations be done at least annually.[13] This examination may be performed by a primary care provider comfortable with this type of assessment, or the patient could be referred to a podiatrist. Once high-risk abnormalities are discovered, a foot examination should be performed several times a year.

The pharmacist is still in an excellent position to screen for insensate feet, as described in unit 2. The pharmacist should share the results of the foot screening with the primary care provider and be alert to any warning symptoms or signs of diabetic foot problems, as listed in **Table 1**.[14] If a pharmacist detects a foot ulcer on a patient with diabetes, the patient should be immediately referred to a physician. Management of a foot ulcer requires skills such as radiological examination, assessment of bacterial cultures, knowledge of antibiotic therapy, debridement, wound care, and evaluation of mechanical stress and circulation. These functions are best performed by a podiatrist, vascular surgeon, or primary care provider who possesses these skills.

Ophthalmology

Diabetic retinopathy is a microvascular complication of diabetes. Nearly 60% of patients with type 2 diabetes will have some degree of retinopathy after 20 years.[15] The following are recommended guidelines for retinopathy screening in type 2 diabetes per the American Diabetes Association:

1. Patients with type 2 diabetes should have an initial dilated and comprehensive eye examination by an ophthalmologist or optometrist shortly after the diabetes diagnosis.
2. Subsequent examinations should be performed annually by an ophthalmologist or optometrist who is knowledgeable and experienced in diagnosing the presence of diabetic retinopathy and is aware of its management. Examinations may be required more frequently if retinopathy progresses.
3. Women with diabetes who are planning pregnancy should have a comprehensive eye examination prior to conception and during the first trimester.
4. Patients with macular edema, severe nonproliferative retinopathy, or proliferative retinopathy should receive prompt care from a knowledgeable and experienced ophthalmologist.
5. Patients who experience vision loss from diabetes should be encouraged to pursue visual rehabilitation.

When you are working with an ambulatory patient with type 2 diabetes, if they should complain of any of the following, you should refer them immediately to their ophthalmologist:

- blurry vision persisting for >1–2 days when not associated with a change in blood glucose;
- sudden loss of vision in one or both eyes; or
- black spots, cobwebs, or flashing lights in field of vision.[16]

Oral and Dental Care

Poorly controlled type 2 diabetes may result in dental complications, such as periodontal disease, tooth decay, xerostomia, candidiasis, and oral peripheral neuropathy.[17] Recommendations for oral and dental care for patients with diabetes include the following:

- practice daily dental hygiene, including flossing and brushing;
- have periodic dental examinations;
- do not smoke or chew tobacco; and
- achieve the best glycemic control possible.[17]

You should inquire about any complaints of redness, foul odor, swelling, or bleeding from the gums, loose teeth, or pain. If these periodontal symptoms develop, or any other dental-related complaints surface, the patient should be referred to the dentist. Remind patients to see their dentist for routine care every 6 months and more frequently if periodontal disease exists.

Table 1. Warning Symptoms and Signs of Diabetic Foot Problems

	Symptoms	Signs
Vascular	Cold feet Intermittent claudication involving calf or foot Pain at rest, especially nocturnal, relieved by dependency	Absent pedal, popliteal, or femoral pulses Femoral bruits Dependent rubor, plantar pallor on elevation Prolonged capillary filling time (>3–4 sec)
Neurological	Sensory: burning, tingling, or crawling sensations; pain and hypersensitivity; cold feet Motor: weakness (foot drop) Autonomic: diminished sweating	Sensory: deficits (vibratory and proprioceptive, then pain and temperature perception); hyperesthesia Motor: diminished to absent deep tendon reflexes (Achilles, then patellar); weakness; sweating
Musculoskeletal	Gradual change in foot shape, sudden painless change in foot shape, with swelling, without history or trauma	Cavus feet with claw toes Drop foot "Rocker-bottom" foot (Charcot's joint) Neuropathic arthropathy
Dermatological	Exquisitely painful or painless wounds Slow-healing or nonhealing wounds or necrosis Skin color changes (cyanosis, redness) Chronic scaling, itching or dry feet Recurrent infections (e.g., paronychia and athlete's foot)	Skin: abnormal dryness; chronic tinea infections; keratotic lesions with or without hemorrhage (plantar or digital), trophic ulcer Hair: diminished or absent Nails: trophic changes; onychomycosis; sublingual ulceration or abscess; ingrown nails with paronychia

Note: Pharmacists who wish to develop the ability to perform these advanced level physical assessments should refer to reference 14.

Urgent Situations for Ambulatory Patients with Type 2 Diabetes

Urgent situations for ambulatory patients with type 2 diabetes aside from those described above are severe hyperglycemia, hypoglycemia, and development of infections. Specifically, patients who develop hyperglycemic hyperosmolar nonketotic syndrome, hypoglycemia, or an infection (in addition to the development of a foot ulcer, as discussed above) require immediate attention. Let's consider these separately.

Hyperglycemic Hyperosmolar Nonketotic Syndrome

Hyperglycemic hyperosmolar nonketotic syndrome (HHNS) is a hyperglycemic metabolic crisis experienced by type 2 diabetes patients and is a life-threatening emergency. HHNS usually occurs in older adults, and 35% of cases are patients previously undiagnosed with type 2 diabetes mellitus. HHNS carries an even higher mortality rate than diabetic ketoacidosis, a form of extreme hyperglycemia associated with type 1 diabetes.

Patients with type 2 diabetes generally still produce enough insulin to prevent the development of ketosis.

Precipitating causes of HHNS include drugs (e.g., corticosteroids and diuretics), therapeutic procedures (e.g., peritoneal dialysis, hemodialysis, and surgical stress), chronic diseases (e.g., renal disease, heart disease, hypertension, old stroke, alcoholism, psychiatric conditions, and loss of thirst), or an acute state (e.g., infection, diabetic gangrene, urinary tract infection, septicemia, extensive burns, gastrointestinal hemorrhage, cerebrovascular accident, myocardial infarction, or pancreatitis).[18]

There are four major clinical features of HHNS:

- severe hyperglycemia (blood glucose >600 mg/dl, but generally between 1000 and 2000 mg/dl);
- absence of or slight ketosis;
- plasma or serum hyperosmolality (>340 mOsm/L); and
- profound dehydration.[18]

Physical signs of HHNS the pharmacist can look for include excessive thirst, altered sensorium (e.g., confusion or coma), and physical signs of severe dehydration (e.g., poor skin turgor, dry mucous membranes, decreased neck vein filling seen from below a patient lying flat, and soft eyeballs).

An occurrence of HHNS is a medical emergency, and patients should be referred directly to the emergency room. Patients found to be in HHNS are generally admitted to an intensive care unit, where the precipitating event is determined and corrected, and life-saving measures are administered, including intravenous fluids, insulin, and potassium and other electrolytes.

It is important for pharmacists to remember that a patient with a seemingly mild case of diabetes, such as an older adult on a low dose of an oral agent, can develop HHNS.

Hypoglycemia

On the other end of the blood glucose spectrum is hypoglycemia, which occurs when there is an imbalance between food intake, diabetes medications, and/or exercise. Decreased oral intake, inappropriate dosing of hypoglycemia-causing medications, increased or unanticipated exercise, and alcohol may precipitate hypoglycemia. Declining organ function (e.g., liver or kidney) that results in drug accumulation and increased hypoglycemic action may also cause hypoglycemia. Although a blood glucose <70 mg/dl is considered to be hypoglycemia, it is difficult to assign an absolute blood glucose value, as some patients are very symptomatic with a blood glucose level of 60 mg/dl, whereas others show few symptoms with a blood glucose level <50 mg/dl.

Hypoglycemic episodes can be mild, meaning the patient is still capable of self-help ("mild" does not imply the episode is inconsequential), or severe, meaning the patient requires help from another. We can divide the symptoms of hypoglycemia into two categories: autonomic and neuroglycopenic. Autonomic symptoms, such as trembling, sweating, and heart palpitations, are due to the hormonal counterregulation that occurs in response to low blood glucose. Neuroglycopenic symptoms occur when glucose levels in the brain and central nervous system are too low to maintain normal function. Milder neuroglycopenic symptoms include difficulty concentrating, slowed thinking, lightheadedness, dizziness, and uncoordination. Severe neuroglycopenic symptoms include lethargy, mental stupor, and unconsciousness.[19]

Patients frequently contact their pharmacist for advice on treating actual or perceived hypoglycemia. It is important to distinguish between the two, as shown by this real example from the author's practice.

MRS. PATTI (ON THE TELEPHONE, CALLING THE PHARMACIST):

"Hello, Dr. Johnson, I wanted to give you a call because I'm very concerned. My blood glucose is 29 mg/dl. What should I do?"

PHARMACIST:

"How do you feel Mrs. Patti?"

MRS. PATTI:

"I feel great, but I'm very worried that my blood sugar is so low."

PHARMACIST:

"Mrs. Patti, I think you should check it again; I'll hold on while you check your glucose. Tell me what you are doing as you go through the process."

MRS. PATTI:

"Okay, let me get my monitor."

Mrs. Patti checks her blood glucose again, describing to the pharmacist each step as she does it.

Mrs. Patti:

"Oh goodness! Now it says 172 mg/dl; I guess it was wrong the first time, huh?"

Pharmacist:

"Well, I suspected you wouldn't be talking normally to me on the telephone if your blood glucose was really 29 mg/dl. If it were really 29 mg/dl, you would probably be unconscious."

Sometimes patients will claim they feel a little shaky and self-treat this perceived hypoglycemia with a very large carbohydrate load (two pieces of pecan pie, just to be safe). The pharmacist should teach the patient to recognize both the autonomic and mild neuroglycopenic warning symptoms of hypoglycemia, advise the patient to check his or her blood glucose, and treat appropriately. Appropriate treatment consists of 15–20 grams of rapid-acting carbohydrate (fruit juice [1/3 cup cranberry, grape, or prune juice or ½ cup apple, pineapple, grapefruit, or orange juice provide 15 g carbohydrate], glucose tablets [5 grams per tablet], or 4 oz cola) if the patient is conscious. If the patient is unconscious or uncooperative, administer parenteral glucagon or intravenous glucose (dextrose 50%). Should a patient become unconscious due to hypoglycemia in the pharmacy or practice setting, ask the patient's companion (if present) if he or she is carrying a rapid-acting glucose product, such as glucose gel. If so, it should be administered immediately. Do not attempt to administer a solid or liquid glucose product to an unconscious patient. If a patient becomes uncooperative or unconscious, the pharmacist should call 911.

Infection

It is important the pharmacist be alert to any signs or symptoms suggestive of an infection in a patient with type 2 diabetes, because infection is a leading cause of HHNS. Common infections seen in patients with diabetes include cutaneous furunculosis and carbuncles, vulvovaginitis, cellulitis, and urinary tract infections. Suspected infections should be referred promptly to the patient's primary care provider. Repeat or relapsing vaginal yeast infections may be due to poor blood glucose control and should be evaluated.

Case Study

Let's return to Mrs. Gonzalez. Review her TPL; does she have complaints or problems that require triage? Are there any referrals to make?

After briefly discussing Mrs. Gonzalez's case with her physician, the plan is for the patient to begin with MNT. The pharmacist has provided some basic literature on meal planning in type 2 diabetes, but Mrs. Gonzalez would benefit most from an appointment with a dietitian. She agrees to this suggestion and is looking forward to meeting with the dietitian.

Dr. Thompson has approved Mrs. Gonzalez for beginning a walking program. She agrees to this as well and plans to join a group of ladies in her neighborhood who walk daily. Mrs. Gonzalez does not feel the need to talk to an exercise physiologist at this time. The pharmacist will educate the patient about precautions with exercise (e.g., footwear selection).

Mrs. Gonzalez wears glasses, and she saw her ophthalmologist about 2 years ago. The pharmacist suggests that she make an appointment to be seen within the next month or two, and Mrs. Gonzalez agrees. She recently had an appointment with her dentist. Because she is not complaining of any symptoms she does not need to be seen by a dentist again at this time. She has a follow-up appointment with Dr. Thompson in a month, at which time he will perform a comprehensive foot screening examination.

Mrs. Gonzalez needs to begin her education in type 2 diabetes, which she will do with Pharmacist Radcliffe. They set up a series of appointments, and the pharmacist provides some reading material for Mrs. Gonzalez.

At this time, Mrs. Gonzalez has no acute complications necessitating referral, such as HHNS, hypoglycemia, or an infection.

Practice Example

It's your turn to practice determining health care needs and the need for referral to other health care providers for a patient with type 2 diabetes. Turn to **Appendix B** and review the TPL for Mr. Jones. What are his health care needs and triage/referral needs at this time?

Some additional information that you will find useful came to light during Mr. Jones' conversation with Pharmacist O'Malley. Dr. Middleton had recommended a dietary plan several years ago when Mr. Jones was diagnosed with hypertension and recommended the diet again in 1997 when Mr. Jones was found to have hypercholesterolemia. Although

Dr. Middleton did not refer Mr. Jones to a dietitian at that time, he did provide some sample diet sheets to Mr. Jones. Even though Mr. Jones emphatically declared he would follow the diet because he did not want to begin medication therapy for his high cholesterol, he failed to follow the diet because he found it too restrictive. On discussion with the pharmacist, Mr. Jones agreed to talk to a dietitian, in an effort to modify his meal plan to both fit his lifestyle and meet his metabolic goals.

Mr. Jones walks half a mile each day to the racetrack. Dr. Middleton has encouraged Mr. Jones to increase his walking to a mile a day. Mr. Jones said he would think about it, but that he did not want to see an exercise physiologist.

Mr. Jones has never had any problems with his vision but has agreed to see an ophthalmologist within the next 2 months. Mr. Jones is morbidly afraid of the dentist and has not had a dental appointment in quite some time. He understands that he needs to be seen, and he claims that he shows good dental hygiene, but he wants to think about whether he's willing to see a dentist.

Health Care Needs

What health care needs did you identify? Mr. Jones has just been diagnosed with type 2 diabetes mellitus, and he has a history of hypertension and hypercholesterolemia. He has evidence of cardiovascular disease and nephropathy. Therefore, we list the following as health care needs:

- adequate control of type 2 diabetes
- adequate control of hypertension
- adequate control of hypercholesterolemia
- prevention or slowing of progression of long-term complications of diabetes
- slowing of progression of cardiovascular disease
- slowing of progression of nephropathy
- prevention or slowing of progression of long-term complications of hypertension and hypercholesterolemia

Mr. Jones has several modifiable risk factors for cardiovascular disease, such as not receiving an aspirin tablet daily, high cholesterol, a history of smoking, and use of alcohol. We can therefore add the following health care need:

- decrease modifiable cardiovascular risk factors

Mr. Jones is supposed to follow a recommended meal plan, but he is not adhering to it. He could also benefit from an enhanced exercise program. We can list these health care needs as follows:

- improve knowledge of diabetes medical nutrition therapy
- improve knowledge of exercise options

The following are additional health care needs:

- improve knowledge of drug therapy and monitoring
- ensure adherence to pharmacologic therapeutic interventions
- prevent adverse effects from drug therapy
- optimize therapy and reduce risk of drug-disease interactions
- avoid interactions of medications with other diseases
- initiate self-monitoring of blood glucose
- initiate peak flow monitoring

Because Mr. Jones is casual about keeping appointments with health care providers, we can add this health care need:

- promote adherence to follow-up medical appointments

Mr. Jones is missing several health maintenance interventions, such as an annual home fecal occult test and an annual rectal/prostate exam. Therefore, we can add one additional health care need:

- screen for and minimize the risk for developing significant comorbid conditions

Triage and Referral Needs

Because Mr. Jones agreed to speak with a dietitian in an effort to match his lifestyle with a suitable diet, the pharmacist will make a referral to a dietitian.

Since Dr. Middleton cleared Mr. Jones to expand his walking program, the pharmacist has encouraged the patient to walk home from the racetrack in addition to walking to the racetrack in the morning. This would increase his daily walk from half a mile to a whole mile.

Mr. Jones has agreed to make an appointment with his ophthalmologist for the near future, but he wants to think about seeing a dentist before making an appointment. The pharmacist makes a note to revisit this topic in the future.

Mr. Jones has a follow-up appointment with Dr. Middleton in 2 months, at which time he will perform a comprehensive foot screening examination.

Mr. Jones needs to begin his education in type 2 diabetes, which he will do with the pharmacist. They set up a series of appointments, and the pharmacist provides some reading material for Mr. Jones. The pharmacist stressed to Mr. Jones the importance of keeping follow-up appointments, and Mr. Jones agreed this education plan was reasonable.

At this time, the only acute need Mr. Jones has

that warrants referral is the fungal infection in the soft pad crease of his little toe. The pharmacist contacts Dr. Middleton, who agrees to a prescription for clotrimazole cream, with instructions to call the office if the infection does not clear within a week to 10 days.

Summary

A patient's health care needs are elements of care required to improve or prevent deterioration of health and well-being. Identification of a patient's health care needs ensure consideration of the patient's entire clinical picture. This is reinforced by the pharmacist's ability to appropriately triage complaints and health problems and refer to appropriate health care providers. These activities complete the circle of pharmaceutical care.

References

1. American Dietetic Association. Identifying patients at risk: ADA's definition for nutrition screening and nutrition assessment. *J Am Diet Assoc* 1994;94:838–9.
2. Tinker LF, Heins JM, Holler HJ. Commentary and translation: 1994 nutrition recommendations for diabetes. *J Am Diet Assoc* 1994;94:507–11.
3. Diabetes Control and Complications Trial Research Group. Expanded role of the dietitian in the Diabetes Control and Complications Trial: implications for clinical practice. *J Am Diet Assoc* 1993;93:758–67.
4. American Diabetes Association. Nutrition recommendations and principles for people with diabetes mellitus (position statement). *Diabetes Care* 1994;17:519–22.
5. American Dietetic Association. Scope of practice for qualified professionals in diabetes care and education. *J Am Diet Assoc* 1995;95:607–8.
6. Leontos C, Splett PL. Nutrition practice guidelines for type 1 diabetes mellitus: development and field testing. *Diabetes Spectrum* 1996;9:128–30.
7. Monk A, Barry B, McClain K, Weaver T, Cooper N, Franz MJ. Practice guidelines for medical nutrition therapy provided by dietitians for persons with non-insulin-dependent diabetes mellitus. *J Am Diet Assoc* 1995;95:999–1006.
8. Expert Panel on Detection, Evaluation, and Treatment of High Blood Cholesterol in Adults. Summary of the second report of the National Cholesterol Education Program (NCEP) expert panel on detection, evaluation, and treatment of high blood cholesterol in adults (Adult Treatment Panel II). *JAMA* 1993;269:3015–23.
9. American Diabetes Association. Nutrition recommendations and principles for people with diabetes mellitus. *Diabetes Care* 1999;22(*Suppl* 1):S42–5.
10. United States Department of Agriculture. The Food Guide Pyramid. http://www2.hqnet.usda.gov/cnpp/pyramid2.htm (accessed December 3, 1998).
11. American Diabetes Association. Diabetes mellitus and exercise. *Diabetes Care* 1999;22(*Suppl* 1):S49–54.
12. Schneider SH, Ruderman N. Use of exercise in the treatment of type 2 diabetes mellitus. *Clinical Diabetes* 1997;15:176–9.
13. American Diabetes Association. Foot care in patients with diabetes mellitus. *Diabetes Care* 1999;22(*Suppl* 1):S54–5.
14. Bates B. *A Guide to Physical Examination and History Taking.* 6th ed. Philadelphia, PA: JB Lippincott;1995.
15. American Diabetes Association. Diabetic retinopathy. *Diabetes Care* 1999;22(*Suppl* 1):S70–3.
16. Kelley DB, editor. *Medical Management of Type 2 Diabetes.* 4th ed. Alexandria, VA: American Diabetes Association; 1998. p.117–8.
17. Finney L, Finney MO, Gonzalez-Campoy JM. Tooth and consequences of diabetes. *Clinical Diabetes* 1997;15:243–4.
18. Kelley DB, editor. *Medical Management of Type 2 Diabetes.* 4th ed. Alexandria, VA: American Diabetes Association;1998. p.122–3.
19. Gonder-Frederick L, Cox DJ, Clarke WL. Helping patients understand and recognize hypoglycemia. *Clinical Diabetes* 1996;14:86–90.

Self-Study Questions

Objective

Define the health care needs of an ambulatory patient with type 2 diabetes.

1. Turn to the case of Ms. McLucas in **Appendix C**. Review her TPL to define her health care needs at this time.

Objective

Explain portions of the pharmacist's care plan for an ambulatory patient with type 2 diabetes that should be managed by health care professionals other than the pharmacist.

2. Explain why medical nutrition therapy should be managed by health care professionals other than a pharmacist.

3. Explain why a comprehensive ophthalmologic examination should be managed by health care professionals other than a pharmacist.

4. Explain why a foot ulcer should be managed by health care professionals other than a pharmacist.

Objective

Explain situations unique to the treatment of ambulatory patients with type 2 diabetes that require immediate attention.

5. Name and describe situations unique to treatment of ambulatory patients with type 2 diabetes that require immediate attention.

Self-Study Answers

1. Ms. McLucas has just been diagnosed with diabetes mellitus, and she has a history of hypertension and hypercholesterolemia. Therefore, we list the following as health care needs:

   - adequate control of type 2 diabetes
   - adequate control of hypertension
   - adequate control of hypercholesterolemia
   - prevention of long-term complications of diabetes
   - prevention of long-term complications of hypertension
   - prevention of long-term complications of hypercholesterolemia

   Ms. McLucas has several modifiable risk factors for cardiovascular disease: she is not receiving an aspirin tablet daily, she has high cholesterol, and she is postmenopausal but is not having hormone replacement therapy. Therefore, we can add another health care need:

   - decrease modifiable cardiovascular risk factors

   Ms. McLucas is supposed to be following a recommended meal plan, but she is only partially adherent to the plan. We can list these health care needs as follows:

   - improve knowledge of diabetes medical nutrition therapy
   - improve knowledge of exercise options
   - ensure adherence to nonpharmacologic therapeutic interventions

   We can also list these needs:

   - educate patient regarding drug therapy and monitoring
   - ensure adherence to pharmacologic therapeutic interventions

   - prevent adverse effects from drug therapy
   - optimize therapy and reduce risk of drug-disease interactions
   - avoid interactions of medications with other diseases
   - initiate self-monitoring of blood glucose

   Ms. McLucas is fairly reliable about health maintenance issues, but we can still list the following health care need:

   - screen for and minimize the risk for developing significant comorbid conditions

2. Dietitians (particularly RDs and CDEs) are specifically trained to assess patients' metabolic, nutritional, and lifestyle parameters; identify and negotiate nutrition goals; design interventions to achieve the individualized goals; and evaluate these outcomes.

3. Patients with diabetes need a dilated and comprehensive eye examination. Pharmacists are not equipped to do this, nor do pharmacists have the educational background to do so.

4. Management of a foot ulcer requires skills such as radiological examination, assessment of bacterial cultures and knowledge of antibiotic therapy, debridement, wound care, and evaluation of mechanical stress and circulation. These functions are best performed by a podiatrist, vascular surgeon, or primary care provider who possesses these skills.

5. Situations that require immediate attention and referral for patients with type 2 diabetes include suspected HHNS, hypoglycemia, and infections.

AMBULATORY PHARMACIST'S CARE PLAN

Patient Rose Gonzalez   Pharmacist Jane Radcliffe   Date 2/20/98

Page 1 of 2

DATE IDENTIFIED	PROBLEM (TPL)	PHARMACOTHERAPEUTIC AND RELATED HEALTH CARE GOAL	RECOMMENDATIONS FOR THERAPY	MONITORING PARAMETER(S)	DESIRED ENDPOINT(S)	MONITORING FREQUENCY
2/20/98	poor control of diabetes					
"	poor control of HTN					
"	poor control of cholest.					
"	not on daily ASA tx					
"	post menopausal s̄ HRT					
"	not receiving calcium tx					
"	Potential of HCTZ to affect DM & chol.					
"	no exercise plan					

AMBULATORY PHARMACIST'S CARE PLAN

Patient **Rose Gonzalez**   Pharmacist **Jane Radcliffe**   Date **2/20/98**

Page 2

DATE IDENTIFIED	PROBLEM (TPL)	PHARMACOTHERAPEUTIC AND RELATED HEALTH CARE GOAL	RECOMMENDATIONS FOR THERAPY	MONITORING PARAMETER(S)	DESIRED ENDPOINT(S)	MONITORING FREQUENCY
2/20/98	no MNT plan					
"	no home BG monitoring					
'	no home BP monitoring					
"	no home fecal test					
"	no influenza vaccine					
"	no monthly breast self-exam					

AMBULATORY PHARMACIST'S CARE PLAN

Patient George Jones   Pharmacist John O'Malley   Date 3-3-98

Page 1 of 3

DATE IDENTIFIED	PROBLEM (TPL)	PHARMACOTHERAPEUTIC AND RELATED HEALTH CARE GOAL	RECOMMENDATIONS FOR THERAPY	MONITORING PARAMETER(S)	DESIRED ENDPOINT(S)	MONITORING FREQUENCY
3/3/98	Sx and BG suggestive of DM. High risk status					
	poor control of hypertension					
	nonadherence to diet					
	h/o med schedule nonadherence					
	Furosemide may worsen lipids					
	smoking history					
	Alcohol use history					

AMBULATORY PHARMACIST'S CARE PLAN

Patient __George Jones__   Pharmacist __John O'Malley__   Date __3-3-98__

Page 2 of 3

DATE IDENTIFIED	PROBLEM (TPL)	PHARMACOTHERAPEUTIC AND RELATED HEALTH CARE GOAL	RECOMMENDATIONS FOR THERAPY	MONITORING PARAMETER(S)	DESIRED ENDPOINT(S)	MONITORING FREQUENCY
3/3/98	h/o non-adherence to flu appts					
	nonadherence to exercise					
	Not doing peak flow monitoring					
	No rectal/prostate exam					
	no home Fecal test					
4/3/98	poor control of diabetes					
	Furosemide may ↑ BG					
	Fungal skin infection on toe					

AMBULATORY PHARMACIST'S CARE PLAN

Patient ___George Jones___   Pharmacist ___John O'Malley___   Date ___3-3-98___

Page 3 of 3

DATE IDENTIFIED	PROBLEM (TPL)	PHARMACOTHERAPEUTIC AND RELATED HEALTH CARE GOAL	RECOMMENDATIONS FOR THERAPY	MONITORING PARAMETER(S)	DESIRED ENDPOINT(S)	MONITORING FREQUENCY
4/3	Insensate feet					
	Not on daily ASA tx					
	Poor control of cholesterol					
	Not doing SMBG					
	No dilated retinal exam					
	No recent dental exam					
	liver dysfunction					

Ambulatory Pharmacist's Care Plan

Patient __Sarah McLucas__   Pharmacist __Alexa Sheffield__   Date __4-23-98__

Page 1 of 2

DATE IDENTIFIED	PROBLEM (TPL)	PHARMACOTHERAPEUTIC AND RELATED HEALTH CARE GOAL	RECOMMENDATIONS FOR THERAPY	MONITORING PARAMETER(S)	DESIRED ENDPOINT(S)	MONITORING FREQUENCY
4/23/98	Poor control of diabetes					
"	Poor control of HTN					
"	Poor control of lipids					
"	Postmenopausal w/o HRT					
"	Not on ASA Qᴰ tx					
"	PPA in Tavist-D may worsen BP & BG					
"	Nonadherence to diet					
"	NSAID may ↑ BP					

AMBULATORY PHARMACIST'S CARE PLAN

Patient **Sarah McLucas**   Pharmacist **Alexa Sheffield**   Date **4-23-98**

Page 2 of 2

DATE IDENTIFIED	PROBLEM (TPL)	PHARMACOTHERAPEUTIC AND RELATED HEALTH CARE GOAL	RECOMMENDATIONS FOR THERAPY	MONITORING PARAMETER(S)	DESIRED ENDPOINT(S)	MONITORING FREQUENCY
4/23/98	Taking Tavist-D year-round					
"	Taking Naprosyn and ibuprofen					
"	Poor control of OA pain					
"	NSAID may ↑ Sxs of GERD					
"	Nonadherence to cholestyramine					
"	No SMBG					
"	No exercise plan					

Identifying Pharmacotherapeutic and Related Health Care Goals for Patients with Type 2 Diabetes

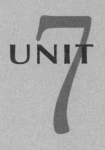

UNIT 7

You have completed the first phase in designing a pharmacist's care plan for an ambulatory patient with type 2 diabetes: identifying a patient's therapy problem list and health care needs. As discussed in unit 5, the goal of pharmaceutical care is to improve a patient's quality of life through achievement of definite therapeutic outcomes. These outcomes are defined as pharmacotherapeutic and related health care goals. Identifying pharmacotherapeutic and related health care goals that address the problems defined in the problem list is the next phase in designing your pharmacist's care plan.

Unit Objectives

After you successfully complete this unit, you will be able to:

- explain factors unique to patients with type 2 diabetes that may influence identifying pharmacotherapeutic and related health care goals, including:
  - disease characteristics of type 2 diabetes,
  - goals established by other health care professionals for ambulatory patients with type 2 diabetes,
  - therapy problems of ambulatory patients with type 2 diabetes, and
  - nondisease factors of ambulatory patients with type 2 diabetes;
- explain the role of patients with type 2 diabetes in determining their therapeutic goals;
- explain the use of guidelines in the specification of pharmacotherapeutic and related health care goals for patients with type 2 diabetes;
- explain realistic limits of treatment outcomes for patients with type 2 diabetes in the ambulatory care setting; and
- specify pharmacotherapeutic and related health care goals for a patient with type 2 diabetes that integrate patient data, disease- and medication-specific information, and ethical and quality-of-life considerations.

Unit Organization

This unit begins with a brief discussion of issues that influence the establishment of pharmacotherapeutic and related health care goals for ambulatory patients

with type 2 diabetes. You will gain appreciation for the role that patients with type 2 diabetes play in determining therapeutic goals for their disease management. After a brief review of findings from recent diabetes outcomes studies, you will be able to justify the use of guidelines in the identification of pharmacotherapeutic and related health care goals for an ambulatory patient with type 2 diabetes. At the conclusion of this unit, you will practice identifying pharmacotherapeutic and related health care goals for patients with type 2 diabetes.

Considerations When Identifying Pharmacotherapeutic and Related Health Care Goals

In identifying pharmacotherapeutic and related health care goals for patients with type 2 diabetes, there are several factors you must consider, including the nature of diabetes itself, health care goals established by other health care providers, patient wishes and concerns, and realistic goals for type 2 diabetes management. Optimally, the pharmacist should work collaboratively with the patient as well as other health care providers to establish goals.

Disease Characteristics of Type 2 Diabetes

When you identify pharmacotherapeutic and related health care goals for treating a disease, you must understand both the normal physiology of the system involved and the pathophysiology of the disease. This understanding is an important consideration in setting pharmacotherapeutic and related health care goals for an ambulatory patient with type 2 diabetes, because the patient's disease characteristics dictate the drug and nondrug therapy regimen and monitoring plan. The goal of treatment is to return the patient to as near to normal physiology as possible. By understanding where the patient is and where you would like him or her to be, the pharmacotherapeutic and related health care goals for a patient with a particular disease become clear. Similarly, in drug therapy selection, knowledge of the pathophysiology of diabetes (e.g., insulin resistance vs. decreased insulin secretion) will lead you to select the most appropriate drug to treat the patient's specific pathophysiology and return the patient to as near normal physiology as possible. By adopting this thought process, this module will never be out of date, even as new drugs for diabetes become available.

Let's consider Mrs. Gonzalez. In her case, type 2 diabetes, hypertension, and hypercholesterolemia and their related complications are the disease characteristics with the greatest effect on Mrs. Gonzalez's pharmacotherapeutic and related health care goals. When assessing the goals for disease control, you must consider these questions:

- Is this disease acute or chronic?
- Are there complications of the disease present?
- Is the disease or its complications amenable to nondrug therapy alone or is drug therapy required?
- What previous therapies has the patient received and were they successful?

Each of Mrs. Gonzalez's conditions are chronic and require therapy to be adequately controlled. For treatment of her type 2 diabetes, nondrug therapy alone may be effective; for treatment of hypertension and hypercholesterolemia, nondrug therapy and drug therapy are required. When establishing goals, it is important to remember that goals for one disease can influence goals for another disease. For example, improving control of Mrs. Gonzalez's blood glucose by weight loss and exercise will also improve her hypertension and hypercholesterolemia.

Health Care Goals Established by Other Health Care Professionals

As a pharmacist, you are a member of a health care team. As discussed in unit 6, you should practice in an *inter*disciplinary rather than *multi*disciplinary fashion. You may not always agree with the approach or plan of action developed by another health care provider, but you can probably develop a plan that will satisfy the team and provide optimal patient care. You should consult the pharmacist's patient database to determine if other health care professionals have goals that will influence yours. You will need to consider these goals when setting pharmacotherapeutic and related health care goals for a patient; if you do not, your plan will most likely fail.

Similarly, as other health care providers set goals for patients, your plan can reinforce these goals. If a patient has proliferative retinopathy and the ophthalmologist suggests follow-up appoint-

ments every 3 months, you can reinforce his or her health care goals by encouraging the patient to keep these appointments.

Therapy Problems

Once you have identified a patient's therapy problems using the Therapy Problem List (TPL) column of the Ambulatory Pharmacist's Care Plan (APCP) you can use this information to set the pharmacotherapeutic and related health care goals. The purpose of establishing patient goals is to ensure that each therapy problem is solved, or at least addressed. When we determine goals for Mrs. Gonzalez and Mr. Jones later in this unit, you will notice that many of their therapy problems are related to their chronic conditions: diabetes, hypertension, and hyperlipidemia.

Nondisease Factors

Many nondisease factors influence pharmacotherapeutic and related health care goals. These may or may not be patient specific. If the patient is elderly or has impaired renal or hepatic function, the pharmacokinetics of drugs may be altered, which may require dosage adjustments or selection of different agents. As discussed in unit 13 of the *Ambulatory Care Clinical Skills Program: Core Module*, other influencing variables may include drug allergies, financial implications, health beliefs, and quality of life and ethical considerations. We will consider health beliefs and readiness to learn in the next section of this unit.

The Role of Patients with Type 2 Diabetes in Determining Their Goals

Patients must have an active part in determining the goals set for them. As a foundation for this active role, patients must understand their diabetes and associated conditions. For example, if a patient does not perceive the seriousness of hypertension because of its asymptomatic presentation, he or she is less likely to adhere to lifestyle modifications that are a nuisance or impair quality of life. Threats and scare tactics are unlikely to persuade an adult to change his or her behavior. The pharmacist's responsibilities in providing this education are described in unit 8.

According to the Health Belief Model, a person's behavior reflects his or her subjective interpretation of a situation.[1] A patient's behavior is influenced by four perceptions:

- How susceptible he or she feels to the negative consequences of the illness
- How the patient perceives the severity of diabetes and its complications
- How the patient perceives the benefits of self-care of diabetes
- How the patient perceives costs of self-care (financial and personal costs)[2]

The patient's health beliefs may be assessed by having him or her respond to a series of questions, indicating agreement or disagreement. Statements used to evaluate the patient's beliefs regarding benefit, cost, severity, and susceptibility of diabetes are shown in **Table 1**.[2] If the patient does not believe that type 2 diabetes is a serious disorder to which he or she is susceptible and that the benefits of self-managing the disease outweigh the costs, the patient will require special attention in diabetes education.

Another valuable assessment in ambulatory patients with type 2 diabetes is determination of their readiness to learn. This is best accomplished by applying the transtheoretical, or stages of change, model.[3] This model consists of five stages: precontemplation, contemplation, preparation, action, and maintenance. The five stages are defined as follows:

- *Precontemplation*—the stage at which there is no intention to change behavior in the foreseeable future.
- *Contemplation*—the stage at which people are aware that a problem exists and are seriously thinking about changing their behavior in the next 6 months.
- *Preparation*—a stage that combines intention and behavioral criteria; people at this stage intend to take action (change behavior) in the next month.
- *Action*—the stage at which people modify their behavior for a period of time from 1 day up to 6 months.
- *Maintenance*—the stage at which people work to prevent relapse; the behavior change in this stage has been consistently maintained for at least 6 months.[3]

You can determine which stage a patient is at for any given behavior (e.g., medication regimen adherence, self-monitoring of blood glucose, or dietary adherence) by presenting the patient with possible responses for that behavior. For example, this question:

Table 1. Statements for Assessing Health Beliefs of Patients with Diabetes

Benefit

- I'll be healthier in later life if I control my diabetes.
- I believe that exercise can help me control my diabetes.
- Controlling my blood sugar will help me avoid heart disease.
- Changing my eating habits would help me control my diabetes.
- Even if I took my medicine as I should, I wouldn't be able to control my diabetes.
- I can control my diabetes if I follow my regimen closely.

Cost

- It will take a lot of effort to control my diabetes.
- I would have to change too many habits to use a meal plan.
- Taking my medication interferes with my daily activities.
- I'm always hungry when I stick to my meal plan.
- It takes a lot of effort to exercise.

Severity

- Diabetes is a serious disease if you don't control it.

Susceptibility

- My diabetes would be worse day-to-day if I did nothing about it.
- I'm more likely to have eye problems if my diabetes control is poor.
- If my diabetes isn't controlled, I'm likely to die sooner.

Source: reprinted with permission from reference 2.

"Do you always follow your exercise plan in the way you were instructed?"

The following are possible responses:

- Yes, I have been for more than 6 months (maintenance).

- Yes, I have been for less than 6 months (action).
- No, but I plan to in the next month (preparation).
- No, but I plan to in the next 6 months (contemplation).
- No, and I do not intend to in the next 6 months (precontemplation).

Intervention strategies for each behavior are geared to the level the patient is currently at or their readiness to change. In unit 8 we will discuss guidelines for applying these stages and processes of change to type 2 diabetes care.

Use of Research-Based Guidelines in Specifying Goals

As we determine pharmacotherapeutic and related health care goals, it is helpful to determine if guidelines exist to assist us. Measures of achieving pharmacotherapeutic and related health care goals are often referred to as *outcomes*. There are three types of outcomes measures we can assess in caring for ambulatory patients with type 2 diabetes: process measures, medical events, and physiological (or metabolic) measures.[4]

Process measures assess adherence to standards of care. For example, did the patient have an annual dilated retinal exam, or an annual comprehensive foot exam? While this information is important, it is difficult to correlate directly to health outcomes.

Recording medical events such as hospitalizations, myocardial infarctions, strokes, amputations,

and cases of blindness yield valuable information. However, these outcomes take years to track.

Metabolic (or physiologic) measures, such as hemoglobin A_{1c}, blood glucose values, lipid values, and blood pressure readings can be obtained easily, are relatively inexpensive, and are linked to definitive health care outcomes. For these reasons, the American Diabetes Association has established normal, goal, and action points for markers of glycemic control, lipid values, and blood pressure, shown in **Table 2**.[5] What evidence do we have that a goal of tight metabolic control, particularly glycemic control, makes a difference in patient outcomes? Guidelines, such as those cited above, are developed as a result of research findings that assess significant, pertinent outcomes such as life or death, the development of diabetes-related complications, and overall patient well-being.

The first large study to evaluate the impact of tight glycemic control in patients with type 1 diabetes was the Diabetes Control and Complications Trial (DCCT), conducted from 1983 to 1993.[6] A total of 1,441 patients with type 1 diabetes were enrolled; half had no complications of diabetes at baseline, and the other half had early microvascular and neurologic complications of diabetes. Within each group (with and without complications), half of the patients continued to receive conventional diabetes therapy (one or two insulin injections per day), while the other half received intensive insulin therapy (three or more insulin injections per day or treatment with an insulin pump) and medical follow-up and monitoring. The goal of intensive treatment was to achieve blood glucose values as close to normal values as possible. During a mean of 6.5 years of follow-up, patients in the intensive

Table 2. Recommendations for Metabolic Control in Nonpregnant Adult Patients with Diabetes[5]

Biochemical Index	Goal	Action Suggested
Average preprandial glucose (mg/dl)	80–120	<80 or >140
Average bedtime glucose (mg/dl)	100–140	<100 or >160
HbA_{1c} (%)	<7%	>8%
Systolic blood pressure (mmHg)	<85	N/A
Diastolic blood pressure (mmHg)	<130	N/A
Total cholesterol (mg/dl)	<200	N/A
LDL cholesterol (mg/dl)	<100	N/A
HDL cholesterol (mg/dl)	>45	N/A
Triglycerides (mg/dl)	<200	N/A

groups achieved a significantly lower median hemoglobin A_{1c} and developed microvascular and neuropathic complications at a significantly lower rate than those in the conventional treatment groups; patients with complications who received intensive therapy had significantly slower progression of their complications. The risk reductions ranged from 35% to >70%.

This is very useful information, but can we directly extrapolate these results to patients with type 2 diabetes? The answer to the effect of tighter blood glucose control in type 2 diabetes came in 1998, when the results of the United Kingdom Prospective Diabetes Study (UKPDS) were released.[7–10] The UKPDS was a very complex study conducted over a 20-year period (1977–1997) that actually consisted of several studies within one. The primary objectives were to determine:

- if lowering the blood glucose to the normal range with any one of several diabetes medications would reduce the likelihood of diabetes-specific complications and the macrovascular events that are the major cause of mortality and severe morbidity in type 2 diabetes,
- whether there is an advantage or disadvantage to any of the diabetes medications used in the study (e.g., do the oral sulfonylurea agents increase cardiovascular mortality, or is insulin atherogenic?), and finally,
- does tight blood pressure control have any benefit on microvascular or cardiovascular outcomes?

The design for this randomized, controlled trial was very complex; patients were initially assigned to either conventional treatment with diet or intensive treatment with either one of three oral sulfonylurea agents or insulin. Patients in the conventional treatment group could progress to drug treatment if needed, and patients started on one of the study medications could have additional agents added if needed. This study design resulted in significant therapeutic overlap between comparison groups. Three aggregate endpoints were used to assess differences between conventional and intensive therapy: any diabetes-related endpoint, diabetes-related death, and all-cause mortality (i.e., death from any cause).

The results of this portion of the trial showed that the hemoglobin A_{1c} was improved in the intensive treatment group (7.0%) over the conventional treatment group (7.9%). There was no difference in hemoglobin A_{1c} between the agents used in the intensive group. Results showed the following:

- Compared to the conventional group, the risk in the intensive group was 12% lower for any diabetes-related endpoint (sudden death, death from hyperglycemia or hypoglycemia, fatal or nonfatal myocardial infarction, angina, heart failure, stroke, renal failure, amputation [of at least one digit], vitreous hemorrhage, retinopathy requiring photocoagulation, blindness in one eye, or cataract extraction). This result was due largely to a 25% risk reduction in microvascular endpoints, including the need for retinal photocoagulation.
- The risk of diabetes-related death (death from myocardial infarction, stroke, peripheral vascular disease, renal disease, hyperglycemia or hypoglycemia, or sudden death) was 10% lower in the intensive group.
- The incidence of all-cause mortality was 6% lower in the intensive group.

The authors concluded that intensive blood glucose control by either the sulfonylurea agents or insulin decreased the risk of microvascular complications but not macrovascular disease in patients with type 2 diabetes. None of the drugs used (chlorpropamide, glibenclamide [glyburide], or insulin) had an adverse effect on cardiovascular outcomes. However, all intensive treatments increased the risk of hypoglycemia and caused weight gain.[7]

The UKPDS also investigated the use of metformin.[8] The goal of this portion of the study was to determine if the use of metformin to achieve tight glycemic control has any advantages or disadvantages. A cohort of 1704 overweight patients (overweight defined as 120% of ideal body weight) were randomized to receive either conventional diet therapy (411 patients), intensive therapy with metformin (342 patients), or intensive therapy with an alternate pharmacologic agent (951 patients). A comparison of the 753 patients assigned to intensive metformin therapy or conventional diet therapy showed a median hemoglobin A_{1c} of 7.4% in the metformin group vs. 8.0% in the conventional group during the 10-year follow-up. Using the same definitions for endpoints described in the DCCT, patients treated with metformin had risk reductions of 32% for any diabetes-related endpoint, 42% for diabetes-related death, and 36% for all-cause mortality. All outcomes achieved statistical significance. A secondary analysis comparing the patients receiving intensive treatment with metformin to overweight patients receiving intensive therapy with oral sulfonylurea agents or insulin showed that the effect of metformin on these endpoints was greater than that achieved by the oral sulfonylurea agents or insulin.

A more troubling analysis is the result from a supplementary study of patients treated with maximum doses of a sulfonylurea who had metformin added to their regimen. This group showed a 96% increased risk of diabetes-related death and a 60% increase in all-cause deaths when compared to patients who continued on present treatment with the sulfonylurea. These outcomes were statistically significant. The authors hypothesized that this finding could be due to chance and performed a meta-analysis of all combined data, showing that the addition of metformin had a comparable effect to that seen with intensive therapy with sulfonylurea or insulin, with a net reduction of 19% in any diabetes-related endpoint.

Another part of the UKPDS evaluated whether tight control of blood pressure (blood pressure <150/85 mmHg) prevented macrovascular and microvascular complications in patients with type 2 diabetes as compared to patients with type 2 diabetes with less tight blood pressure control (blood pressure <180/105 mmHg).[9] Patients in the tight blood pressure control group were treated with either captopril or atenolol as first agents, although 29% of patients required three or more hypotensive agents to control their blood pressure. The use of captopril or atenolol was avoided, if possible, in the group maintaining less tight control. Patients in the tight blood pressure control group achieved an average blood pressure of 144/82 mmHg vs. 154/87 mmHg in the conventional arm. Patients in the tight control group had a risk reduction of 24% in diabetes-related endpoints, 32% decrease in diabetes-related deaths, 44% decrease in strokes, 56% decrease in heart failure, and 37% reduction in microvascular endpoints (largely because of a reduced risk of retinal photocoagulation). As you recall, patients in the major UKPDS blood glucose control group showed a 12% decreased risk of diabetes-related endpoints and a 25% decrease in microvascular disease. Patients in the blood pressure intensive group also had a 34–47% reduced risk of retinopathy progression.

Conclusions from an analysis of the patients started on atenolol vs. captopril as initial therapy showed that both agents were similarly effective in reducing diabetic complications. Neither drug was shown to have any specific beneficial or deleterious effect; however, patients receiving atenolol gained more weight (3.4 kg) than patients receiving captopril (1.6 kg), which suggests that the blood pressure reduction in itself may be more important than the treatment used.[10]

While the UKPDS raises as many questions as it answers, the results of the study generally support the concept that improved metabolic control positively affects outcomes in patients with type 2 diabetes. Tight blood glucose control reduces the risk of microvascular complications; results were inconclusive concerning effect on cardiovascular outcomes, although the lack of adverse cardiovascular outcomes related to treatments is positive. Tight blood pressure control is as important, possibly more so, than tight blood glucose control. Ultimately, a goal of strict metabolic and blood pressure control along with early treatment should give significantly improved outcomes in patients with type 2 diabetes.

The efficacy of metformin compared with other monotherapeutic agents in obese patients is striking. The findings associated with adding metformin to the medication therapy of a patient already receiving an oral sulfonylurea are of concern, but may be a consequence of the investigator's analytical strategy. While this area requires additional study, the use of metformin in combination with an oral sulfonylurea agent should not be precluded in appropriate patients unless we have more convincing evidence to the contrary.

The UKPDS and the DCCT study evaluated the achievement of "hard" outcomes: life or death, occurrence rates of complications, and surrogate markers such as hemoglobin A_{1c} and blood pressure. What about the economic benefits and quality of life associated with improved glycemic control? These shorter-term benefits have been recently documented in a major clinical trial evaluating 569 patients with type 2 diabetes.[11] Patients were randomized to receive either diet and placebo or diet and glipizide therapy. Outcomes that were followed included change from baseline in glucose and hemoglobin A_{1c} levels, symptom distress, quality of life, and economic indicators.

After 12 weeks, the mean hemoglobin A_{1c} and fasting blood glucose levels were statistically different in the intervention group (7.5% and 126 mg/dl, respectively) from those achieved in the placebo group (9.3% and 168 mg/dl, respectively). Quality of life differences for symptom distress, general perceived health, cognitive functioning, and the overall visual analog scale were significantly more favorable in the glipizide group. Favorable economic outcomes were reported in the glipizide group, including higher retained employment, productive capacity, less absenteeism, fewer bed days, and fewer restricted-activity days. The authors concluded that improved glycemic control in type 2 diabetes is associated with substantial short-term symptomatic, quality of life, and economic benefits.[11]

In summary, we are practicing in an era of evidence-based medicine. In using established guidelines (such as those provided by the American Diabetes Association) to establish pharmacotherapeutic and health care goals, it is important for you to be familiar with the evidence supporting these recommendations. Knowing the research supporting these guidelines will make you a more creditable member of the health care team and make your therapeutic recommendations more likely to be accepted. For an in-depth review of these studies, please see references 6–11.

Realistic Limits of Treatment Outcomes for Patients with Type 2 Diabetes

As discussed in unit 13 of the *Ambulatory Care Clinical Skills Program: Core Module*, the ambulatory care setting is different from the acute care setting. You will have less access to all the health care professionals involved or to all the information you would like to have. In addition, you cannot cure type 2 diabetes; it is a chronic disease that at best can only be controlled. Finally, ambulatory care practice settings vary in the amount of monitoring that is feasible. Some practices are structured to allow more physical assessment and have equipment to do laboratory testing. In other practice settings assessment and testing are less feasible, requiring the pharmacist to obtain this data from other sources.

Another consideration in establishing realistic goals for treatment outcomes for ambulatory patients with type 2 diabetes are the financial and personal costs associated with meeting guidelines and suggested goals for diabetes management. While we have reviewed the evidence supporting tight blood glucose and blood pressure control, you must create a balance sheet for each individual patient to assess the cost of attaining these goals. For example, on the positive side you can list an improved chance of preventing complications related to type 2 diabetes, improved life expectancy, and improved quality of life. On the negative side you can list the

inconvenience of treatment and monitoring, more frequent visits with health care providers resulting in higher occupational absences, higher out-of-pocket costs, and possible adverse effects of drug therapy. Pharmacotherapeutic and related health care goals must be individualized for patients.

Case Study

Let us return to the case of Mrs. Gonzalez and develop her pharmacotherapeutic and related health care goals. Her APCP is found in **Appendix A**. Her first three problems are poor control of type 2 diabetes, hypertension, and hypercholesterolemia. The corresponding pharmacotherapeutic and related health care goals are to improve control of these conditions as well as prevent complications associated with these chronic diseases. As the care plan continues to develop, you will see how the pharmacist will make recommendations for therapy for each of these problems, identify monitoring parameters to ensure the goal is met, and specify desired endpoints. As research discussed in this unit has shown, achievement of target glycemic and blood pressure goals delays or prevents the complications of type 2 diabetes.

The next identified therapy problem is that Mrs. Gonzalez is postmenopausal, but is not receiving hormone replacement therapy. Because Mrs. Gonzalez has not vocalized any specific complaints at this time (e.g., hot flashes or vaginal dryness), the pharmacist has identified a goal of reducing the risk of postmenopausal symptoms. Another and probably more important aspect of hormone replacement therapy in this patient is the cardiovascular protection it affords, which is even more important since she was diagnosed with type 2 diabetes.

Another important intervention to reduce Mrs. Gonzalez's risk of cardiovascular complications is the initiation of daily aspirin therapy. The goal is accordingly listed.

Pharmacist Radcliffe also identified a potential drug-induced complication, hydrochlorothiazide-induced hyperglycemia and hypercholesterolemia. The goal is to avoid worsened blood glucose and lipid control.

Mrs. Gonzalez is not presently following an exercise or diet plan, so the pharmacist has developed goals for starting and adhering to each. Although Mrs. Gonzalez's calcium intake may increase because of her dietary changes, she still requires supplemental calcium. The goal for this therapy problem is to reduce her risk for developing osteoporosis.

Mrs. Gonzalez also needs to learn two new skills: self-monitoring her blood glucose and blood pressure monitoring. The pharmacist has noted the goal for her to learn and regularly perform these procedures.

The last three problems and related goals pertain to Mrs. Gonzalez's health maintenance. The pharmacist has recorded the need to perform annual home fecal occult blood testing, receipt of an annual influenza vaccine, and monthly breast self-examinations.

Review **Appendix A** to see how these goals were recorded on the APCP for Mrs. Gonzalez.

Practice Example

It's your turn to practice developing pharmacotherapeutic and related health care goals for an ambulatory patient with type 2 diabetes. Turn to the APCP for Mr. Jones that is completed through the therapy problem list (**Appendix B**). Using this form, complete the column for pharmacotherapeutic and related health care goals. When you are finished, refer to the APCP for Mr. Jones in **Appendix C**. Compare your plan to the completed one; if you have any deficiencies you may want to review this unit or the corresponding units in the *Ambulatory Care Clinical Skills Program: Core Module*.

Summary

The third phase of a pharmacist's care plan is to establish pharmacotherapeutic and related health care goals. You must set goals to address identified problems and to meet each health care need. To determine these goals, you must integrate various influences: disease characteristics, goals of other health care professionals, therapy problems, nondisease factors, patient preferences, and inherent limits in the ambulatory care setting.

References

1. Becker MH, Janz NK. The health belief model applied to understanding diabetes regimen compliance. *Diabetes Educ* 1985;11(1):41–7.
2. Rubin RR. Psychosocial Assessment. In: Funnell MM, Hunt C, Kulkarni K, Rubin RR, Yarborough PC, editors. *A Core Curriculum for Diabetes Educators*, 3rd ed. Chicago, IL: American Association of Diabetes Educators; 1998. p. 89–91.
3. Prochaska JO, DiClemente CC, Norcross JC. In search of how people change: applications to addictive behavior. *Diabetes Spectrum* 1993;6(1):25–33.
4. Riddle MC. A_{1c} is our best outcome measures: let's use it. *Clinical Diabetes* 1996; 14:79–82.
5. American Diabetes Association. Standards of medical care for patients with diabetes mellitus. *Diabetes Care* 1999;22(*Suppl* 1):S32–41.
6. The Diabetes Control and Complications Trial Research Group. The effect of intensive treatment of diabetes on the development and progression of long-term complications in insulin-dependent diabetes mellitus. *N Engl J Med* 1993; 329:977–86.
7. UK Prospective Diabetes Study (UKPDS) Group. Intensive blood-glucose control with sulphonylureas or insulin compared with conventional treatment and risk of complications in patients with type 2 diabetes (UKPDS 33). *Lancet* 1998; 352:837–53.
8. UK Prospective Diabetes Study (UKPDS) Group. Effect of intensive blood-glucose control with metformin on complications in overweight patients with type 2 diabetes (UKPDS 34). *Lancet* 1998; 352:854–65.
9. UK Prospective Diabetes Study Group. Tight blood pressure control and risk of macrovascular and microvascular complications in type 2 diabetes: UKPDS 38. *Br Med J* 1998; 317:703–13.
10. UK Prospective Diabetes Study Group. Efficacy of atenolol and captopril in reducing risk of macrovascular and microvascular complications in type 2 diabetes: UKPDS 39. *Br Med J* 1998; 317:713–20.
11. Testa MA, Simonson DC. Health economic benefits and quality of life during improved glycemic control in patients with type 2 diabetes mellitus. *JAMA* 1998; 280:1490–6.

Self-Study Questions

Objective

Explain factors unique to ambulatory patients with type 2 diabetes that may influence identifying pharmacotherapeutic and related health care goals, including:

- *disease characteristics of type 2 diabetes*
- *goals established by other health care professionals for ambulatory patients with type 2 diabetes*
- *therapy problems of ambulatory patients with type 2 diabetes*
- *nondisease factors of ambulatory patients with type 2 diabetes*

1. Explain why disease characteristics of type 2 diabetes need to be considered when establishing pharmacotherapeutic and related health care goals for an ambulatory patient with type 2 diabetes.

2. Explain why goals established by other health care professionals caring for the patient need to be considered when establishing pharmacotherapeutic and related health care goals for an ambulatory patient with type 2 diabetes.

3. Explain why the patient's quality of life needs to be considered when making decisions on pharmacotherapeutic and related health care goals for an ambulatory patient with type 2 diabetes.

Objective

Explain the role of patients with type 2 diabetes in determining their therapeutic goals.

4. Explain the role of an ambulatory patient with type 2 diabetes in determining his or her therapeutic goals.

5. Explain why an ambulatory patient with type 2 diabetes should have a role in determining his or her therapy goals.

6. Explain why the patient's health beliefs are important in determining the therapy goals.

Objective

Explain the use of guidelines in the specification of pharmacotherapeutic and related health care goals for ambulatory patients with type 2 diabetes.

7. Explain the use of recommended guidelines in the specification of pharmacotherapeutic and related health care goals for an ambulatory patient with type 2 diabetes.

8. Explain the importance of guidelines for glycemic control in the specification of pharmacotherapeutic and related health care goals for an ambulatory patient with type 2 diabetes.

9. Explain the importance of guidelines for blood pressure control in the specification of pharmacotherapeutic and related health care goals for an ambulatory patient with type 2 diabetes.

Objective

Explain realistic limits of treatment outcomes for ambulatory patients with type 2 diabetes in the ambulatory care setting.

10. Explain the realistic limits of treatment outcomes for an ambulatory patient with type 2 diabetes.

11. Explain why the chronic nature of type 2 diabetes is a factor in identifying realistic treatment outcomes for an ambulatory patient with type 2 diabetes.

12. Explain why the ambulatory care practice setting may be a factor in identifying realistic treatment outcomes when caring for an ambulatory patient with type 2 diabetes.

Objective

Specify pharmacotherapeutic and related health care goals for a patient with type 2 diabetes that integrate patient-specific data, disease- and medication-specific information, and ethical and quality-of-life considerations.

13. Identify appropriate pharmacotherapeutic and related health care goals for Ms. McLucas and record these goals on the pharmacist's care plan in **Appendix D**.

Self-Study Answers

1. An understanding of the pathophysiology of type 2 diabetes will help the pharmacist to establish appropriate pharmacotherapeutic and related health care goals and select the most appropriate drug therapy. Understanding the chronic nature of diabetes and the probability of complication development also assists in establishing goals and selecting nondrug and drug therapy options.

2. You must consider the goals established by other health care professionals caring for the patient so you can reinforce their goals and develop a plan that will satisfy the entire team and benefit the patient.

3. The patient's quality of life is an important consideration when setting pharmacotherapeutic and related health care goals. If the lifestyle modifications required to reach the goal impair the patient's quality of life, the patient is less likely to adhere to the plan. The goal of pharmaceutical care is to achieve the best therapeutic outcomes while improving the patient's quality of life.

4. The patient should have an active role in determining the goals of therapy. To achieve this active role, the patient must be knowledgeable about type 2 diabetes and his or her other diseases.

5. If a patient with type 2 diabetes is not involved in establishing goals to manage his or her disease, he or she may not comply with treatments consistent with those goals. You must assess both the patient's health beliefs regarding type 2 diabetes as well as the patient's readiness to learn.

6. Patients who feel they are susceptible to the negative consequences of type 2 diabetes, that these consequences can be severe, and that the benefits of self-care outweigh the financial and personal costs of self-care are more likely to adhere to treatments used to meet the established goals.

7. Recommended guidelines based on results of clinical trials can be useful in determining pharmacotherapeutic and related health care goals for an ambulatory patient with type 2 diabetes because the guidelines set goals that have proven successful in achieving positive therapeutic outcomes.

8. Clinical trials have demonstrated the potential benefits of improved blood glucose control in preventing the development or progression of complications associated with type 2 diabetes. If the pharmacist sets pharmacotherapeutic and related health care goals based on the guidelines developed subsequent to these clinical trials, it would seem reasonable that the patient would also enjoy these beneficial outcomes.

9. Clinical trials have demonstrated the potential benefits of tight blood pressure control in preventing the development or progression of complications associated with type 2 diabetes. If the pharmacist sets pharmacotherapeutic and related health care goals based on the guidelines developed subsequent to these clinical trials, it would seem reasonable that the patient would also enjoy these beneficial outcomes.

10. Realistic limits of treatment outcomes for an ambulatory patient with type 2 diabetes include the inability to cure type 2 diabetes through currently available treatments, an incomplete database, less access to other involved health care professionals, practice site limitations, and the costs involved in achieving near-euglycemia.

11. Diabetes is a chronic disease. Therefore, the goal of therapy is limited to controlling the disease and preventing the development or progression of associated complications. In addition, the chronic nature of type 2 diabetes requires that the majority of the care be provided on an outpatient visit. Generally, the outpatient pharmacist will have less information than colleagues in acute-care practice and less access to other health care professionals involved in the patient's care, because of different locations.

12. The ambulatory care setting where the pharmacist practices may not be equipped to perform physical assessment or have the appropriate equipment to obtain laboratory data. The pharmacist may need to rely on other health care professionals for this information.

13. Refer to the APCP for Ms. McLucas in **Appendix E**. If there are discrepancies between the health care goals you listed and those given by the author, you may want to review this unit or the corresponding units in the *Ambulatory Care Clinical Skills Program: Core Module*.

AMBULATORY PHARMACIST'S CARE PLAN

Patient Rose Gonzalez   Pharmacist Jane Radcliffe   Date 2/20/98

Page 1 of 2

DATE IDENTIFIED	PROBLEM (TPL)	PHARMACOTHERAPEUTIC AND RELATED HEALTH CARE GOAL	RECOMMENDATIONS FOR THERAPY	MONITORING PARAMETER(S)	DESIRED ENDPOINT(S)	MONITORING FREQUENCY
2/20/98	poor control of diabetes	Improve diabetes control; prevent complications.				
=	poor control of HTN	Improve BP control; prevent complications.				
=	poor control of cholest.	Improve lipid control; prevent complications.				
=	Not on daily ASA tx	↓ risk CV complic. of diabetes				
=	post menopausal s̄ HRT	↓ risk post-men. Sxs/↓risks of postmenopause				
=	Not receiving calcium tx	↓ risk for osteoporosis				
=	Potential of HCTZ to affect DM & chol.	Avoid worsened BG & lipid control				
=	no exercise plan	start & adhere to regular exercise program.				

AMBULATORY PHARMACIST'S CARE PLAN

Patient __Rose Gonzalez__   Pharmacist __Jane Radcliffe__   Date __2/20/98__

Page 2 of 2

DATE IDENTIFIED	PROBLEM (TPL)	PHARMACOTHERAPEUTIC AND RELATED HEALTH CARE GOAL	RECOMMENDATIONS FOR THERAPY	MONITORING PARAMETER(S)	DESIRED ENDPOINT(S)	MONITORING FREQUENCY
2/20/98	no MNT plan	start & adhere to MNT plan.				
"	no home BG monitoring	learn & regularly perform SMBG				
"	no home BP monitoring	learn & regularly perform BP measurements				
"	no home fecal test	perform annual home fecal blood test				
"	no influenza vaccine	receive annual influenza vaccine				
"	no monthly breast self-exam	learn & regularly perform exam				

AMBULATORY PHARMACIST'S CARE PLAN

Patient George Jones Pharmacist John O'Malley Date 3-3-98

Page 1 of 3

DATE IDENTIFIED	PROBLEM (TPL)	PHARMACOTHERAPEUTIC AND RELATED HEALTH CARE GOAL	RECOMMENDATIONS FOR THERAPY	MONITORING PARAMETER(S)	DESIRED ENDPOINT(S)	MONITORING FREQUENCY
3/3/98	SX and BG suggestive of DM. High risk status					
	poor control of hypertension					
	nonadherence to diet					
	h/o med schedule nonadherence					
	Furosemide may worsen lipids					
	smoking history					
	Alcohol use history					

AMBULATORY PHARMACIST'S CARE PLAN

Patient George Jones   Pharmacist John O'Malley   Date 3-3-98

Page 2 of 3

DATE IDENTIFIED	PROBLEM (TPL)	PHARMACOTHERAPEUTIC AND RELATED HEALTH CARE GOAL	RECOMMENDATIONS FOR THERAPY	MONITORING PARAMETER(S)	DESIRED ENDPOINT(S)	MONITORING FREQUENCY
3/3/98	h/o non-adherence to flu appts					
	nonadherence to exercise					
	Not doing peak flow monitoring					
	No rectal/ prostate exam					
	no home Fecal test					
4/3/98	poor control of diabetes					
	Furosemide may ↑ BG					
	Fungal skin infection on toe					

AMBULATORY PHARMACIST'S CARE PLAN

Patient ___George Jones___   Pharmacist ___John O'Malley___   Date ___3-3-98___

Page 3 of 3

DATE IDENTIFIED	PROBLEM (TPL)	PHARMACOTHERAPEUTIC AND RELATED HEALTH CARE GOAL	RECOMMENDATIONS FOR THERAPY	MONITORING PARAMETER(S)	DESIRED ENDPOINT(S)	MONITORING FREQUENCY
4/3	Insensate feet					
	Not on daily ASA tx					
	Poor control of cholesterol					
	Not doing SMBG					
	No dilated retinal exam					
	No recent dental exam					
	liver dysfunction					

AMBULATORY PHARMACIST'S CARE PLAN

Patient ___George Jones___   Pharmacist ___John O'Malley___   Date ___3-3-98___

Page 1 of 3

DATE IDENTIFIED	PROBLEM (TPL)	PHARMACOTHERAPEUTIC AND RELATED HEALTH CARE GOAL	RECOMMENDATIONS FOR THERAPY	MONITORING PARAMETER(S)	DESIRED ENDPOINT(S)	MONITORING FREQUENCY
3/3/98	Sx and BG suggestive of DM. High risk status	Rule in/out DM. Determine cause of high BG and nocturia				
	poor control of hypertension	Improve BP control; Prevent complications				
	nonadherence to diet	start and adhere to prescribed meal plan				
	h/o med schedule nonadherence	adherence to medication regimen				
	Furosemide may worsen lipids	Avoid worsened lipid profile				
	smoking history	Stop smoking				
	Alcohol use history	Stop alcohol use				

AMBULATORY PHARMACIST'S CARE PLAN

Patient George Jones   Pharmacist John O'Malley   Date 3-3-98

Page 2 of 3

DATE IDENTIFIED	PROBLEM (TPL)	PHARMACOTHERAPEUTIC AND RELATED HEALTH CARE GOAL	RECOMMENDATIONS FOR THERAPY	MONITORING PARAMETER(S)	DESIRED ENDPOINT(S)	MONITORING FREQUENCY
3/3/98	h/o non-adherence to flu appts	Adherence to flu appt. scheduling				
	nonadherence to exercise	start and adhere to exercise plan				
	Not doing peak flow monitoring	Learn and perform peak flow monitoring regularly				
	No rectal/prostate exam	Annual rectal prostate exam				
	no home fecal test	Home fecal blood test q 6 months				
4/3/98	poor control of diabetes	Improve control; prevent complications				
	Furosemide may ↑ BG	Avoid worsened BP control				
	Fungal skin infection on toe	Eliminate fungal toe infection				

AMBULATORY PHARMACIST'S CARE PLAN

Patient ___George Jones___   Pharmacist ___John O'Malley___   Date ___3-3-98___

Page 3 of 3

DATE IDENTIFIED	PROBLEM (TPL)	PHARMACOTHERAPEUTIC AND RELATED HEALTH CARE GOAL	RECOMMENDATIONS FOR THERAPY	MONITORING PARAMETER(S)	DESIRED ENDPOINT(S)	MONITORING FREQUENCY
4/3	Insensate feet	Absence of infection trauma, ulcerations				
	Not on daily ASA tx	↓ risk CV complications 2° to diabetes				
	Poor control of cholesterol	Improve control, prevent complications				
	Not doing SMBG	Learn and perform regular SMBG				
	No dilated retinal exam	Annual dilated retinal exam				
	No recent dental exam	Dental exam q 6 months				
	liver dysfunction	monitor liver function				

AMBULATORY PHARMACIST'S CARE PLAN

Patient ___Sarah McLucas___   Pharmacist ___Alexa Sheffield___   Date ___4-23-98___

Page 1 of 2

DATE IDENTIFIED	PROBLEM (TPL)	PHARMACOTHERAPEUTIC AND RELATED HEALTH CARE GOAL	RECOMMENDATIONS FOR THERAPY	MONITORING PARAMETER(S)	DESIRED ENDPOINT(S)	MONITORING FREQUENCY
4/23/98	Poor control of diabetes					
"	Poor control of HTN					
"	Poor control of lipids					
"	Postmenopausal w/o HRT					
"	Not on ASA QD tx					
"	PPA in Tavist-D may worsen BP & BG					
"	Nonadherence to diet					
"	NSAID may ↑ BP					

AMBULATORY PHARMACIST'S CARE PLAN

Patient __Sarah McLucas__   Pharmacist __Alexa Sheffield__   Date __4-23-98__

Page 2 of 2

DATE IDENTIFIED	PROBLEM (TPL)	PHARMACOTHERAPEUTIC AND RELATED HEALTH CARE GOAL	RECOMMENDATIONS FOR THERAPY	MONITORING PARAMETER(S)	DESIRED ENDPOINT(S)	MONITORING FREQUENCY
4/23/98	Taking Tavist-D year-round					
"	Taking naprosyn and ibuprofen					
"	Poor control of OA pain					
"	NSAID may ↑ Sx's of GERD					
"	Nonadherence to cholestyramine					
"	No SMBG					
"	No exercise plan					

AMBULATORY PHARMACIST'S CARE PLAN

Patient **Sarah McLucas**   Pharmacist **Alexa Sheffield**   Date **4-23-98**

Page 1 of 2

DATE IDENTIFIED	PROBLEM (TPL)	PHARMACOTHERAPEUTIC AND RELATED HEALTH CARE GOAL	RECOMMENDATIONS FOR THERAPY	MONITORING PARAMETER(S)	DESIRED ENDPOINT(S)	MONITORING FREQUENCY
4/23/98	Poor control of diabetes	Improve control of diabetes; prevent complications				
"	Poor control of HTN	Improve control of HTN; prevent complications				
"	Poor control of lipids	Improve control of hypercholesterolemia; prevent complications				
"	Postmenopausal w/o HRT	Eliminate post-menopausal Sxs and ↓ assoc risks (CV and ↓ osteoporosis)				
"	Not on ASA QD tx	Prevent cardiovascular complications				
"	PPA in Tavist-D may worsen BP & BG	Avoid worsened BP and BG control				
"	Nonadherence to diet	Adhere to prescribed diet				
"	NSAID may ↑ BP	Avoid worsened BP control				

AMBULATORY PHARMACIST'S CARE PLAN

Patient __Sarah McLucas__   Pharmacist __Alexa Sheffield__   Date __4-23-98__

Page 2 of 2

DATE IDENTIFIED	PROBLEM (TPL)	PHARMACOTHERAPEUTIC AND RELATED HEALTH CARE GOAL	RECOMMENDATIONS FOR THERAPY	MONITORING PARAMETER(S)	DESIRED ENDPOINT(S)	MONITORING FREQUENCY
4/23/98	Taking Tavist-D yearround	Control seasonal allergic rhinitis SXs				
"	Taking naprosyn and ibuprofen	Avoid duplicate tx				
"	Poor control of OA pain	Control pain Preserve/increase functional status				
"	NSAID may ↑ SXs of GERD	Avoid SXs of GERD				
"	Nonadherence to cholestyramine	Control hypercholest.				
"	No SMBG	Regular SMBG				
"	No exercise plan	Adhere to exercise plan				

Designing a Therapy Regimen for Patients with Type 2 Diabetes

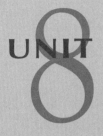

In the previous unit you learned how to identify pharmacotherapeutic and related health care goals for patients with type 2 diabetes. In this unit you will learn the next phase: how to design a therapy regimen based on these goals and your patient's health care needs. The process used to design the therapy regimen was shown in Figure 1 of unit 14 in the *Ambulatory Care Clinical Skills Program: Core Module*. Now that you have identified pharmacotherapeutic and related health care goals, you will prioritize them and develop recommendations to achieve them. A therapy regimen is a listing of recommendations to achieve the pharmacotherapeutic and related health care goals you have established for the patient. These recommendations will be documented on the ambulatory pharmacist's care plan (APCP).

You will also learn how to design a patient-specific education plan for an ambulatory patient with type 2 diabetes. You will learn which topics should be covered in a diabetes educational program, the educational process, factors to consider in planning your educational approach, and sources of educational materials.

Unit Objectives

After you successfully complete this unit, you will be able to:

- explain how patient-related concerns unique to ambulatory patients with type 2 diabetes may influence the design of their therapy regimen;
- explain the use of treatment guidelines in the design of therapy regimens for ambulatory patients with type 2 diabetes;
- explain education needs unique to ambulatory patients with type 2 diabetes;
- explain factors unique to ambulatory patients with type 2 diabetes that affect the approaches used for education, including patient-specific factors;
- state potential education resources used to meet an ambulatory diabetes patient's educational needs so the patient may successfully participate in the pharmacist's care plan;
- design a therapy regimen (including patient-specific education) that meets the pharmacotherapeutic and related health care goals established for an ambulatory patient with type 2 diabetes, integrates patient-specific

disease and drug information as well as ethical and quality of life issues, and considers pharmacoeconomic principles.

Unit Organization

To begin, this unit describes factors that influence the design of a therapy regimen for ambulatory patients with type 2 diabetes. The process of designing or selecting a patient-specific educational program for ambulatory patients with type 2 diabetes will then be discussed. Next, selection of the most appropriate therapeutic agents and the use of treatment guidelines are explained. Last, a case study will be used to illustrate how to design a therapy regimen for an ambulatory patient with type 2 diabetes, followed by a practice opportunity.

Factors That Influence Design of a Therapy Regimen

Patient-Related Aspects

In unit 7 you learned about the Health Belief Model, which states that a person's behavior reflects his or her subjective interpretation of a situation. Another important consideration for the pharmacist is to be aware that patients with type 2 diabetes have many fears. Hendricks et al. reference the following story to illustrate this point:

A man whose sister had died from complications of diabetes was unable to overcome fear when he was diagnosed with diabetes. He was convinced that what happened to his sister would happen to him. He didn't share his fear with his medical team. Their view of him was that he was an otherwise healthy person who could manage his disease with all of the latest technology and education. He took classes and bought the blood monitoring device and never used either the information or the tools. He was so fearful he would die soon anyway that he did nothing to prevent that from happening. And his daily life was lived in desperation as he ate extravagantly, drank heavily, and smoked cigarettes with the full knowledge that he was courting disaster. Fear became the power in control of his life.[1,2]

Fear of diabetes is a major concern for patients with type 2 diabetes; the most feared complications are amputation and retinopathy.[1] Fear contributes greatly to the stress associated with having diabetes. Pharmacists developing care plans and educational plans for patients with type 2 diabetes must be familiar with these fears to better enable the patient to engage in appropriate self-care of his or her disease. If patient fears are not assessed and dealt with, patients may follow the course of the patient in the story described above. In the Hendricks study,[1] 20 patients with type 2 diabetes were surveyed and asked the question, "What is your greatest fear about having diabetes?" Responses suggestive of acute complications included "stress" and "losing control." Most responses suggested that long-term complications were the greater area of concern, with comments primarily related to diabetic complications (e.g., "going blind," "kidney failure," "amputations," "stroke," "loss of vision," and "neuropathy"). However, many of those surveyed testified to the usefulness of knowledge of the disease in combating fear, such as:

> The more I read the more I learn about all the side effects of diabetes. This knowledge makes me more fearful, yet this same knowledge helps me want to be in as much control as possible of the disease.[1]

Implications for the pharmacist developing care plans and educational programs for patients with type 2 diabetes include the need to confront patient fears directly and gear educational efforts accordingly. Patients should be made aware of the data regarding the effect of enhanced blood glucose control and advances in the management of diabetes complications, should they occur. It is important to reinforce the need to adhere to prescribed therapies (drug and nondrug) and to maintain follow-up appointments with health care providers.

Another patient-related factor that can influence design of the therapy regimen for ambulatory patients with type 2 diabetes is the presence of a disability, such as visual impairment, amputation, or other limitation that affects the patient's ability to provide self-care (e.g., accurately draw up an insulin dose or read blood glucose monitor results). One example from the author's practice is: A home care nurse contacted the author for recommendations on insulin storage and administration for a bed-bound patient who lived alone. The patient had a bilateral amputation of both legs above the knees; also, an earlier stroke resulted in the inability to use one arm. Prefilled insulin syringes were recommended. The patient was able to retrieve her prefilled insulin

syringe from her bedside table, remove the cap with her teeth, self-inject, and dispose of the syringe in the bedside container. This is an extreme example, but physical disabilities must be considered.

Another example from the author's practice involves a patient with impaired vision. While teaching the patient to self-inject insulin, the patient obligingly pinched up a skin fold on her thigh, but jabbed the needle into her thumb instead, because of her poor vision. It is important for pharmacists to recognize the need for and to recommend aids that are available to visually-impaired patients, such as syringe magnifiers, insulin measurement aids, needle guides and insulin vial stabilizers for patients who inject insulin, and blood glucose monitor attachments with voice synthesizer components.

An important consideration that may influence design of the therapy regimen for an ambulatory patient with type 2 diabetes is the level of patient satisfaction with treatment. As stated earlier in this module, a patient's quality of life is a major consideration in establishing pharmacotherapeutic and related health care goals; a dissatisfied patient is less likely to adhere to therapeutic recommendations. The Diabetes Treatment Satisfaction Questionnaire (DTSQ) was designed to measure satisfaction with diabetes treatment regimens. The status version of the DTSQ is shown in **Figure 1**.[3] The answers to this series of questions will give insight into a patient's satisfaction with his or her current type 2 diabetes treatment. The questionnaire is designed for self-administration, is quick to complete, and provides a total score of satisfaction with treatment.

A second survey, the DTSQ change version, was designed to address the possible occurrence of a ceiling effect when treatment is altered.[4] For example, a patient may believe that he or she is completely satisfied with current therapy, but a change in therapy (e.g., from regular insulin to insulin lispro or from an agent in one therapeutic class to another) may bring improved satisfaction. However, until the patient experiences the benefits of the changed therapy, he or she has no reason to believe that the current treatment could be improved and no means to rate this improved satisfaction if the highest rating has already been chosen on a previous questionnaire. By using a scale that includes phrases such as "much more satisfied now" and "much less convenient," the DTSQ change version allows a comparison of treatment regimens. If you wish to use these instruments in your practice,

The following questions concern your diabetes treatment (including insulin, tablets, and/or diet) and your experience over the past few weeks. Please answer each question by circling a number on each of the scales.

1.   How satisfied are you with your current treatment?

very satisfied   6   5   4   3   2   1   0   very dissatisfied

2.   How often have you felt that your blood sugars have been unacceptably high recently?

most of the time   6   5   4   3   2   1   0   none of the time

3.   How often have you felt that your blood sugars have been unacceptably low recently?

most of the time   6   5   4   3   2   1   0   none of the time

4.   How convenient have you been finding your treatment to be recently?

very convenient   6   5   4   3   2   1   0   very inconvenient

5.   How flexible have you been finding your treatment to be recently?

very flexible   6   5   4   3   2   1   0   very inflexible

6.   How satisfied are you with your understanding of your diabetes?

very satisfied   6   5   4   3   2   1   0   very dissatisfied

7.   Would you recommend this form of treatment to someone else with your kind of diabetes?

Yes, I would   6   5   4   3   2   1   0   No, I would
definitely   definitely not
recommend the   recommend the
treatment   treatment

8.   How satisfied would you be to continue with your present form of treatment?

very satisfied   6   5   4   3   2   1   0   very dissatisfied

Please make sure that you have circled one number on each of the scales.

Figure 1. Diabetes Treatment Satisfaction Questionnaire (DTSQ)
Source: reprinted with permission from reference 3.

Table 1. Factors to Consider in Designing a Therapy Regimen

Drug-Related Factors	Patient-Related Factors	Non–patient-Related Factors
Efficacy	Age	Reimbursement for therapy to health care setting
Safety	Gender	Availability of therapy
Cost	Renal function	Policies of practice sites
Formulary issues	Hepatic function	Ethical considerations
Drug regimen	Concurrent illness	
Dose and dosing frequency	Known hypersensitivity or adverse reactions	
Route of administration	Therapy costs	
Dosage form	Health beliefs	
Mode of administration	Living environment	
Length of therapy	Quality of life	

you should contact Dr. Clare Bradley, Department of Psychology, Royal Holloway, University of London, for permission as well as the most current version of the survey.

Treatment Guidelines

As discussed in unit 14 of the *Ambulatory Care Clinical Skills Program: Core Module*, guidelines are an important tool in patient care; however, they must be interpreted and applied with consideration of regional and patient-specific circumstances. Guidelines developed by the American Diabetes Association[5] for the pharmacologic management of

type 2 diabetes (**Figure 2**) allow for individualization based on the factors listed in **Table 1**, which must be considered in designing a therapy regimen. Appropriate use of guidelines also requires you to be aware of how current they are in view of possible advances in the management of diabetes. For example, the guidelines shown in Figure 2 do not include repaglinide, a new oral hypoglycemic agent used to treat diabetes. Application of these guidelines will be addressed later in this unit.

Finally, you should realize that most treatment protocols for diabetes are not aimed at women with preexisting or gestational diabetes. If you are

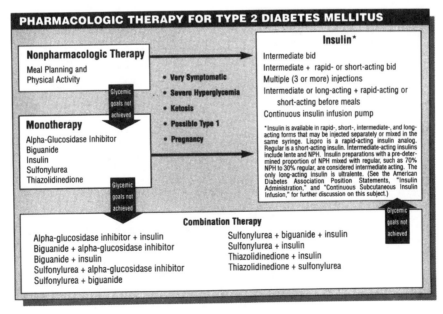

Figure 2. Pharmacologic therapy for managing type 2 diabetes mellitus
Source: reprinted with permission from reference 5.

Table 2. Order of Priorities for Treatment of Adults with Diabetic Dyslipidemia

I. LDL cholesterol lowering[a]
    First choice
        HMG-CoA reductase inhibitor (statin)
    Second choice
        Bile acid binding resin (resin) or fenofibrate

II. HDL cholesterol raising
    Behavioral interventions such as weight loss, increased physical activity and smoking cessation may be useful
    Glycemic control
    Difficult except with nicotinic acid, which is relatively contraindicated, or fibrates

III. Triglyceride lowering
    Glycemic control first priority
    Fibric acid derivative (gemfibrozil, fenofibrate)
    Statins are moderately effective at high dose in hypertriglyceridemic subjects who also have high LDL cholesterol

IV. Combined hyperlipidemia
    First choice
        Improve glycemic control plus high dose statin
    Second choice
        Improve glycemic control plus statin[b] plus fibric acid derivative[b] (gemfibrozil, fenofibrate)
    Third choice
        Improve glycemic control plus resin plus fibric acid derivative (gemfibrozil, fenofibrate)
        Improve glycemic control plus statin[b] plus nicotinic acid[b] (glycemic control must be monitored carefully)

[a]Decision for treatment of high LDL cholesterol before elevated triglyceride is based on clinical trial data indicating safety as well as efficiency of the available agents.
[b]The combination of the statins with nicotinic acid and especially with gemfibrozil or fenofibrate may carry an increased risk of myositis. Refer to ADA guidelines for recommendations for patients with triglyceride levels >400 mg/dl.

Source: reprinted with permission from reference 10.

involved in the care of pregnant women who have or develop diabetes, you should refer to appropriate references. Bear in mind that women in this situation should be started on insulin therapy if nonpharmacologic interventions are insufficient to control blood glucose.[6–9]

Other useful guidelines in caring for patients with type 2 diabetes include recommendations for the treatment of hypercholesterolemia and hypertension in a patient with diabetes. **Table 2** shows the preferred order for managing dyslipidemias in patients with diabetes, and the recommended drug selection.[10] *The Sixth Report of the Joint National Committee on Prevention, Detection, Evaluation and Treatment of High Blood Pressure* is an evidence-based, consensus report that describes the most contemporary approach to hypertension control.[11] Applications of these suggested guidelines to patients with type 2 diabetes will be discussed later in this unit.

Don't forget to recommend treatments for other diabetes-related complications, such as gastroparesis (e.g., recommend metoclopramide or cisapride) or painful peripheral neuropathy (e.g., recommend a tricyclic antidepressant or anticonvulsant agent).

Case Study

Let's consider the case of Mrs. Gonzalez. Included in **Appendix A** is a survey Mrs. Gonzalez completed, which Pharmacist Radcliffe will use to assess Mrs. Gonzalez's health beliefs about type 2 diabetes. Pharmacist Radcliffe reviews the answers and discusses them with Mrs. Gonzalez as follows.

PHARMACIST:
"Mrs. Gonzalez, I see you have several question marks on this survey. Why do you have questions marks about diet, exercise, and controlling your sugar?"

MRS. GONZALEZ:
"Well, I know diabetes is a serious disease, but I'm not sure it can be controlled."

PHARMACIST:
"Mrs. Gonzalez, do you have any fears about diabetes?"

MRS. GONZALEZ, now moved to tears:
"Yes, I'm afraid I'm going to die. But before I die, all sorts of awful things are going to happen to me. My cousin Emmanuel had his leg cut off, and he went blind. I'm too young for this; I just don't know what I'm going to do!"

PHARMACIST:

"Mrs. Gonzalez, your cousin is an extreme example of what can happen with diabetes. But the truth is that we have convincing evidence that modifying your diet, exercising, taking medications if required, and following all the advice your health care team gives you will go a long, long way in preventing diabetes complications. You've been examined very thoroughly by Dr. Thompson, and you have no complications at this time. It's true we can't cure diabetes, high blood pressure, or high cholesterol, but we can work to control them. Dr. Thompson and I will be right here for you, as will the rest of the people involved in your care. Do you understand what I'm telling you?"

MRS. GONZALEZ:

"Do you have any other patients who have been able to control their sugar and pressure and not have these complications?"

PHARMACIST:

"Absolutely! Do you know who has the biggest impact on whether you develop complications?"

MRS. GONZALEZ:

"No, who?"

PHARMACIST:

"You do! You're the captain of this team; myself, Dr. Thompson, the dietitian I've referred you to, your ophthalmologist, and the dentist are all here to help you by giving you the tools you need to do a good job. I know you can do it, but the proof is in doing it."

MRS. GONZALEZ:

"Well, I'm glad you're so confident in me. I guess, if it's up to me, I'll just buckle down and do it. But, you're sure you'll be available if I need to call with questions right?"

PHARMACIST:

"Absolutely."

In this example, Mrs. Gonzalez appreciates the severity of type 2 diabetes and her susceptibility to diabetes-related complications. However, her greatest fear is that she will end up like her cousin, and she isn't sure that interventions can alter her course. The discussion with the pharmacist helped allay her fears to some extent. With self-monitoring of blood glucose, Mrs. Gonzalez will achieve greater peace of mind by being able to observe her blood glucose decrease; decreases in blood pressure and cholesterol values will also relieve her fears. As she develops a care plan for Mrs. Gonzalez, the pharmacist may consult treatment protocols designed for the management of patients with diabetes, such as the ones shown in **Figure 2** and **Table 2**. Because Mrs. Gonzalez is just starting interventions, it probably would not be very useful to administer the Diabetes Treatment Satisfaction Questionnaire now. This can be administered in a month or two, when she is a little further along in following a prescribed treatment plan (either pharmacologic or nonpharmacologic).

Designing and Selecting Patient-Specific Education

Education is a significant part of diabetes management. As discussed previously, the vast majority of diabetes management is provided by the patient. For the patient to provide good self-care, he or she will require education in type 2 diabetes. The goals of patient-specific education are to prevent problems from occurring and to solve problems if they occur. Prevention of problems is accomplished with proactive education, which teaches patients what they need to know to avoid problems with their medications, conditions, and nondrug therapy. For example, a well-educated patient with diabetes knows prospectively how to deal with sick days and how to avoid dire consequences such as development of Hyperglycemic Hyperosmolar Nonketotic Syndrome (HHNS). As discussed earlier in this unit, the better patients are educated, the less fearful they are of diabetes.

The National Certification Board for Diabetes Educators (NCBDE), located in Chicago, Illinois, offers diabetes educator certification. The telephone number of NCBDE is 1-847-228-9795. After you have accumulated at least 1,000 hours of direct diabetes patient education experience that meet all criteria, you may be eligible to sit for the Certified Diabetes Educator examination. If you are successful, you may use the credential CDE as part of your title; in some states, having the CDE will help you receive reimbursement for diabetes education. You may want to obtain a Candidate Handbook prior to your eligibility so you can read what will be required.

Educational Content

The American Diabetes Association coordinated a task force in 1993 charged with revising the standards for diabetes patient education. Representatives from several diabetes organizations worked together to develop the "National Standards for Diabetes Self-Management Education Programs."[12] The guidelines cover the structure, process, and outcomes necessary for programs recognized by the American Diabetes Association. One aspect of these guidelines is a description of the curriculum that should be part of a quality diabetes self-management education program. According to these guidelines, based on the needs of the target population, the program shall be capable of offering instruction in the following content areas:

a. Diabetes overview
b. Stress and psychosocial adjustment
c. Family involvement and social support
d. Nutrition
e. Exercise and activity
f. Medications
g. Monitoring and use of results
h. Relationship among nutrition, exercise, medication, and blood glucose levels
i. Prevention, detection, and treatment of acute complications
j. Prevention, detection, and treatment of chronic complications
k. Foot, skin, and dental care
l. Behavior change strategies, goal setting, risk factor reduction, and problem solving
m. Benefits, risks, and management options for improving glucose control.
n. Preconception care, pregnancy, and gestational diabetes
o. Use of health care system and community resources

Some of these educational objectives have already been addressed in previous units. An in-depth discussion of each of these content areas is beyond the scope of this module; the reader is referred to several excellent resources, which will be discussed later in this unit.

Educational Process

Unit 16 of the *Ambulatory Care Clinical Skills Program: Core Module* gave an excellent overview of the educational process. You may want to refer back to that unit to refresh your memory. We have already defined the content that is important in diabetes education. Obviously, some aspects of the recommended content will not be pertinent to all patients (e.g., preconception care, pregnancy, and gestational diabetes topics would not be relevant for a male patient or a woman past child-bearing age).

It is obvious that you cannot teach all 15 content areas in one educational session. You should break the educational process into manageable pieces. Decide how many sessions you will schedule with the patient, generally anywhere from four to eight sessions initially, and schedule regular follow-up sessions to assess metabolic control and retention of knowledge. Even if you develop a schedule of sessions and topics, your agenda needs to be flexible enough to accommodate the patient's most critical needs. For example, not all patients will need to learn to monitor their blood glucose at the first session. Many patients, like Mrs. Gonzalez, have been asymptomatic of their diabetes and will be treated initially with nonpharmacologic interventions; therefore, the risk of developing hypoglycemia before the second educational session is low. Conversely, patients who are very symptomatic and are started on hypoglycemic therapy need to be taught the signs and symptoms of hypoglycemia and how to deal with them. Patients should always be educated about their medications, including potential adverse effects. Patients receiving drugs to treat diabetes that may cause hypoglycemia should be aware of the signs and symptoms of hypoglycemia, what is considered a low blood glucose value, and what they should do if hypoglycemia occurs. One example of a medication education sheet for patients with diabetes is shown in **Figure 3**.[13] If you are referring a patient to a dietitian, you may only need to offer basic instructions on diet therapy that will suffice until the patient consults with the dietitian. Also, many principles can be introduced at the first educational session and assessed and reinforced at subsequent sessions. Topics such as use of health care system and community resources can probably be saved for later sessions.

As you consider implementing diabetes education in your practice, you will have to consider several variables. Is your patient population all type 2 patients or mostly type 2 patients with a handful of type 1 patients? Will you conduct individual patient counseling sessions or hold group classes? How many sessions will be required to complete your educational checklist (either individually or in classes)?

As you learned in the *Ambulatory Care Clinical*

Questions To Ask About Your Diabetes Medicines

Ask these questions when your doctor prescribes a medicine. Write the answers in pencil so that you can make changes if your doctor changes your medicines.

When do I take the medicine—before a meal, with a meal, or after a meal?

_____

How often should I take the medicine?

_____

Should I take the medicine at the same time every day?

_____

What should I do if I forget to take my medicine?

_____

What side effects may happen?

_____

_____

What should I do if I get side effects?

_____

_____

Figure 3. Medication Planning Forms for People with Diabetes

My Diabetes Medicines

Fill in this record about your diabetes medicines with the help of your doctor or diabetes teacher. Write this in pencil so you can make changes when your doctor makes changes in your diabetes medicines.

The names of the diabetes medicines (insulin or pills) I take are:

_____

I take _____ (name of diabetes medicine) _____ times a day.
At (time)_____ I take (amount)_____.
At (time)_____ I take (amount)_____.
At (time)_____ I take (amount)_____.

I take _____ (name of diabetes medicine) _____ times a day.
At (time)_____ I take (amount)_____.
At (time)_____ I take (amount)_____.
At (time)_____ I take (amount)_____.

I take _____ (name of diabetes medicine) _____ times a day.
At (time)_____ I take (amount)_____.
At (time)_____ I take (amount)_____.
At (time)_____ I take (amount)_____.

I should call my doctor or diabetes teacher if I have these problems with my diabetes medicines:

_____
_____

I should call my doctor or diabetes teacher if my blood glucose is too low or too high for several days.
Too low is _____ mg/dl for _____ days.
Too high is _____ mg/dl for _____ days.

My blood sugar should be between _____mg/dl and _____mg/dl before my first meal of the day.

My blood sugar should be between _____mg/dl and _____mg/dl 1–2 hours after a meal.

My blood sugar is too low at _____mg/dl.

My blood sugar is too high at _____mg/dl.

My hemoglobin A_{1c} should be _____%.

Figure 3. Amedication Planning Forms for People with Diabetes (cont.)
Source: reprinted from reference 13.

Skills Program: Core Module, there are several patient factors that influence your educational process, including the patient's level of education, cognitive ability, and language comprehension, as well as any vision, hearing, other physical limitations, and age.[14]

In addition to these factors, you must appreciate that people have different learning styles. Some prefer to read about how to perform a task, and some would rather have it explained to them. Other learning styles include use of visual materials, numerical presentation, graphic directions, and demonstration. Some aspects of diabetes education obviously favor use of one learning style over another. For example, drawing up and injecting insulin or self-monitoring blood glucose is probably best taught by explanation and demonstration. Most people probably learn best when more than one learning style and teaching strategy is used. Some useful teaching strategies include: lecture, discussion, demonstration, print materials, audiovisuals, role-playing, game playing, computer simulations, and case reviews.

One last factor that you need to consider in planning your educational program is the patient's readiness to learn each behavior you are teaching. You learned how to assess readiness to learn in unit 7. Your educational strategy must be based on the patient's stage of readiness to learn whatever content you are planning to teach; if you do not do this, your educational intervention is likely to be less than effective. **Table 3** lists some educational treatment suggestions based on the patient's stage of readiness.[15]

Educational Resources

In selecting educational resources, you should consider resources for your own professional development as well as resources directed for patient education use. Refer to **Table 4** for a description of available resources. You are encouraged to contact the American Diabetes Association and the American Association of Diabetes Educators for a catalog of available products.

Additional diabetes educational resources may be obtained from pharmaceutical manufacturers and on the Internet. Pharmaceutical manufacturers provide some excellent diabetes educational materials, but without a guarantee of continued availability. In many ways, you are better off developing your educational program using materials that you can reproduce with permission or sources unlikely to discontinue product availability.

A large amount of education information is available on the Internet; recommended sites are listed in **Table 5**.

Regardless of which educational materials you select, be sure to refer to Figure 1 in unit 16 of the *Ambulatory Care Clinical Skills Program: Core Module*, which is a checklist for evaluating written, audio, and audiovisual educational materials. This checklist will allow you to best match educational resources to your patients and their special needs.

Case Study

As discussed in previous units, one of the pharmacist's first interventions with Mrs. Gonzalez is to set up a diabetes education program. Important elements of diabetes patient education are to assess what the patient knows prior to the educational intervention and then reassess after the session. For each educational topic, the pharmacist should develop objectives, which can be documented as taught, and subsequently assessed. For example, if the topic was acute complications, the pharmacist may have five specific goals:

- State symptoms of hypoglycemia.
- State two reasons why blood glucose could be low.
- Describe two actions to properly treat hypoglycemia.
- State two reasons why blood glucose could be high.
- Describe two actions to take when blood glucose is above acceptable level.

As each competency objective is taught, the pharmacist should note the date taught and the result (e.g., not applicable, achieved outcome, requires assistance, needs instruction, or declines instruction). In subsequent sessions the pharmacist can provide additional instruction and assess retention of knowledge for those competencies where the outcome was noted to have been achieved. For example, Pharmacist Radcliffe could ask Mrs. Gonzalez, "Could you tell me three symptoms of hypoglycemia?" to reassess Mrs. Gonzalez's knowledge in this area. Just as technique in self-monitoring blood glucose requires repeated assessment (e.g., every 6 months), so does diabetes education.

Let's return to the case of Mrs. Gonzalez (**Appendix A**) and develop an educational program for the first session, to begin meeting her education needs. Her first need was to be educated about what the diagnosis of diabetes means. Earlier in this unit

Table 3. General Guidelines for Applying Stages and Processes of Change to Diabetes Care

Stage of Readiness	Key Factors Associated with Movement to Next Stage	Treatment Do's	Treatment Don'ts
Precontemplation	Increased information and awareness, emotional acceptance	Provide personalized information. Allow patient to express emotion about his or her disease.	Do not assume patient has knowledge or expect that providing information will automatically lead to behavior change. Do not ignore patient's emotional adjustment to the disease, which could override ability to process relevant information.
Contemplation	Increased confidence in one's ability to adopt recommended behaviors	Encourage support networks. Give positive feedback about a patient's abilities. Help to clarify ambivalence about adopting behavior and emphasize expected benefits.	Do not ignore potential impact of family members, caregivers, and others on patient's ability to comply. Do not be alarmed or critical of a patient's ambivalence.
Preparation	Resolution of ambivalence, firm commitment, and specific action plan	Encourage patient to set specific, achievable goals (e.g., walk briskly for 15 min at least 3 times a week). Reinforce small changes that patient may have already achieved.	Do not recommend general behavioral changes (e.g., "Get more exercise"). Do not refer to small changes as "not good enough."
Action	Behavioral skill training and social support	Refer to education program for self-management skills. Provide self-help materials.	Do not refer patients to "information-only" classes.
Maintenance	Problem-solving skills and social and environmental support	Encourage patient to anticipate and plan for potential difficulties (e.g., maintaining dietary changes on vacation). Collect information about local resources (e.g., support groups and shopping guides). Encourage patient to "recycle" if he or she has a lapse or relapse.	Do not assume that initial action means permanent change. Do not be discouraged or judgmental about a lapse or relapse.

Source: reprinted with permission from reference 15.

Table 4. Suggested Educational Resources

Resource	Intended Audience	Content	Available Format	Publisher/ Source
A Core Curriculum for Diabetes Educators, 3rd edition	Health care professionals	Resource for diabetes educator; contains useful strategies for working with patients	Book	American Association of Diabetes Educators, (800) 338-DMED, www.aadenet.org
Diabetes Education Programs: Evaluating for Success	Health care professionals and organizations	Provides information for organizations in the process of developing or evaluating a diabetes education program	Book	American Association of Diabetes Educators, (800) 338-DMED, www.aadenet.org
Medical Management of Type 2 Diabetes, 4th edition	Health care professionals	A complete overview of type 2 diabetes and its management	Book	American Diabetes Association, 1-800-ADA-ORDER, www.diabetes.org
Therapy for Diabetes Mellitus and Related Disorders, 3rd edition	Health care professionals	A complete overview of every aspect of diabetes	Book	American Diabetes Association, 1-800-ADA-ORDER, www.diabetes.org
Diabetes Education Goals	Health care professionals	Direction on how to assess, plan, and evaluate patient education and counseling programs	Book	American Diabetes Association, 1-800-ADA-ORDER, www.diabetes.org
"Right From the Start, Type 2 Version" (1998 edition)	Patients with type 2 diabetes mellitus	A resource book for patients with type 2 diabetes	Booklet	American Diabetes Association, 1-800-ADA-ORDER, www.diabetes.org
Facilitating Lifestyle Changes: A Resource Manual	Health care professionals	Provides instruments to use during educational encounters to facilitate life-style change through a four-step model: assessment, goal setting, intervention, and evaluation	Book	American Diabetes Association, 1-800-ADA-ORDER, www.diabetes.org
Life with Diabetes: A Series of Teaching Outlines	Health care professional	A comprehensive curriculum for diabetes educators that covers all recommended content areas. Recommends teaching methods with pertinent content outline, material needed, and evaluation and documentation guidelines.	Book	American Diabetes Association, 1-800-ADA-ORDER, www.diabetes.org

Note: Both organizations have many more educational resources available, which are described in detail at their Internet Web site.

Table 5. Diabetes Information Web Sites

URL	Site
http://www.diabetes.org	American Diabetes Association
http://www.joslin.harvard.edu	Joslin Diabetes Center
http://www.niddk.nih.gov	National Institute of Diabetes and Digestive and Kidney Diseases
http://www.mdcc.com	Diabetes Monitor
http://www.pslgroup.com/DIABETES.htm	Doctor's Guide to Diabetes Information and Resources
http://www.cruzio.com/~mendosa/faq.htm	On-Line Resources for Diabetes

you read a conversation between Mrs. Gonzalez and the pharmacist during which several of Mrs. Gonzalez's fears about diabetes surfaced. As part of this education session, it would be important to discuss facts about controlling type 2 diabetes. Clearly, Mrs. Gonzalez has misconceptions about type 2 diabetes that the pharmacist can clear up. The approach Pharmacist Radcliffe chose was to discuss the issue with Mrs. Gonzalez and provide a copy of the education booklet "Right from the Start," about type 2 diabetes. As Pharmacist Radcliffe explained what type 2 diabetes is, she pointed out sections of the book and illustrations that supported this discussion. At the end of this interactive session, she asked Mrs. Gonzalez to repeat the key points and asked if she had any questions. Pharmacist Radcliffe gave Mrs. Gonzalez a reading assignment in her booklet and instructed her to be prepared to review and discuss the reading at the next session.

Mrs. Gonzalez's next need is to learn to use a blood glucose monitor. The pharmacist explained features of blood glucose monitors, and Mrs. Gonzalez and the pharmacist worked together to select the most appropriate monitor. The content of the education should include all the items on the blood glucose monitor teaching checklist discussed in unit 3 of this module. The pharmacist demonstrated how to perform the blood glucose assessment, had the patient check her own glucose, and explained each step. The pharmacist also discussed the accompanying literature for checking a blood glucose value and pointed out the abbreviated user's guide that walks the patient through the process step by step. Pharmacist Radcliffe also asked Mrs. Gonzalez to review the videotape that came with the blood glucose monitor when she goes home. Assessment would be by patient demonstration and review of her self-monitoring records.

Mrs. Gonzalez has an appointment with the dietitian in a few days, so Pharmacist Radcliffe only needed to answer basic questions Mrs. Gonzalez had about diet. The final educational need was to understand the interrelationship between food, exercise, and blood glucose control. Pharmacist Radcliffe explained to Mrs. Gonzalez that weight loss that results from diet and exercise would benefit her blood pressure control and dyslipidemia. This was done verbally and by pointing out examples in her workbook. Assessment will be by patient interview at the next session by asking her to interpret her log book and explain blood glucose readings. The education program for Mrs. Gonzalez is shown in **Appendix A**.

Designing the Therapy Regimen

Therapy Selection

Consider the American Diabetes Association algorithm of pharmacologic therapy for the management of patients with type 2 diabetes (**Figure 2**). Patients are initially treated with nonpharmacologic therapy (meal planning and physical activity). When should pharmacological agents be used in the treatment of type 2 diabetes? Bearing in mind that therapeutic decision making in type 2 diabetes is guided by glycemic control (see **Table 6** for recommended glycemic control goals),[16] it seems reasonable that if nonpharmacologic interventions have been given an adequate trial (e.g., 3 months) and the glycemic goal has not been achieved or the patient's biochemical markers are in the "additional action suggested" column, pharmacological therapy should be started. However, this is a patient-specific decision affected by several variables, including:

- demographic characteristics (e.g., age, gender, race, and socioeconomic status);

Table 6. Glycemic Control for People with Diabetes

Biochemical Index	Normal	Goal	Additional Action Suggested
Average preprandial glucose (mg/dl)[a]	<110	80–120	<80 >140
Average bedtime glucose (mg/dl)[a]	<120	100–140	<100 >160
HbA$_{1c}$ (%)	<6	<7	>8

The values shown are by necessity generalized to the entire population of individuals with diabetes. Patients with comorbid diseases, the very young, older adults, and others with unusual conditions or circumstances may warrant different treatment goals. The values are for nonpregnant adults. "Additional action suggested" depends on individual patient circumstances. Such actions may include enhanced diabetes self-management education, comanagement with a diabetes team, referral to an endocrinologist, change in pharmacological therapy, initiation of or increase in SMBG, or more frequent contact with the patient. HbA$_{1c}$ is referenced to a nondiabetic range of 4.0–6.0% (mean 5.0%, S.D. 0.5%).
[a]Measurement of capillary blood glucose.

Source: reprinted with permission from reference 16.

- resources (e.g., access to health care, self-care skills, finances/health insurance, and family support); and
- health/disease status (e.g., coexisting diseases and complications of diabetes).[17]

Even though a patient may begin pharmacological therapy after 3 months, continued adherence to medical nutrition therapy and an exercise plan should be stressed to the patient.

An additional consideration is that some patients (such as those with symptoms of hyperglycemia, those patients undergoing surgery, and patients with ketosis) require prompt pharmacological therapy at the time of diagnosis or first visit. As shown in the treatment algorithm, some patients may require insulin therapy at the onset of diabetes, including patients who are:

- very symptomatic,
- severely hyperglycemic,
- ketotic,
- possibly type 1, or
- pregnant.

Another consideration in deciding when to begin pharmacologic treatment is how high the patient's blood glucose and hemoglobin A$_{1c}$ are at the time of evaluation. The higher these values, the less likely nonpharmacologic interventions and lifestyle modifications will be sufficient to meet the therapeutic goal. While this is an individualized

decision for each case, the pharmacist may be inclined to recommend instituting both nonpharmacologic and pharmacologic therapy, or to follow closely patients who insist they will adhere to lifestyle modifications.

With the exceptions and considerations noted above, patients who have not responded satisfactorily to nonpharmacologic therapy should be started on one medication approved for the management of type 2 diabetes. The agents that are available include:

- α-glucosidase inhibitor (acarbose and miglitol);
- biguanide (metformin);
- insulin;
- thiazolidinedione (rosiglitazone);
- sulfonylurea (chlorpropamide, tolbutamide, tolazamide, acetohexamide, glyburide; glipizide, and glimepiride); and
- meglitinide (repaglinide).

Note that repaglinide has come on the market since the treatment algorithm shown in **Figure 2** was published. Both the oral sulfonylurea agents and repaglinide can be considered insulin secretogogues.

We are fortunate to have this many medications to select from in the treatment of type 2 diabetes. Just a handful of years ago, the choices were limited to oral sulfonylurea agents or insulin (or both). **Table 7** contains a comparison of monotherapeutic

Table 7. Comparison of Monotherapeutic Agents Used to Treat Type 2 Diabetes

Agent	Mechanism of Action	Efficacy	Contraindications	Precautions/Comments
Acarbose	Reversibly inhibits intestinal α-glucosidase enzyme, causing diminished and delayed glucose absorption after a meal, resulting in reduced postprandial plasma glucose levels.	Decreases FPG 16–20 mg/dl. Decreases PPG ~50 mg/dl. Decreases HbA_{1c} 0.5–1.0%.	Do not use in patients with gastrointestinal pathophysiologic changes such as cirrhosis, inflammatory bowel disease, colonic ulceration, partial intestinal obstruction, disorders of digestion or absorption, or conditions that may deteriorate secondary to increased gas formation. Do not use in patients with a known hypersensitivity or allergy to the drug or any of its components.	Rarely, may increase serum transaminases; check every 3 months for the first year and periodically thereafter. Not recommended for use by patients with a serum creatinine >2.0 mg/dl. Poorly absorbed; causes GI distress (abdominal pain, diarrhea, and flatulence). Does not cause weight gain or hypoglycemia (as monotherapy; may cause hypoglycemia when used in combination with other antidiabetes medications such as sulfonylureas or insulin). Take with first bite of a meal. Treat hypoglycemia with glucose tablets (not sucrose). Useful in patients with primarily elevated postprandial hyperglycemia.
Insulin	Exogenous administration of insulin.	Dose to response (unlimited effect on FPG and HbA_{1c}).	Contraindicated during episodes of hypoglycemia and in patients sensitive to an excipient.	Diet, level of exercise, illness, concomitant medications, and pregnancy may alter insulin requirements. Allows for flexible dosing. Requires injection. Rapid-acting insulin (e.g., Lispro) is usually injected closer to mealtime than other insulins. Causes hypoglycemia and weight gain.

Agent	Mechanism of Action	Efficacy	Contraindications	Precautions/Comments
Metformin	Primary mechanism is to decrease hepatic glucose output. Secondary mechanism is to enhance tissue sensitivity to insulin action.	Decreases FPG 60–70 mg/dl. Decreases HbA$_{1c}$ 1.5–2.0%.	Do not use in patients with a known hypersensitivity or allergy to the drug or any of its components. Contraindications include: * impaired renal function (serum creatinine $\geq$1.5 mg/dl in men, $\geq$1.4 mg/dl in women, glomerular filtration rate <70 ml/min); * symptomatic congestive heart failure requiring pharmacological treatment; * chronic liver disease (liver transaminases greater than three-fold above upper limit of normal); * elderly ($\geq$80 years old) patients (may be used if creatinine clearance is >70 ml/min); * pregnancy; * lactation; * type 1 diabetes; * patients with alcohol dependency or history of excessive alcohol intake; and * acute or chronic metabolic acidosis including diabetic ketoacidosis (with or without coma).	Lactic acidosis may occur (rare; three cases in 100,000 patient years). Suspend therapy during surgical procedures. Metformin should be temporarily discontinued in patients undergoing radiologic studies involving intravascular administration of iodinated contrast materials (may acutely alter renal function). Assess renal function before initiation of therapy and at least annually thereafter. Does not cause hypoglycemia (as monotherapy; may cause hypoglycemia when used in combination with other antidiabetes medications such as sulfonylureas or insulin). Does not cause weight gain (may cause modest weight loss). Adverse effects predominantly gastrointestinal (e.g., diarrhea, nausea, vomiting, abdominal bloating, flatulence, and anorexia). Favorable effect on lipid profile. Useful in overweight, insulin-resistant patients.
Miglitol	Reversibly inhibits intestinal α-glucosidase enzyme, causing diminished and delayed glucose absorption after a meal, resulting in reduced postprandial plasma glucose levels.	Decreases PPG 57–64 mg/dl. Decreases HbA$_{1c}$ 0.7–0.8%.	Do not use in patients with gastrointestinal pathophysiologic changes such as cirrhosis, inflammatory bowel disease, colonic ulceration, partial intestinal obstruction, disorders of digestion or absorption, or conditions that may deteriorate secondary to increased gas formation.	Does not cause weight gain or hypoglycemia (as monotherapy; may cause hypoglycemia when used in combination with other antidiabetes medications such as sulfonylureas or insulin).

continued on next page

Table 7. Comparison of Monotherapeutic Agents Used to Treat Type 2 Diabetes (cont.)

Agent	Mechanism of Action	Efficacy	Contraindications	Precautions/Comments
Miglitol (cont.)			Do not use in patients with a known hypersensitivity or allergy to the drug or any of its components. Do not use in patients in diabetic ketoacidosis.	Unabsorbed carbohydrates cause abdominal pain, diarrhea, and flatulence. Treat hypoglycemia with glucose tablets (not sucrose). Useful in patients with primarily elevated postprandial hyperglycemia. Take with first bite of a meal. Dosage adjustment is not recommended for renal impairment. Increase in liver enzymes has not been noted.
Repaglinide	Rapid-acting nonsulfonylurea; insulin secretogogue.	Decreases FPG by 60–70 mg/dl. Decreases HbA_{1c} by 1.7%.	Patients with diabetic ketoacidsosis (with or without coma). Type 1 diabetes. Do not use in patients with a known hypersensitivity or allergy to the drug or any of its components.	Dosage may require adjustment in patients with renal impairment/failure. Dose with caution in patients with impaired liver function. Causes hypoglycemia and weight gain. Take before each meal; flexible dosing (skip a meal, delete dose; add a meal, add a dose). May be preferred agent in leaner type 2 patients, particularly if symptomatic.
Rosiglitazone	Primary effect is to increase sensitivity to insulin in muscle and adipose tissue. An additional effect is to inhibit hepatic gluconeogenesis.	Decreases FPG 25–55 mg/dl. Decreases HbA_{1c} up to ~1.0%.	Patients with ALT >2.5 times the upper limit of normal should not begin rosiglitazone therapy. Do not use in patients with a known hypersensitivity or allergy to the drug or any of its components.	Does not cause hypoglycemia (as monotherapy). Because of structural similarity to troglitazone, liver enzyme monitoring is required before treatment, every 2 months for the first 12 months and periodically

Agent	Mechanism of Action	Efficacy	Contraindications	Precautions/Comments
Rosiglitazone (cont.)				thereafter. If ALT levels are mildly elevated (1–2.5 times upper limit of normal) during therapy, continuation of therapy should proceed with caution and appropriate close clinical and laboratory follow-up. If ALT level exceeds three or more times the upper limit of normal, recheck levels; if consistent, therapy should be discontinued. Rosiglitazone may result in resumption of ovulation in premenopausal, anovulatory women with insulin resistance. May decrease hemoglobin and hematocrit. Use with caution in patients with edema and CHF. May increase LDL cholesterol and HDL cholesterol.
Sulfonylureas	Primary effect is to stimulate the release of insulin from the pancreas; secondary effect is to improve tissue sensitivity to insulin; reduced hepatic insulin extraction.	Decreases FPG by 50–60 mg/dl. Decreases HbA_{1c} by 1–2%.	Patients with diabetic ketoacidsosis (with or without coma). Type 1 diabetes. Do not use in patients with a known hypersensitivity or allergy to the drug or any of its components.	Dosage may require adjustment in patients with renal impairment/failure. Dose with caution in patients with impaired liver function. Causes hypoglycemia (especially in elderly; especially in combination with chlorpropamide and glyburide). Causes weight gain. May be preferred in leaner type 2 patients, particularly if symptomatic.

agents used to treat type 2 diabetes.[18-28]

There are several considerations in the initial selection of a therapeutic agent for a patient with type 2 diabetes. For most patients just diagnosed with type 2 diabetes, any of the monotherapeutic agents could potentially be used. One primary consideration is that of efficacy. For example, the α-glucosidase inhibitors (acarbose and miglitol) are less effective than other agents in lowering fasting plasma glucose and hemoglobin A_{1c} but are particularly effective in patients with postprandial hyperglycemia as their predominant glucose abnormality. The α-glucosidase inhibitors have a relatively slow onset due to the necessary titration period to reduce gastrointestinal side effects.

In obese patients it may be preferable to select an agent that does not cause weight gain, such as an α-glucosidase inhibitor or metformin. Metformin was shown to be particularly efficacious in the UKPDS; it may even produce a modest weight loss. Metformin is probably more efficacious than an α-glucosidase inhibitor as monotherapy, and it has a favorable effect on the lipid profile. Obesity, particularly central adiposity, is indicative of insulin resistance, for which metformin would be a useful agent. However, metformin cannot be used in patients with renal impairment or with risk factors for lactic acidosis (see **Table 7**).

The thiazolidinedione group of drugs (troglitazone and rosiglitazone) are also useful in reducing insulin resistance. Although troglitazone was initially approved as monotherapy, the Food and Drug Administration announced changes to labeling and recommended uses of troglitazone in June 1999 as a result of reported cases of hepatotoxicity following troglitazone therapy. Per those recommendations, troglitazone should be limited to patients not adequately controlled by other therapy and should not be used as initial single agent therapy in the treatment of type 2 diabetes (it may be used in combination with sulfonylureas and metformin). Monitoring should include liver function tests before therapy, monthly during the first year of therapy, and quarterly thereafter.

Two additional thiazolidinediones have recently been introduced. Rosiglitazone (Avandia) has been approved for use as monotherapy adjunctively with diet and exercise or in combination with metformin therapy. In clinical studies of almost 5,000 patients, representing 3600 patient years of exposure, rosiglitazone has not resulted in drug-induced hepatotoxicity or increased liver enzyme levels.

Because rosiglitazone is structurally similar to troglitazone, and postmarketing surveillance may provide new information regarding rosiglitazone safety, it is recommended that liver enzymes be evaluated frequently during therapy (refer to **Table 7**). Pioglitazone (Actos) is currently being evaluated by the Food and Drug Administration.

The remaining monotherapeutic options are insulin or the insulin secretogogues: sulfonylurea agents and repaglinide. Insulin is generally reserved for patient presentations described previously in this unit (e.g., very symptomatic, severely hyperglycemic, ketotic, possibly type 1, or pregnant). The sulfonylurea agents and repaglinide are equally efficacious, are effective within 1 week, and share similar adverse effects. Second-generation sulfonylurea agents are dosed once per day and may be increased to twice-daily dosing. Repaglinide is dosed with each meal. Dosing three or more times per day may either cause an adherence problem or be beneficial for patients who require flexibility. You may also consider selecting an insulin secretogogue over other oral agents if a patient is without significant excess body weight or is fairly symptomatic at presentation.

Application of these patient- and agent-specific variables are shown in **Figure 4** (pages 266–7), an expanded version of the American Diabetes Association pharmacologic recommendations.[4,19,29] Patients whose diabetes did not respond to oral monotherapy should receive combination oral therapy, then oral therapy in combination with insulin, and finally insulin therapy. Several approved or frequently studied oral combination regimens as well as suggested regimens for oral therapy in combination with insulin are listed in **Figure 4**. For example, combining insulin with a sulfonylurea has proven useful in achieving glycemic goals, while minimizing weight gain and hypoglycemia.[30-32] One common regimen is termed BIDS (bedtime insulin, daytime sulfonylurea) and includes administration of insulin prior to bedtime as well as a daily dose of a sulfonylurea. Insulin may also be used in combination with other oral antidiabetic medications.[30-39] An example of adding bedtime insulin to a sulfonylurea regimen is:

> If the patient is receiving the maximum dose of a sulfonylurea, add 5–10 units of NPH insulin SQ at 10:00 p.m. to the regimen. Patients must be proficient at home blood glucose monitoring, and should assess their fasting blood glucose every morning. Titrating to a therapeutic fasting blood glucose,

increase the evening NPH by up to 5 units every 4–7 days. As the fasting blood glucose approached goal (e.g., 160–180 mg/dl) increase the NPH by 2–4 units every 4–7 days, and as the fasting blood glucose approaches 140 mg/dl, increase the insulin dose by 1–2 units every 4–7 days.[40] This combination strategy is beneficial because the evening insulin dose works to decrease hepatic glucose production, leading to better-controlled fasting blood glucose, and the daytime administered sulfonlyurea continues to stimulate pancreatic insulin secretion in response to meals.[41]

Patients who do not achieve acceptable blood glucose control with combined insulin–oral therapy regimens (with two, three, or possibly four medications) generally require full insulin therapy. Several possible regimens are listed in **Figure 4**, including intermediate-acting insulin (e.g., NPH insulin), administered twice a day (30 minutes before breakfast and 30 minutes before dinner); intermediate-acting insulin plus short- or rapid-acting insulin (regular or Lispro), administered twice a day (15–30 minutes before breakfast and 15–30 minutes before dinner); multiple injections per day (such as short- or rapid-acting insulin prior to each meal with NPH or Ultralente once or twice daily); or continuous insulin infusion via pump therapy.[41]

Preferred agents in the management of hypertension in patients with diabetes include the angiotensin-converting enzyme (ACE) inhibitors, alpha blockers, calcium channel blockers, and possibly diuretics.[11] ACE inhibitors (e.g., lisinopril and enalapril) have been shown to decrease the progression of diabetic nephropathy, improve insulin sensitivity, and have a neutral effect on the lipid profile.[42–44] ACE inhibitors are also useful in patients with a history of congestive heart failure. Patients who develop a cough with ACE inhibitor therapy may benefit from an ACE-II antagonist (losartan or valsartan). Alpha blockers (prazosin) have been shown to improve insulin sensitivity and to have a beneficial effect on the lipid profile.

The calcium channel blockers (nondihydropyridines [e.g., diltiazem and verapamil] and dihydropyridines [e.g., nifedipine, amlodipine, and felodipine]) are lipid neutral and do not interfere with blood glucose control. Nondihydropyridine calcium channel blockers may improve diabetic nephropathy by decreasing proteinuria and microalbuminuria.[45,46] However, because of cardiac concerns, short-acting formulations of the calcium channel blockers are not recommended.[47–50] A

recent trial compared nisolidipine (a long-acting dihydropyridine calcium channel blocker) with enalapril in preventing or slowing the progression of diabetic complications.[51] Results showed that treatment with nisolidipine was associated with a higher incidence of fatal and nonfatal myocardial infarctions (risk ratio 9.5). It is unclear if this result was due to the adverse effect of nisolidipine, the cardioprotective effect of enalapril, or a combination of both. While this area deserves further research, it seems reasonable to favor ACE inhibitors in this situation.

Diuretics have been shown to be effective in lowering blood pressure and are synergistic with ACE inhibitors. The thiazide diuretics are preferred antihypertensive agents, while the loop diuretics are preferred in congestive heart failure and preferred over thiazides as renal function worsens. Be aware that diuretics may adversely affect the lipid profile and blood glucose control.[7]

Finally, beta-adrenergic blocking agents are associated with adverse effects on peripheral blood flow and may prolong hypoglycemia and mask hypoglycemic symptoms, but they have been shown to be cardioprotective and performed favorably in the UKPDS (patients received atenolol vs. captopril as initial therapy; results showed they were similarly effective in reducing diabetic complications).[52–54]

Case Study

Turn to the APCP in **Appendix A** that has been completed through the "Recommendations for Therapy" column for Mrs. Gonzalez. To improve her control of diabetes (and also positively affect her hypertension and hypercholesterolemia), the recommendation is to institute nonpharmacologic interventions such as diet and exercise. With a hemoglobin A_{1c} of 10.2% and glucose values ranging from 184 to 242 mg/dl, Pharmacist Radcliffe considered recommending pharmacologic therapy at this time as well. However, the patient insisted she had a lot of room to improve her diet and exercise, and wanted to wait to begin drug therapy to treat her type 2 diabetes. The patient presented a similar argument for beginning drug therapy for management of her elevated LDL cholesterol, but the pharmacist explained that it is unlikely that dietary interventions would reduce the LDL cholesterol >25 mg/dl. The pharmacist decided to recommend atorvastatin 10 mg by mouth daily to the physician.

The pharmacist also recommended discontinuing the hydrochlorothiazide and beginning lisinopril

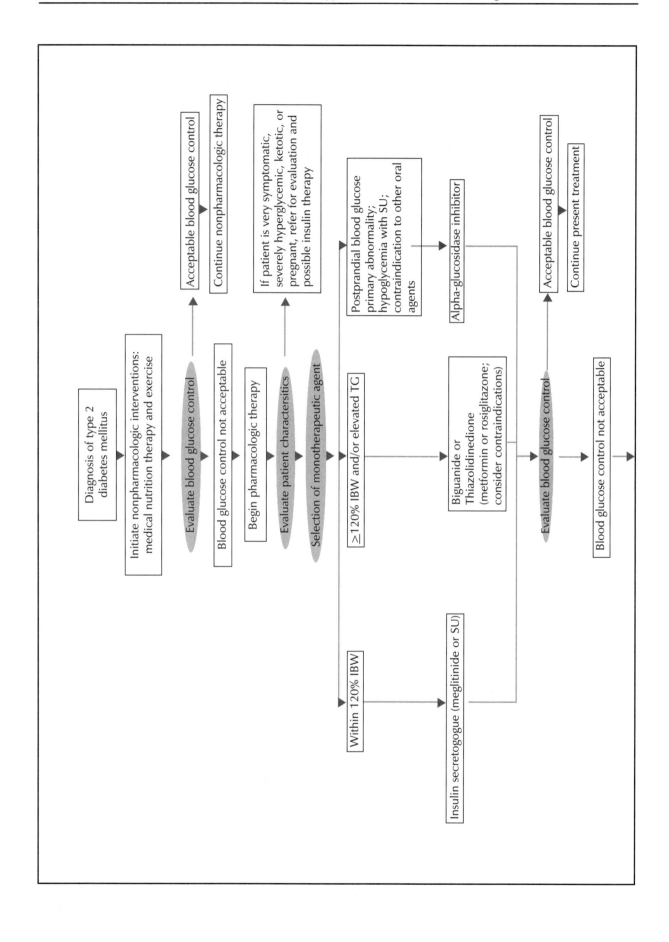

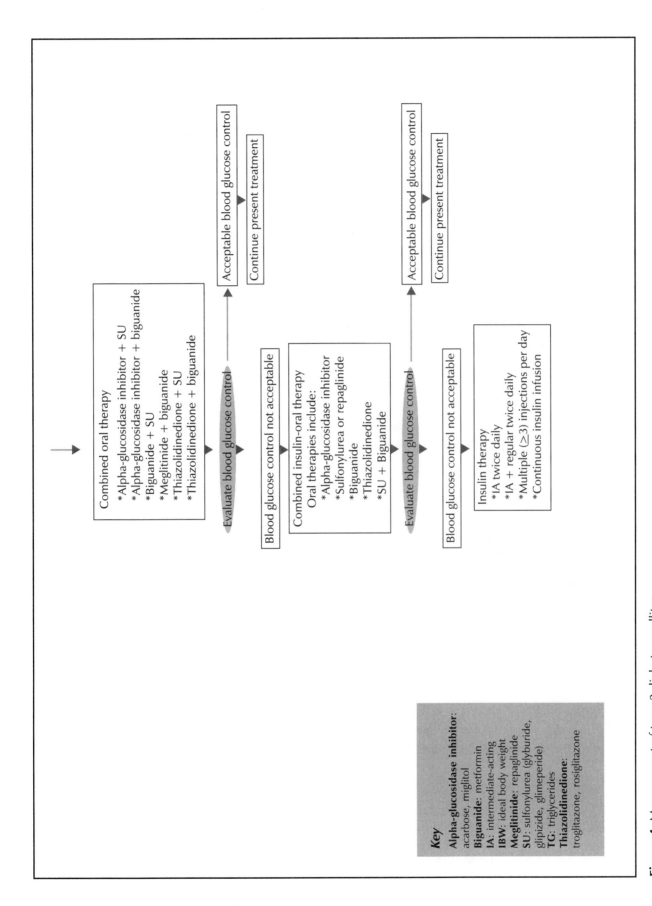

Figure 4. Management of type 2 diabetes mellitus
Source: adapted from references 5, 19, and 29.

10 mg by mouth daily instead. As described above, hydrochlorothiazide may increase blood glucose, and ACE inhibitors are preferred antihypertensive agents in patients with diabetes. If the patient is very successful with her nonpharmacologic interventions, the pharmacist may be able to recommend decreasing or discontinuing the lisinopril therapy.

The pharmacist also recommended beginning conjugated estrogen and progestin therapy, calcium supplementation, and one enteric coated aspirin daily. The pharmacist will work with the patient to select and learn to use a blood glucose monitor and blood pressure cuff, provide home fecal occult blood test cards, encourage the patient to receive an influenza vaccine in the fall, and make an appointment with her primary care physician for information on monthly breast self-examination.

Practice Example

Turn to the case of Mr. Jones in **Appendix B**. Review his database and Diabetes Health Beliefs form. You will notice from Mr. Jones' Diabetes Health Beliefs form that he appreciates the benefits of good blood glucose control, thinks diabetes can be severe, and is susceptible to the effects of diabetes. However, it is clear that he does not value a meal plan, nor does he find it likely he will follow one. On further discussion about type 2 diabetes, Mr. Jones indicates he isn't particularly frightened about any aspect of diabetes. Although he's willing to talk to a dietitian, he states that he is unlikely to make major changes in his diet. The main issue is his erratic and frequently missed mealtimes. He is willing to try to cut back on high-fat food items, but he does not anticipate that his erratic meal pattern will change.

Drawing on the skills you have learned, develop the "Recommendations for Therapy" on Mr. Jones' APCP, develop an educational program for Mr. Jones, and complete the blank "Medication Planning Form for People with Diabetes" for the recommendation to begin repaglinide. When you are done, compare your answers to those described in the next section and in **Appendix C**.

Mr. Jones has many pharmacotherapeutic and related health care goals. With the data collected on March 3, 1998, the pharmacist has identified that the patient is at risk for developing type 2 diabetes and has signs and symptoms suggestive of the disease. The recommendation is to refer Mr. Jones to his primary physician for confirmation of type 2 diabetes. In addition, Mr. Jones has a history of poor control of cholesterol, per patient report. The pharmacist recommends medical nutrition therapy and referral to a dietitian.

As discussed in unit 5 of this module, the pharmacist felt that Mr. Jones might benefit from switching his antihypertensive agent from furosemide to lisinopril, which does not increase blood glucose. Glucose intolerance was noted at the time of Mr. Jones' initial contact; also, lisinopril is a favorable agent in patients with glucose intolerance and potential diabetes when microalbuminuria is noted (as in this case). The initial dose of lisinopril is based on the patient's creatinine clearance. Mr. Jones' creatinine clearance calculates to 39 ml/min, as follows:

He is 5'8", actual body weight 109 kg, ideal body weight 68.4 kg.

Using the creatinine clearance equation discussed in unit 3 of this module:

$$\text{Cl}_{cr} \text{ (for males) ml/min} = \frac{(140 - \text{age})(\text{body weight in kg})}{(\text{SrCr})(72 \text{ kg})}$$

$$= \frac{(140 - 66)(68.4)}{(1.8)(72)}$$

$$= 39 \text{ ml/min}$$

The starting dose of lisinopril for patients with a creatinine clearance of ≥ 30 ml/min is 10 mg per day. Patients with a creatinine clearance between 10 and 30 ml/min should be started at 5 mg per day; those with a creatinine clearance <10 ml/min should begin at 2.5 mg per day.

Other recommendations from the first contact with Mr. Jones include nicotine replacement and smoking cessation counseling, counseling on the risks associated with alcohol use, instructions on the importance of exercise, instructions on peak flow monitoring, provision of home fecal occult blood test cards, and general counseling on medication regimen adherence and the importance of following recommendations for follow-up appointments with health care professionals.

When additional blood tests and physical assessment results became available in April, the pharmacist made additional recommendations. Mr. Jones is diagnosed with type 2 diabetes, and he is symptomatic. Given his high hemoglobin A_{1c} (11.6%) and blood glucose values ranging from 190 to 258 mg/dl, it is unlikely that dietary interventions alone will be sufficient to control Mr. Jones' blood glucose. Refer to the type 2 diabetes management flow chart shown in **Figure 4**. Mr. Jones' blood glucose abnormalities are not limited to postprandial hyperglycemia, therefore, acarbose is unlikely to have a significant effect. It would be reasonable to consider metformin or rosiglitazone, given that Mr. Jones is >120% of his ideal body weight. Unfortunately, Mr. Jones has renal dysfunction, a contraindication for metformin, as well as hepatic dysfunction, a contraindication to rosiglitazone. It is important for the reader to critically evaluate new medications as they become available for the management of type 2 diabetes and appreciate any differences in side effects and dosing considerations. For example, when pioglitazone becomes available, the pharmacist will need to evaluate its effect on liver function (if any). What remains is a choice between a sulfonylurea agent or repagalinide for Mr. Jones (or insulin). Both the sulfonlyurea agents and meglitinide may cause hypoglycemia. While the sulfonlyurea agents are less expensive, the pharmacist recommends repaglinide for Mr. Jones because of his erratic meal pattern. He agrees to take repaglinide prior to each meal, but he cannot promise that his meals will occur more regularly.

When the pharmacist received the results of the fasting lipid profile from March 30, 1998, he noted that Mr. Jones' LDL cholesterol is 229 mg/dl. As discussed, it is unlikely that dietary adherence will lower the LDL cholesterol >25 mg/dl, and the patient is clearly >25 mg/dl above his LDL cholesterol goal (<100 mg/dl). Therefore, on 4/3/98 the pharmacist added to the recommendations to begin cholestyramine 4 g twice daily. As you recall and can see in **Table 2**, the first choice of therapy for treating an elevated LDL cholesterol in a patient with diabetes is use of an HMG-CoA reductase inhibitor. Unfortunately, Mr. Jones has pre-existing liver disease, as evidenced by elevated liver enzymes. The next choice is a bile-acid sequestrant, which has been shown to lower the LDL cholesterol by 15–30%. The pharmacist recommended beginning Questran Light 4 g (1 scoop) twice daily, which, when combined with better glycemic control and dietary fat restriction, should move Mr. Jones closer to his LDL cholesterol goal. The pharmacist needed to provide significant patient education concerning the use of cholestyramine for Mr. Jones, particularly in light of his history of therapy nonadherence. Because cholestyramine increases the risk of constipation, the pharmacist advised Mr. Jones to purchase Metamucil and begin treatment if constipation occurred.

The pharmacist recommended clotrimazole cream for the fungal skin infection on Mr. Jones'

toe, recommended one enteric coated aspirin daily, provided referrals to the ophthalmologist and dentist, and instructed Mr. Jones on home blood glucose monitoring.

Summary

In this unit you have learned a great deal about factors that influence design of a therapy regimen for ambulatory patients with type 2 diabetes, including fear of complications, physical disabilities, health beliefs, and satisfaction with treatment. You learned about the existence of treatment guidelines for type 2 diabetes and the need to individualize the guidelines for each patient. When selecting a monotherapeutic diabetes medication, there are many variables to consider. Selecting a medication to treat type 2 diabetes is just one part of developing therapeutic recommendations in caring for patients with type 2 diabetes; you must also consider comorbid states and other health-related needs.

As a pharmacist it is logical for you to serve as a diabetes educator. Patients with type 2 diabetes frequently interact with their pharmacist, and these opportunities may be used to benefit the patient and pharmacist.

References

1. Hendricks LE, Hendricks RT. Greatest fears of type 1 and type 2 patients about having diabetes: implications for diabetes educators. *The Diabetes Educator* 1998;24:168–73.

2. Feste C. *The Physician Within*. 2nd ed. Minneapolis, MN: Chronimed Publishing; 1993.

3. Bradley C, editor. *Handbook of Psychology and Diabetes: A Guide to Psychological Measurement in Diabetes Research and Practice*: Chur, Switzerland: Harwood Academic Publishers; 1995. Diabetes Treatment Satisfaction Questionnaire (DTSQ), p. 115.

4. Bradley C. Diabetes treatment satisfaction questionnaire: change version for use alongside status version provides appropriate solution where ceiling effects occur. *Diabetes Care* 1999;22:530–2.

5. American Diabetes Association: ADA 1998 Clinical Practice Recommendations At-a-Glance, Tri-fold Pocket Chart. Catalog number, 5905-02; Alexandria, VA: American Diabetes Association, 1998.

6. American Diabetes Association. *Medical Management of Pregnancy Complicated by Diabetes*. 2nd ed. Alexandria, VA: American Diabetes Association; 1995.

7. Carr DB, Gabbe S. Gestational diabetes: detection, management and implications. *Clinical Diabetes* 1998;16:4–11.

8. Sullivan BA, Henderson ST, Davis JM. Gestational diabetes. *J Am Pharm Assoc* 1998;38:364–71.

9. American Pharmaceutical Association Diabetes Mellitus Panel. American Pharmaceutical Association drug treatment protocols: management of gestational diabetes mellitus and impaired glucose tolerance during pregnancy. *J Am Pharm Assoc* 1998;38:307–16.

10. American Diabetes Association. Management of dyslipidemia in adults with diabetes. *Diabetes Care* 1999;22(*Suppl* 1):S56–9.

11. The Sixth Report of the Joint National Committee on Prevention, Detection, Evaluation, and Treatment of High Blood Pressure. *Arch Intern Med* 1997;157:2413–2446.

12. American Diabetes Association. National standards for diabetes self-management education programs and American Diabetes Association review criteria. *Diabetes Care* 1999;22(*Suppl* 1):S111–4.

13. "Medication Planning Forms for People with Diabetes." http://www.niddk.nih.gov/health/diabetes/pubs/med/forms.htm. Accessed Jan. 30, 1999.

14. Williams AS. Teaching nonvisual diabetes self-care: choosing appropriate tools and techniques for visually impaired individuals. *Diabetes Spectrum* 1997;10:128–34.

15. Curry SJ. Commentary (on "In search of how people change: applications to addictive behaviors"). *Diabetes Spectrum* 1993;6:34–5.

16. American Diabetes Association. Standards of medical care for patients with diabetes mellitus. *Diabetes Care* 1999;22(*Suppl* 1):S32–41.

17. American Diabetes Association. The pharmacological treatment of hyperglycemia in NIDDM (consensus statement). *Diabetes Care* 1996;19(*Suppl* 1):S54–61.

18. Oates JA, Wood AJJ. Oral hypoglycemic agents. *N Eng J Med* 1989;321:1231–45.

19. White JR. The pharmacological reduction of blood glucose in patients with type 2 diabetes mellitus. *Clinical Diabetes* 1998;16:58–69.

20. Scheen AJ, Lefebvre PJ. Oral antidiabetic agents. *Drugs* 1998;56:225–36.

21. Elson DF, Meredith M. Therapy for type 2 diabetes mellitus. *Wis Med J* 1998;49–54.

22. Wang F. Focus on repaglinide. *Formulary* 1998;33:409–23.

23. Goldberg RB, Einhorn D, Lucas CP, et al. A randomized placebo-controlled trial of repaglinide in the treatment of type 2 diabetes. *Diabetes Care.* 1998;21:1897–1903.

24. Martin AE, Montgomery PA. Acarbose: an α-glucosidase inhibitor. *Am J Health-Syst Pharm* 1996;53:2277–90.

25. Wildasin EM, Skaar DJ, Kirchain WR, Hulse M. Metformin, a promising oral antihyperglycemic for the treatment of noninsulin-dependent diabetes mellitus. *Pharmacotherapy* 1997;17:62–73.

26. Cusi K, DeFonzo RA. Metformin: a review of its metabolic effects. *Diabetes Rev* 1998;6:89–131.

27. Schwartz S, Raskin P, Fonseca, Graveline JF for the Troglitazone and Exogenous Insulin Study Group. Effect of troglitazone in insulin-treated patients with type II diabetes mellitus. *N Eng J Med* 1998;338:861–6.

28. Johnson MD, Campbell LK, Campbell RK. Troglitazone: review and assessment of its role in the treatment of patients with impaired glucose tolerance and diabetes mellitus. *Ann Pharmacother* 1998;32:337–48.

29. Oki JC, Isley WL. Rethinking new and old diabetes drugs for type 2 disease. *Pract Diabetology* 1997;27–40.

30. Koivisto VA. Insulin therapy in type II diabetes. *Diabetes Care* 1993;16(*Suppl* 3):29–39.

31. Johnson JL, Wolf SL, Kabadi UM. Efficacy of insulin and sulfonylurea combination therapy in type II diabetes. *Arch Int Med* 1996;156:259–64.

32. Pugh JA, Wagner ML, Sawyer J, Ramirez G, Tuley M, Friedberg SJ. Is combination sulfonylurea and insulin therapy useful in NIDDM patients? *Diabetes Care* 1992;15:953–9.

33. Schwartz S, Raskin P, Fonseca V, Graveline JF, for the Troglitazone and Exogenous Insulin Study Group. Effect of troglitazone in insulin-treated patients with type II diabetes mellitus. *NEJM* 1998;338:861-6.

34. Buse JB, Gumbiner B, Mathias NP, Nelson DM, Faja BW, Whitcomb RW, for the Troglitazone and Exogenous Insulin Study Group. Troglitazone use in insulin-treated type 2 diabetic patients. *Diabetes Care* 1998;21:1455–61.

35. Giugliano D, Auatraro A, Consoli G, Minei A,

Ceriello A, De Rosa N, D'Onofrio F. Metformin for obese, insulin-treated diabetic patients: improvement in glycaemic control and reduction of metabolic risk factors. *Eur J Clin Pharmacol* 1993;44:107–12.

36. Bergenstal R, Johnson M, Whipple D, Noller D, Boyce K, Roth L, Upham P, Fish L, Debold R. Advantages of adding metformin to multiple dose insulin therapy in type 2 diabetes (Abstract). *Diabetes* 47(*Suppl* 1):A89, 1998.

37. Chiasson JL, Josse RG, Hunt JA, Palmason C, Rodger NW, Ross SA, Ryan EA, Tan MH, Wolever TMS. The efficacy of acarbose in the treatment of patients with non-insulin-dependent diabetes mellitus. *Ann Intern Med* 1994;121:928–35.

38. Kelley DE, Magner J, Kroll A, Taylor T. Efficacy and safety of acarbose in patients with type 2 diabetes inadequately controlled with insulin therapy (Abstract). *Diabetes* 1998;47(*Suppl* 1):348.

39. Coniff RF, Shapiro JA, Seaton TB, Hoogwerf FJ, Hunt JA. A double-blind placebo-controlled trial evaluating the safety and efficacy of acarbose for the treatment of patients with insulin-requiring type 2 diabetes. *Diabetes Care* 1995;18:928–32.

40. Riddle MC, DeFronzo RA. Combination therapy: insulin-sulfonylurea and insulin-metformin. In: DeFronzo RA, editor. *Current Therapy of Diabetes Mellitus*. St. Louis, MO: Mosby;1998. p.117–21.

41. Skyler JS. Insulin therapy in type 2 diabetes mellitus. In: DeFronzo RA, editor. *Current Therapy of Diabetes Mellitus*. St. Louis, MO: Mosby; 1998. p. 108–16.

42. Lewis EJ, Hunsicker LG, Bain RP, Rohde RD, for the Collaborative Study Group. The effect of anogiotensin-converting-enzyme inhibition on diabetic nephropathy. *N Engl J Med* 1993;329:1456–62.

43. Ravid M, Lang R, Rachmani R, Lishner M. Long-term renoprotective effect of angiotensin-converting eynzme inhibition in non-insulin dependent diabetes mellitus: a 7-year follow-up study. *Arch Intern Med* 1996;156:286–9.

44. Kasiske BL, Kalil RNS, Ma JZ, Liao M, Keane WF. Effect of antihypertensive therapy on the kidney in patients with diabetes: a meta-reression analysis. *Ann Intern Med* 1993;118:129–38.

45. Bakris GL, Copley JB, Vicknair N, Sadler R, Leurgans S. Calcium channel blockers versus other antihypertensive therapies on progression of NIDDM associated nephropathy. *Kidney Int* 1996;50:1641–50.

46. Velussi M, Brocco E, Frigato F, et al. Effects of cilazapril and amlodipine on kidney function in hypertensive NIDDM patients. *Diabetes* 1996;45:216–22.

47. Grossman E, Merrerli FH, Grodzicki T, Kowey P. Should a moratorium be placed on sublingual nifedipine capsules given for hypertensive emergencies and pseudoemergencies? *JAMA* 1996;276:1328–31.

48. Furberg CD, Psaty BM, Meyer JV. Nifedipine: dose-related increase in mortality in patients with coronary heart disease. *Circulation* 1995;92:1326–31.

49. Ad Hoc Subcommittee of the Liaison Committee of the World Health Organization and the International Society of Hypertension. Effects of calcium antagonists on the risks of coronary heart disease, cancer and bleeding. *J Hypertens* 1997;15:105–15.

50. Psaty BM, Furberg CD. Clinical implications of the WHO/ISH statement on calcium antagonists. *J Hypertens* 1997;15:1197–1200.

51. Estacio RO, Jeffers BW, Hiatt WR, Biggerstaff SL, Gifford N, Schrier RW. The effect of nisoldipine as compared with enalapril on cardiovascular outcomes in patients with non-insulin-dependent diabetes and hypertension. *N Engl J Med* 1998;338:645–52.

52. Curb JD, Pressel SL, Cutler JA, et al. For the Systolic Hypertension in the Elderly Program Cooperative Research Group. Effect of diuretic-based antihypertensive treatment on cardiovascular disease risk in older diabetic patients with isolated systolic hypertension. *JAMA* 1996;276:1886–92.

53. Shorr RI, Ray WA, Daugherty JR, Griffin MR. Antihypertensives and the risk of serious hypoglycemia in older persons using insulin or sulfonylureas. *JAMA* 1997;278:40–3.

54. U.K. Prospective Diabetes Study Group. Efficacy of atenolol and captopril in reducing risk of macrovascular and microvascular complications in type 2 diabetes: UKPDS 39. *Br Med J* 1998;317:713–20.

Self-Study Questions

Objective

Explain how patient-related concerns unique to ambulatory patients with type 2 diabetes may influence the design of their therapy regimen.

1. Explain how patient-related concerns unique to an ambulatory patient with type 2 diabetes may influence the design of his or her therapy regimen.

2. Explain why the patient's fears need to be considered when making decisions on the design of his or her therapy regimen.

3. Explain why a patient's disabilities need to be considered when making decisions on the design of his or her therapy regimen.

Objective

Explain the use of treatment guidelines in the design of therapy regimens for ambulatory patients with type 2 diabetes.

4. Explain the use of treatment guidelines in the design of a therapy regimen for an ambulatory patient with type 2 diabetes.

5. Explain guidelines for the treatment of dyslipidemia in patients with type 2 diabetes.

6. Explain how the American Diabetes Association guidelines and other guidelines allow for the individualization of treatment of a patient with type 2 diabetes.

Objective

Explain education needs unique to ambulatory patients with type 2 diabetes.

7. List the common education needs unique to ambulatory patients with type 2 diabetes.

8. Explain the need for ambulatory patients with type 2 diabetes to be educated on proper foot care.

9. Explain the need for ambulatory patients with type 2 diabetes to be educated on exercise.

Objective

Explain factors unique to ambulatory patients with type 2 diabetes that affect the approaches used for education, including patient-specific factors.

10. Explain how the best approach to education for an ambulatory patient with type 2 diabetes may be determined.

Objective

State potential education resources used to meet an ambulatory diabetes patient's educational needs so that the patient may successfully participate in the pharmacist's care plan.

11. List potential patient-specific education resources that meet a diabetes patient's needs for learning.

Objective

Design a therapy regimen (including patient-specific education) that meets the pharmacotherapeutic and related health care goals established for an ambulatory patient with type 2 diabetes, integrates patient-specific disease and drug information as well as ethical and quality-of-life issues, and considers pharmacoeconomic principles.

12. Refer to the case of Ms. McLucas, in **Appendix D**. Building on the APCP form provided, design a recommended therapeutic plan and an educational plan for the patient.

Self-Study Answers

1. The patient may hold health beliefs or fears about diabetes that preclude his or her adherence to therapeutic recommendations. The patient may also have disabilities (physical or psychological) that may make plan implementation difficult. Finally, the patient's satisfaction plays a large role in adherence; therefore, treatment satisfaction as well as quality of life should be evaluated as the treatment regimen changes.

2. Patients who hold specific fears about diabetes (e.g., amputation and blindness) may be overwhelmed and feel that trying to control their disease is useless. Studies have shown that patients who are better educated about their diabetes feel more in control of their disease.

3. The patient's physical and other limitations must be considered when designing the therapy regimen because they may affect the patient's ability to provide self-care or may require use of a special educational approach. For example, a patient with decreased vision may not be able to monitor his or her blood glucose or draw up or inject insulin. Special equipment such as a blood glucose monitor with voice synthesizer and insulin measurement aids can be recommended in this instance. A patient with visual impairment may also require different types of patient education materials and approaches.

4. Treatment guidelines help the practitioner establish therapeutic recommendations. The pharmacist must assure currency of the guidelines and remember to individualize recommendations for the patient.

5. One common abnormality found in an ambulatory patient with type 2 diabetes who has concomitant dyslipidemia is elevated LDL cholesterol. According to the American Diabetes Association recommendations, the first choice for treating this would be use of an HMG-CoA reductase inhibitor (statin). If there are contradindications to HMG-CoA reductase inhibitor use, consider a bide acid binding resin.

Another common dyslipidemic finding is hypertriglyceridemia. Fortunately, improved glycemic control alone will lower the triglyceride level. If this is insufficient, the patient may benefit from a fibric acid derivative (particularly if the hypertriglyceridemia is isolated) or an HMG-CoA reductase inhibitor if both the triglycerides and LDL cholesterol are elevated.

For patients who have a low HDL cholesterol, encourage behavioral interventions such as weight loss and increased activity as well as improving glycemic control.

6. Treatment guidelines for the management of type 2 diabetes allow for individualization by considering patient-related variables such as body weight, glycemic control patterns, concomitant diseases that influence drug therapy, and preference for dosing regimen (see **Figure 4**).

7. a. Diabetes overview
   b. Stress and psychosocial adjustment
   c. Family involvement and social support
   d. Nutrition
   e. Exercise and activity
   f. Medications
   g. Monitoring and use of results
   h. Relationship among nutrition, exercise, medication, and blood glucose levels
   i. Prevention, detection, and treatment of acute complications
   j. Prevention, detection, and treatment of chronic complications
   k. Foot, skin, and dental care
   l. Behavior change strategies, goal setting, risk factor reduction, and problem solving
   m. Benefits, risks, and management options for improving glucose control
   n. Preconception care, pregnancy, and gestational diabetes
   o. Use of health care system and community resources

8. As discussed in previous units and highlighted in this unit as an education need, ambulatory patients with diabetes should be well-educated on proper foot care inspection to reduce amputations that arise from improper care.

Patients with diabetes may develop neuropathy, losing protective sensation in their feet. Should the patient have an injury that goes unnoticed, it can quickly become a more serious problem.

9. Patients with type 2 diabetes should follow a routine exercise plan, such as walking 3–5 days per week. This will enhance insulin-mediated glucose utilization and blood glucose control.

10. It is important to consider the patient's readiness to learn when designing the education program. The patient's stage of readiness will guide you in selecting what type of education strategy to use.

11. Resources may be obtained from the American Diabetes Association (e.g., "Right from the Start") or the American Association of Diabetes Educators (e.g.,"Life with Diabetes").

12. Refer to the completed APCP and education program for Ms. McLucas (**Appendix E**).

Diabetes Health Beliefs

Patient **Rose Gonzalez**   Date **2/27/98**

STATEMENT	Agree	Disagree
BENEFIT		
I'll be healthier in later life if I control my diabetes.	✓	
I believe that exercise can help me control my diabetes.	?	
Controlling my blood glucose will help me avoid heart disease.	?	
Changing my eating habits would help me control my diabetes.	?	
Even if I took my medicine as I should, I wouldn't be able to control my diabetes.	✓	
I can control my diabetes if I follow my regimen closely.		✓
COST		
It will take a lot of effort to control my diabetes.	✓	
I would have to change too many habits to use a meal plan.		✓
Taking my medication interferes with my daily activities.		✓
I'm always hungry when I stick to my meal plan.	?	
It takes a lot of effort to exercise.	✓	
SEVERITY		
Diabetes is a serious disease if you don't control it.	✓	
SUSCEPTIBILITY		
My diabetes would be worse day-to-day if my control is poor.	✓	
I'm more likely to have eye problems if my control is poor.	✓	
If my diabetes isn't controlled, I'm likely to die sooner.	✓	

Patient Education Program for Mrs. Gonzalez

Goals:

1. To educate Mrs. Gonazlez about diabetes mellitus and the importance of blood glucose control.
2. To educate Mrs. Gonzalez about uncontrolled hypertension and hypercholesterolemia and potential complications.
3. To educate Mrs. Gonzalez on the importance of health maintenance.

Educational Objective	*Date Taught*	*Outcome*	*Follow-up Required?*
1. Mrs. Gonzalez will understand what diabetes mellitus is, including: -basic pathophysiology -the role of blood glucose control -potential complications of diabetes -signs and symptoms of hyperglycemia			
2. Mrs. Gonzalez will understand the role of hypertension and hypercholesterolemia and complications of each, which may interact with and worsen complications of diabetes.			
3. Mrs. Gonzalez will understand the role of hormone replacement therapy and daily aspirin therapy as part of her therapeutic regimen.			
4. Mrs. Gonzalez will understand how to properly evaluate blood glucose and will monitor blood glucose as recommended.			
5. Mrs. Gonzalez will understand how to properly monitor blood pressure and will monitor blood pressure as recommended.			
6. Mrs. Gonzalez will understand the importance of adherence to dietary recommendations for control of diabetes, hypertension, and hypercholesterolemia.			
7. Mrs. Gonzalez will understand the importance of adherence to an exercise program for control of diabetes, hypertension, and hyper-cholesterolemia.			
8. Mrs. Gonzalez will understand the importance of performing annual home fecal occult blood tests and monthly breast self-examinations.			

Educational Objective	Date Taught	Outcome	Follow-up Required?

9. Mrs. Gonzalez will understand the importance of follow-up with health care providers, including the ophthalmologist, dentist, pharmacist, and primary care provider.

10. Mrs. Gonzalez will understand the importance of taking her medications as prescribed and at the recommended times.

11. Mrs. Gonzalez will recognize adverse effects of her medications and what action to take should they occur.

12. Mrs. Gonzalez will understand the importance of and demonstrate good technique for foot and skin inspection.

Outcome:

1. Patient restated content correctly/performed task acceptably well.
2. Patient needs reinforcement of content or performance of task.
3. Patient cannot or will not restate content correctly or perform task.

Content:

Content will depend on Mrs. Gonzalez' current understanding of the above issues. Educational content will fill in gaps in her knowledge base.

Delivery Methods:

Method is verbal for all objectives. Provided video on introduction to diabetes mellitus. Provided book, *Right from the Start*, on type 2 diabetes. Demonstrated blood glucose and blood pressure monitoring.

Evaluation of Effectiveness:

1. Patient interview for health beliefs, restate content when requested, adherence to recommended follow-up
2. Demonstrate use of blood glucose monitoring; demonstrate foot and skin inspection
3. Refill records for medications and metabolic control

AMBULATORY PHARMACIST'S CARE PLAN

Patient ___Rose Gonzalez___   Pharmacist ___Jane Radcliffe___   Date ___2/20/98___

Page 1 of 2

DATE IDENTIFIED	PROBLEM (TPL)	PHARMACOTHERAPEUTIC AND RELATED HEALTH CARE GOAL	RECOMMENDATIONS FOR THERAPY	MONITORING PARAMETER(S)	DESIRED ENDPOINT(S)	MONITORING FREQUENCY
2/20/98	poor control of diabetes	Improve diabetes control ; prevent complications.	Institute non-pcol interventions (diet & exercise)			
"	poor control of HTN	Improve BP control; prevent complications.	As above, plus rec. Δ to lisinopril 10 mg QD			
"	poor control of cholest.	Improve lipid control; prevent complications.	nonpcol interventions & Atorvastatin 10 mg			
"	not on daily ASA tx	↓ risk CV complic. of diabetes	Rec. EC ASA 325 mg QD			
"	post menopausal s̄ HRT	↓ risk post-men. SXs/↓ risks of postmenopause	Rec. conjugated estrogen/progestin			
"	not receiving calcium tx	↓ risk for osteoporosis	Rec calcium carbonate 500 mg TID			
"	Potential of HCTZ to affect DM & chol.	Avoid worsened BG & lipid control	D/C HCTZ			
"	no exercise plan	start & adhere to regular exercise program.	Begin regular walking program			

AMBULATORY PHARMACIST'S CARE PLAN

Patient __Rose Gonzalez__   Pharmacist __Jane Radcliffe__   Date __2/20/98__

Page 2 of 2

DATE IDENTIFIED	PROBLEM (TPL)	PHARMACOTHERAPEUTIC AND RELATED HEALTH CARE GOAL	RECOMMENDATIONS FOR THERAPY	MONITORING PARAMETER(S)	DESIRED ENDPOINT(S)	MONITORING FREQUENCY
2/20/98	no MNT plan	start & adhere to MNT plan.	refer to RD— follow meal plan			
''	no home BG monitoring	learn & regularly perform SMBG	select & explain use of BG monitor			
''	no home BP monitoring	learn & regularly perform BP measurements	select and explain use of BP cuff			
''	no home fecal test	perform annual home fecal blood test	Provide home fecal blood test cards			
''	no influenza vaccine	receive annual influenza vaccine	Receive flu vaccine Fall 98			
''	no monthly breast self-exam	learn & regularly perform exam	refer to primary physician for exam technique			

Diabetes Health Beliefs

Patient **George Jones**   Date **4/3/98**

STATEMENT	Agree	Disagree
BENEFIT		
I'll be healthier in later life if I control my diabetes.	✓	
I believe that exercise can help me control my diabetes.	✓	
Controlling my blood glucose will help me avoid heart disease.	✓	
Changing my eating habits would help me control my diabetes.		✓
Even if I took my medicine as I should, I wouldn't be able to control my diabetes.		✓
I can control my diabetes if I follow my regimen closely.	✓	
COST		
It will take a lot of effort to control my diabetes.		✓
I would have to change too many habits to use a meal plan.	✓	
Taking my medication interferes with my daily activities.		✓
I'm always hungry when I stick to my meal plan.	✓	
It takes a lot of effort to exercise.		✓
SEVERITY		
Diabetes is a serious disease if you don't control it.	✓	
SUSCEPTIBILITY		
My diabetes would be worse day-to-day if my control is poor.	✓	
I'm more likely to have eye problems if my control is poor.	✓	
If my diabetes isn't controlled, I'm likely to die sooner.	✓	

AMBULATORY PHARMACIST'S CARE PLAN

Patient __George Jones__   Pharmacist __John O'Malley__   Date __3-3-98__

Page 1 of 3

DATE IDENTIFIED	PROBLEM (TPL)	PHARMACOTHERAPEUTIC AND RELATED HEALTH CARE GOAL	RECOMMENDATIONS FOR THERAPY	MONITORING PARAMETER(S)	DESIRED ENDPOINT(S)	MONITORING FREQUENCY
3/3/98	Sx and BG suggestive of DM. High risk status	Rule in/out DM. Determine cause of high BG and nocturia				
	poor control of hypertension	Improve BP control;				
		Prevent complications				
	nonadherence to diet	start and adhere to prescribed meal plan				
	h/o med schedule nonadherence	adherence to medication regimen				
	Furosemide may worsen lipids	Avoid worsened lipid profile				
	smoking history	Stop smoking				
	Alcohol use history	Stop alcohol use				

AMBULATORY PHARMACIST'S CARE PLAN

Patient ___George Jones___   Pharmacist ___John O'Malley___   Date ___3-3-98___

Page 2 of 3

DATE IDENTIFIED	PROBLEM (TPL)	PHARMACOTHERAPEUTIC AND RELATED HEALTH CARE GOAL	RECOMMENDATIONS FOR THERAPY	MONITORING PARAMETER(S)	DESIRED ENDPOINT(S)	MONITORING FREQUENCY
3/3/98	h/o nonadherence to f/u appts	Adherence to f/u appt. scheduling				
	nonadherence to exercise	start and adhere to exercise plan				
	Not doing peak flow monitoring	Learn and perform peak flow monitoring regularly				
	No rectal/prostate exam	Annual rectal prostate exam				
	no home fecal test	Home fecal blood test q 6 months				
4/3/98	poor control of diabetes	Improve control; prevent complications				
	Furosemide may ↑ BG	Avoid worsened BP control				
	Fungal skin infection on toe	Eliminate fungal toe infection				

AMBULATORY PHARMACIST'S CARE PLAN

Patient __George Jones__   Pharmacist __John O'Malley__   Date __3-3-98__

Page 3 of 3

DATE IDENTIFIED	PROBLEM (TPL)	PHARMACOTHERAPEUTIC AND RELATED HEALTH CARE GOAL	RECOMMENDATIONS FOR THERAPY	MONITORING PARAMETER(S)	DESIRED ENDPOINT(S)	MONITORING FREQUENCY
4/3	Insensate feet	Absence of infection trauma, ulcerations				
	Not on daily ASA tx	↓ risk CV complications 2° to diabetes				
	Poor control of cholesterol	Improve control, prevent complications				
	Not doing SMBG	Learn and perform regular SMBG				
	No dilated retinal exam	Annual dilated retinal exam				
	No recent dental exam	Dental exam q 6 months				
	liver dysfunction	monitor liver function				

Questions To Ask About Your Diabetes Medicines

Ask these questions when your doctor prescribes a medicine. Write the answers in pencil so that you can make changes if your doctor changes your medicines.

When do I take the medicine—before a meal, with a meal, or after a meal?

_____

How often should I take the medicine?

_____

Should I take the medicine at the same time every day?

_____

What should I do if I forget to take my medicine?

_____

What side effects may happen?

_____

_____

What should I do if I get side effects?

_____

_____

My Diabetes Medicines

Fill in this record about your diabetes medicines with the help of your doctor or diabetes teacher. Write this in pencil so you can make changes when your doctor makes changes in your diabetes medicines.

The names of the diabetes medicines (insulin or pills) I take are:

_____

I take _____ (name of diabetes medicine) _____ times a day.
At (time)_____ I take (amount)_____.
At (time)_____ I take (amount)_____.
At (time)_____ I take (amount)_____.

I take _____ (name of diabetes medicine) _____ times a day.
At (time)_____ I take (amount)_____.
At (time)_____ I take (amount)_____.
At (time)_____ I take (amount)_____.

I take _____ (name of diabetes medicine) _____ times a day.
At (time)_____ I take (amount)_____.
At (time)_____ I take (amount)_____.
At (time)_____ I take (amount)_____.

I should call my doctor or diabetes teacher if I have these problems with my diabetes medicines:

_____
_____

I should call my doctor or diabetes teacher if my blood glucose is too low or too high for several days.
Too low is _____ mg/dl for _____ days.
Too high is _____ mg/dl for _____ days.

My blood sugar should be between _____mg/dl and _____mg/dl before my first meal of the day.

My blood sugar should be between _____mg/dl and _____mg/dl 1–2 hours after a meal.

My blood sugar is too low at _____mg/dl.

My blood sugar is too high at _____mg/dl.

My hemoglobin A_{1c} should be _____%.

AMBULATORY PHARMACIST'S CARE PLAN

Patient George Jones   Pharmacist John O'Malley   Date 3-3-98

Page 1 of 3

DATE IDENTIFIED	PROBLEM (TPL)	PHARMACOTHERAPEUTIC AND RELATED HEALTH CARE GOAL	RECOMMENDATIONS FOR THERAPY	MONITORING PARAMETER(S)	DESIRED ENDPOINT(S)	MONITORING FREQUENCY
3/3/98	SX and BG suggestive of DM. High risk of DM status	Rule in/out DM. Determine cause of high BG and nocturia	Refer to primary physician—await results			
	poor control of hypertension	Improve BP control; Prevent complications	D/C furosemide Begin lisinopril 10 mg q AM			
	nonadherence to diet	start and adhere to prescribed meal plan	Referral to dietitian			
	h/o med schedule nonadherence	adherence to medication regimen	Provide written instructions			
	Furosemide may worsen lipids	Avoid worsened lipid profile	Rec d/c furosemide. Begin lisinopril			
	smoking history	Stop smoking	Nicotine replacement and counseling. Pt. refuses at this time			
	Alcohol use history	Stop alcohol use	↓ or stop alcohol use Pt. refuses at this time			

AMBULATORY PHARMACIST'S CARE PLAN

Patient ___George Jones___   Pharmacist ___John O'Malley___   Date ___3-3-98___

Page 2 of 3

DATE IDENTIFIED	PROBLEM (TPL)	PHARMACOTHERAPEUTIC AND RELATED HEALTH CARE GOAL	RECOMMENDATIONS FOR THERAPY	MONITORING PARAMETER(S)	DESIRED ENDPOINT(S)	MONITORING FREQUENCY
3/3/98	h/o nonadherence to flu appts	Adherence to flu appt. scheduling	Counsel pt.			
	nonadherence to exercise	start and adhere to exercise plan	Counsel pt.			
	Not doing peak flow monitoring	Learn and perform peak flow monitoring regularly	Instruct pt. on peak flow monitoring			
	No rectal/ prostate exam	Annual rectal prostate exam	Refer to PCP. Pt. refuses at this time			
	no home fecal test	Home fecal blood test q 6 months	Provide home fecal test cards. Pt. refuses at this time			
	poor control of diabetes	Improve control; prevent complications	Rec. repaglinide 0.5 mg before meals			
4/3/98	Furosemide may ↑ BG	Avoid worsened BP control	Rec d/c furosemide Begin lisinopril			
	Fungal skin infection on toe	Eliminate fungal toe infection	Rec. Lotrimin cream to affected area BID for 7-10 days			

AMBULATORY PHARMACIST'S CARE PLAN

Patient __George Jones__   Pharmacist __John O'Malley__   Date __3-3-98__

Page 3 of 3

DATE IDENTIFIED	PROBLEM (TPL)	PHARMACOTHERAPEUTIC AND RELATED HEALTH CARE GOAL	RECOMMENDATIONS FOR THERAPY	MONITORING PARAMETER(S)	DESIRED ENDPOINT(S)	MONITORING FREQUENCY
4/3	Insensate feet	Absence of infection trauma, ulcerations	Daily self-inspection Quarterly exam			
	Not on daily ASA tx	↓ risk CV complications 2° to diabetes	Rec EC ASA 325 mg QD			
	Poor control of cholesterol	Improve control, prevent complications	Refer for MNT Rec. cholestyramine 4 g BID			
	Not doing SMBG	Learn and perform regular SMBG	Instruct on SMBG			
	No dilated retinal exam	Annual dilated retinal exam	Refer to ophthalmologist			
	No recent dental exam	Dental exam q 6 months	Refer to dentist			
	liver dysfunction	monitor liver function	monitor LFTs			

Questions To Ask About Your Diabetes Medicines

Ask these questions when your doctor prescribes a medicine. Write the answers in pencil so that you can make changes if your doctor changes your medicines.

Mr. George Jones

When do I take the medicine—before a meal, with a meal, or after a meal?

15 minutes before each meal

How often should I take the medicine?

Only before each meal. If you skip a meal, skip the Prandin. For an extra meal, take an extra Prandin.

Should I take the medicine at the same time every day?

Before each meal, whenever that is.

What should I do if I forget to take my medicine?

Wait until before the next meal.

What side effects may happen?

Low blood glucose (hypoglycemia) ⇒ shaky, nervous, sweaty, hard time concentrating

What should I do if I get side effects?

Eat 5-6 Lifesavers or drink 1/2 cup juice

Check your blood sugar first; record this in your logbook.

My Diabetes Medicines

Fill in this record about your diabetes medicines with the help of your doctor or diabetes teacher. Write this in pencil so you can make changes when your doctor makes changes in your diabetes medicines.

The names of the diabetes medicines (insulin or pills) I take are:

__Prandin (repaglinide)_____

I take __Prandin_____ (name of diabetes medicine) __3__ times a day.
At (time)_____ I take (amount)_____.   One tablet 15 minutes
At (time)_____ I take (amount)_____.   before each meal.
At (time)_____ I take (amount)_____.

I take _____ (name of diabetes medicine) _____ times a day.
At (time)_____ I take (amount)_____.
At (time)_____ I take (amount)_____.
At (time)_____ I take (amount)_____.

I take _____ (name of diabetes medicine) _____ times a day.
At (time)_____ I take (amount)_____.
At (time)_____ I take (amount)_____.
At (time)_____ I take (amount)_____.

I should call my doctor or diabetes teacher if I have these problems with my diabetes medicines:
___shaky, sweaty, nervous, hungry, light-headed___
___confused, hardtime thinking, angry -___
___symptoms of low blood glucose___
I should call my doctor or diabetes teacher if my blood glucose is too low or too high for several days.
Too low is __<80__ mg/dl for __2-3__ days.
Too high is __>200__ mg/dl for __2-3__ days.   After 7-10 days of therapy

My blood sugar should be between ____80____ mg/dl and ____140____ mg/dl before my first meal of the day.

My blood sugar should be between ____120____ mg/dl and ____160____ mg/dl 1–2 hours after a meal.

My blood sugar is too low at _____less than 80_____ mg/dl.

My blood sugar is too high at _____more than 200_____ mg/dl.

My hemoglobin A^{1c} should be _____less than 8_____ %.

If you have any questions,
call me at 555-RX4U.

John O'Malley
Pharmacist

Education Program for Mr. George Jones

Goals:

1. To educate Mr. Jones about diabetes mellitus and the importance of blood glucose control.
2. To educate Mr. Jones about uncontrolled hypertension and hypercholesterolemia and potential complications.
3. To educate Mr. Jones on monitoring and management of asthma.
4. To educate Mr. Jones on importance of health maintenance.
5. To educate Mr. Jones on importance of, and techniques to improve, health care compliance.

Educational Objective	*Date Taught*	*Outcome*	*Follow-up Required?*
1. Mr. Jones will understand what diabetes mellitus is, including: - basic pathophysiology - the role of blood glucose control - potential complications of diabetes - signs and symptoms of hyperglycemia.			
2. Mr. Jones will understand the role of hypertension and hypercholesterolemia and the complications of each, which may interact with and worsen complications of diabetes.			
3. Mr. Jones will understand how to properly perform peak flow monitoring and administer albuterol at appropriate times.			
4. Mr. Jones will understand how to properly evaluate blood glucose and will monitor blood glucose as recommended.			
5. Mr. Jones will understand the importance of adherence to dietary recommendations for control of diabetes, hypertension, and hypercholesterolemia.			
6. Mr. Jones will understand the importance of adherence to an exercise program for control of diabetes, hypertension, and hypercholesterolemia.			
7. Mr. Jones will understand the importance of performing annual home fecal occult blood tests.			
8. Mr. Jones will understand the importance of follow-up with health care providers, including the ophthalmologist, dentist, pharmacist, and primary care provider.			

Educational Objective	*Date Taught*	*Outcome*	*Follow-up Required?*

9. Mr. Jones will understand the importance
   of taking his medications as prescribed
   and at the recommended times.

10. Mr. Jones will recognize adverse effects
    of his medications, particularly hypoglycemia,
    and what action to take should the effects occur.

11. Mr. Jones will understand the
    importance of and demonstrate
    appropriate foot and skin inspection skills.

Outcome:

1. Patient restated content correctly/performed task acceptably well.
2. Patient needs reinforcement of content or performance of task.
3. Patient cannot/will not restate content correctly or perform task.

Content:

Content will depend on Mr. Jones' current understanding of the above issues. Educational content will fill in gaps in his knowledge base.

Delivery Methods:

Delivery methods are verbal for all objectives. Video was provided on introduction to diabetes mellitus. Book, *Right from the Start*, on type 2 diabetes, was provided. Written materials on repaglinide (see copy attached) was provided. Demonstration was given for blood glucose and peak flow monitoring.

Evaluation of Effectiveness:

1. Patient interview for health beliefs, restate content when requested, adherence to recommended follow-up
2. Demonstrated use of peak flow and blood glucose monitoring; demonstrated foot and skin inspection
3. Refill records for repaglinide and metabolic control

AMBULATORY PHARMACIST'S CARE PLAN

Patient Sarah McLucas   Pharmacist Alexa Sheffield   Date 4-23-98

Page 1 of 2

DATE IDENTIFIED	PROBLEM (TPL)	PHARMACOTHERAPEUTIC AND RELATED HEALTH CARE GOAL	RECOMMENDATIONS FOR THERAPY	MONITORING PARAMETER(S)	DESIRED ENDPOINT(S)	MONITORING FREQUENCY
4/23/98	Poor control of diabetes	Improve control of diabetes; prevent complications				
"	Poor control of HTN	Improve control of HTN; prevent complications				
"	Poor control of lipids	Improve control of hypercholesterolemia; prevent complications				
"	Postmenopausal w/o HRT	Eliminate post-menopausal Sxs and ↓ assoc risks (CV and osteoporosis)				
"	Not on ASA Qd tx	Prevent cardiovascular complications				
"	PPA in Tavist-D may worsen BP & BG	Avoid worsened BP and BG control				
"	Nonadherence to diet	Adhere to prescribed diet				
"	NSAID may ↑ BP	Avoid worsened BP control				

Ambulatory Pharmacist's Care Plan

Patient __Sarah McLucas__   Pharmacist __Alexa Sheffield__   Date __4-23-98__

Page 2 of 2

DATE IDENTIFIED	PROBLEM (TPL)	PHARMACOTHERAPEUTIC AND RELATED HEALTH CARE GOAL	RECOMMENDATIONS FOR THERAPY	MONITORING PARAMETER(S)	DESIRED ENDPOINT(S)	MONITORING FREQUENCY
4/23/98	Taking Tavist→ year-round	Control seasonal allergic rhinitis SXs				
"	Taking naprosyn and ibuprofen	Avoid duplicate tx				
"	Poor control of OA pain	Control pain Preserve/increase functional status				
"	NSAID may ↑ SXs of GERD	Avoid SXs of GERD				
"	Nonadherence to cholestyramine	Control hypercholest.				
"	No SMBG	Regular SMBG				
"	No exercise plan	Adhere to exercise plan				

AMBULATORY PHARMACIST'S CARE PLAN

Patient **Sarah McLucas**   Pharmacist **Alexa Sheffield**   Date **4-23-98**

Page 1 of 2

DATE IDENTIFIED	PROBLEM (TPL)	PHARMACOTHERAPEUTIC AND RELATED HEALTH CARE GOAL	RECOMMENDATIONS FOR THERAPY	MONITORING PARAMETER(S)	DESIRED ENDPOINT(S)	MONITORING FREQUENCY
4/23/98	Poor control of diabetes	Improve control of diabetes; prevent complications	Refer to dietitian for meal planning			
"	Poor control of HTN	Improve control of HTN; prevent complications	Refer to dietitian for meal planning			
"	Poor control of lipids	Improve control of hypercholesterolemia; prevent complications	d/c cholestyramine Rec fluvastatin 20 mg q PM			
"	Postmenopausal w/o HRT	Eliminate post-menopausal SXs and ↓ assoc risks (CV and osteoporosis)	Rec. conj. estrogen 0.625 mg QD and medroxyprogesterone 2.5 mg QD			
"	Not on ASA QD tx	Prevent cardiovascular complications	Rec EC ASA 325 mg QD			
"	PPA in Tavist-D may worsen BP & BG	Avoid worsened BP and BG control	D/C Tavist-D Rec loratidine 10 mg QD w/ seasonal symptoms			
"	Nonadherence to diet	Adhere to prescribed diet	Refer to dietitian			
"	NSAID may ↑ BP	Avoid worsened BP control	D/C NSAIDS Rec acetaminophen up to 4 g QD			

AMBULATORY PHARMACIST'S CARE PLAN

Patient __Sarah McLucas__   Pharmacist __Alexa Sheffield__   Date __4-23-98__

Page 2 of 2

DATE IDENTIFIED	PROBLEM (TPL)	PHARMACOTHERAPEUTIC AND RELATED HEALTH CARE GOAL	RECOMMENDATIONS FOR THERAPY	MONITORING PARAMETER(S)	DESIRED ENDPOINT(S)	MONITORING FREQUENCY
4/23/98	Taking Tavist-D year-round	Control seasonal allergic rhinitis SXs	D/C Tavist-D take loratidine only w/seasonal SX			
"	Taking naprosyn and ibuprofen	Avoid duplicate tx	D/C Naprosyn and ibuprofen			
"	Poor control of OA pain	Control pain Preserve/increase functional status	Rec. Acetaminophen up to 4 g QD and re-evaluate			
"	NSAID may ↑ SXs of GERD	Avoid SXs of GERD	D/C Naprosyn			
"	Nonadherence to cholestyramine	Control hypercholest.	D/C cholestyramine Begin fluvastatin tx			
"	No SMBG	Regular SMBG	Instruct on self-monitoring			
"	No exercise plan	Adhere to exercise plan	Daily walk			

Education Program for Ms. McLucas

Goals:

1. To educate Ms. McLucas about diabetes mellitus and the importance of blood glucose control.
2. To educate Ms. McLucas about uncontrolled hypertension and hypercholesterolemia and potential complications.
3. To educate Ms. McLucas on the importance of health maintenance.

Educational Objective	*Date Taught*	*Outcome*	*Follow-up Required?*
1. Ms. McLucas will understand what diabetes mellitus is, including: - basic pathophysiology - the role of blood glucose control - potential complications of diabetes - signs and symptoms of hyperglycemia			
2. Ms. McLucas will understand the role of hypertension and hypercholesterolemia and the complications of each, which may interact with and worsen complications of diabetes.			
3. Ms. McLucas will understand the role of hormone replacement therapy and daily aspirin therapy as part of her therapy regimen.			
4. Ms. McLucas will understand how to properly evaluate blood glucose and will monitor it as recommended.			
5. Ms. McLucas will understand the importance of adherence to dietary recommendations for control of diabetes, hypertension, and hypercholesterolemia.			
6. Ms. McLucas will understand the importance of adherence to an exercise program for control of diabetes, hypertension, and hypercholesterolemia.			
7. Ms. McLucas will understand the importance of performing annual home fecal occult blood tests.			
8. Ms. McLucas will understand the importance of follow-up with health care providers, including the ophthalmologist, dentist, pharmacist, and primary care provider.			

Educational Objective	Date Taught	Outcome	Follow-up Required?
9. Ms. McLucas will understand the importance of taking her medications as prescribed and at the recommended times (including "prn" seasonal allergy medications).			
10. Ms. McLucas will recognize adverse effects of her medications, and what action to take should the effects occur.			
11. Ms. McLucas will understand the importance of and demonstrate good technique for foot and skin inspection.			

Outcome:

1. Patient restated content correctly/performed task acceptably well.
2. Patient needs reinforcement of content or performance of task.
3. Patient cannot/will not restate content correctly or perform task.

Content:

Content will depend on Ms. McLucas' current understanding of the above issues. Educational content will fill in gaps in her knowledge base.

Delivery Methods:

Delivery methods are verbal for all objectives. Video on introduction to diabetes mellitus. Book, *Right from the Start*, on type 2 diabetes, was provided. Demonstration was given for blood glucose monitoring.

Evaluation of Effectiveness:

1. Patient interview for health beliefs, restate content when requested, adherence to recommended follow-up
2. Demonstrated use of blood glucose monitoring; demonstrated foot and skin inspection
3. Refill records for medications and metabolic control

Designing a Monitoring Plan for Patients with Type 2 Diabetes

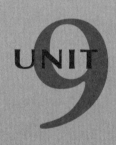
UNIT 9

In unit 8 you learned how to design a therapeutic regimen for an ambulatory patient with type 2 diabetes. The next step in the pharmacotherapeutic process is the development of a monitoring plan that allows you to track your patient's progress and the outcomes of your therapy recommendations. To provide optimal therapy (e.g., pharmaceutical care) you need to know whether the desired outcomes have been achieved.

Unit Objectives

After you successfully complete this unit, you will be able to:

- state the customary monitoring parameters for medication regimens commonly prescribed for ambulatory patients with type 2 diabetes;
- determine monitoring parameters that will measure achievement of pharmacotherapeutic goals for ambulatory patients with type 2 diabetes;
- determine monitoring parameters that will measure achievement of related health care goals for ambulatory patients with type 2 diabetes;
- determine desired endpoints for monitoring parameters in the treatment of ambulatory patients with type 2 diabetes;
- describe factors that influence the frequency and timing of parameter measurement in monitoring plans for ambulatory patients with type 2 diabetes; and
- design a monitoring plan for a regimen for an ambulatory patient with type 2 diabetes that effectively evaluates achievement of pharmacotherapeutic and related health care goals.

Unit Organization

In this unit you will learn to specify monitoring parameters, endpoints, and frequency of monitoring for the therapy of an ambulatory patient with type 2 diabetes. You then learn how this information is incorporated into a monitoring plan, considering treatment guidelines when available.

Unique Issues in Monitoring Therapy for Ambulatory Patients with Type 2 Diabetes

Determining Parameters to Measure Achievement of Pharmacotherapeutic Goals

As you learned in unit 15 of the *Ambulatory Care Clinical Skills Program: Core Module*, there are several considerations in selecting parameters to measure the achievement of pharmacotherapeutic goals, including drug characteristics; therapeutic efficacy and adverse effects of regimen; physiological changes in the patient; practicality, availability, and cost of monitoring; patient adherence; and follow-up on referrals. In the management of ambulatory patients with type 2 diabetes, these may be applied and considered specifically in several different categories, such as metabolic control, behavioral interventions, quality of life, complications, and adverse drug effects and interactions.

Metabolic Control

Parameters that assess a patient's degree of glycemic control include hemoglobin A_{1c} and results from self-monitoring of blood glucose (e.g., fasting, preprandial, postprandial, and bedtime blood glucose values; take particular note of trends). Other monitoring parameters include a patient's blood pressure and lipid profile (i.e., total cholesterol, LDL cholesterol, HDL cholesterol, and triglycerides).

Behavioral Interventions

Nonadherence to therapy is a major health care concern. If patients do not take their medications, it is not very likely they will meet their therapeutic goals. Therefore, patient adherence is an important monitoring parameter, both at the start of therapy and throughout. You can ask the patient to explain how he or she takes medication and how many doses he or she has missed in the past week. Reviewing refill information and doing a tablet or capsule count help assess medication adherence. Try to use more than one technique to assess medication adherence. Other behavioral interventions that require monitoring include adherence to a blood glucose self-monitoring regimen and a good technique when using the blood glucose monitor.

Quality of Life

In unit 8 we discussed use of the Diabetes Treatment Satisfaction Questionnaire (DTSQ), which assesses the patient's overall treatment satisfaction, including convenience and flexibility of current diabetes treatment, control of blood glucose values, and whether the patient would recommend the same form of treatment to another patient with the same level of severity of diabetes. Application and assessment of this instrument as a monitoring parameter will be demonstrated in a future unit.

Complications

Patients with diabetes should be monitored for the development of both acute complications, such as hypoglycemia and hyperglycemia (including hyperglycemic hyperosmolar nonketotic syndrome [HHNS]), and chronic complications, such as macrovascular complications (e.g., cerebral and coronary atherosclerosis and peripheral vascular disease), microvascular complications (e.g., retinopathy and nephropathy), neuropathic complications (including autonomic and sensorimotor complications), and mixed vascular/neuropathic complications. Monitor for complications by asking the patient if he or she has experienced any of these complications, by reviewing the patient's medical record, by conversing with the patient's primary care provider, and by monitoring events such as hospitalization, emergency room admission, amputation, and myocardial infarction.

Adverse Drug Reactions/Drug Interactions

As pharmacists, we are trained to thoroughly assess a patient for the development of drug-induced adverse effects or drug interactions. Table 2 in unit 5 lists common adverse effects associated with medications used to treat diabetes, and patients must be assessed *prospectively* on a regular basis for the development of these adverse effects. For example, if you were following a patient receiving acarbose, you would ask the patient if he or she had experienced any abdominal pain, diarrhea, or flatulence. If the acarbose were used in combination with an antidiabetes medication that causes hypoglycemia, you would ask if the patient had experienced any subjective symptoms of hypoglycemia (dizziness, shakiness, palpitations, sweating, or difficulty concentrating). Objective data you would monitor would include liver enzymes and the patient's hematocrit. It is very important to stress that these monitoring parameters must be identified at the inception of the care plan. Do not assume you will notice when a side effect occurs. If you don't make a note to monitor for a particular potential adverse effect, the patient may not associate the effect with the medication and will fail to describe what he or she is experiencing. Diabetes medication drug interactions are reviewed in Tables 3–6 in unit 5.

Determining Parameters to Measure Achievement of Related Health Care Goals

In addition to establishing monitoring parameters for achievement of pharmacotherapeutic goals, the pharmacist must similarly address how to monitor achievement of related health care goals, such as behavioral modification with diet and exercise, and health maintenance issues specific to diabetes, such as an annual ophthalmic and podiatric examination and a semiannual dental examination. Monitoring may begin with interviewing the patient. Did the patient see the referent? Has the patient been adherent to the referent's plan? For example, did the patient see the dietitian he or she was referred to? If so, what plan did the dietitian suggest? Follow this through to the outcome goal of the intervention; for example, what is the patient's weight and body mass index?

To monitor whether a patient implements an exercise program, ask the patient about adherence to the plan, assess the patient's daily or weekly exercise regimen, and track the patient's blood pressure and heart rate.

Regarding foot care, ask the patient if he or she is checking his or her feet daily, and following through with the recommended plan.

Remember that some monitoring parameters are appropriate for more than one goal. For example, monitoring the blood pressure may reflect the patient's adherence to their medication regimen, medical nutrition therapy, and exercise plan.

Determining Desired Endpoints for Monitoring Parameters

Now that you've identified what parameters you would like to follow to measure achievement of pharmacotherapeutic and related health care goals, you need to identify what those values or responses should be. For example, what hemoglobin A_{1c} would be acceptable for a patient with diabetes? Recommended guidelines are useful in evaluating the parameters you are monitoring (see **Table 1**). The American Diabetes Association states that a normal

Table 1. Recommendations for Metabolic Control in Nonpregnant Adult Patients with Diabetes

Monitoring Parameter	Goal Values	Values at Which Intervention Is Suggested
Average preprandial glucose (mg/dl)	80–120	<80 or >140
Average bedtime glucose (mg/dl)	100–140	<100 or >160
HbA$_{1c}$ (%)	<7%	>8%
Systolic blood pressure (mmHg)	<85	N/A
Diastolic blood pressure (mmHg)	<130	N/A
Total cholesterol (mg/dl)	<200	N/A
LDL cholesterol (mg/dl)	<100	N/A
HDL cholesterol (mg/dl)	>45	N/A
Triglycerides (mg/dl)	<200	N/A

Source: data from reference 1.

hemoglobin A$_{1c}$ is <6%, a goal hemoglobin A$_{1c}$ for a patient with diabetes is <7%, and that an intervention is suggested with a hemoglobin A$_{1c}$ of ≥8%. Therefore, using guidelines can be quite useful. However, bear in mind that suggested therapeutic endpoints are not patient specific. For example, if you can work with a patient to lower his or her hemoglobin A$_{1c}$ from 12.6% to 10.2%, you are making progress toward your ultimate goal, and no amount of improvement should be discounted. Likewise, some patients develop hypoglycemia easily, and therefore should not set normal glucose as a goal. As discussed in the *Ambulatory Care Clinical Skills Program: Core Module*, patient-specific factors should be considered in establishing endpoints, as well as drug characteristics, efficacy, and toxicity.

The characteristics of diabetes medications should be considered in setting your endpoint values. For example, if it is unlikely a patient will gain further blood glucose improvement from nonpharmacologic interventions, and the patient's hemoglobin A$_{1c}$ is still 10.4%, the patient is unlikely to achieve a hemoglobin A$_{1c}$ of <8% with only acarbose therapy. Acarbose will lower the hemoglobin A$_{1c}$ approximately 0.5–1.0% when used alone.

Factors Influencing Frequency and Timing of Parameter Measurements

In unit 15 of the *Ambulatory Care Clinical Skills Program: Core Module*, you learned that three factors

influence monitoring frequency: specific needs of the patient, details of the therapy, and cost and practicality of monitoring. We will use monitoring parameters for glycemic control to illustrate how these factors determine frequency and timing of parameter measurement.

Specific Needs of the Patient

One specific patient need is a level of metabolic control. For example, a diabetes patient with a fasting blood glucose of 280 mg/dl who is exhibiting symptoms requires more frequent self-monitoring of blood glucose than a patient with a fasting blood glucose <120 mg/dl.

How closely a patient is trying to control his or her blood glucose also determines the frequency of monitoring. For example, a highly motivated patient with type 2 diabetes who counts carbohydrates and adjusts insulin therapy based on preprandial blood glucose values would self-monitor more frequently than a patient controlled with nonpharmacologic interventions and who demonstrates good response.

Patients prone to frequent episodes of hypoglycemia, particularly with impaired warning symptoms, will probably self-monitor blood glucose more frequently than patients who seldom or never experience symptoms of hypoglycemia.

Defined endpoints are discussed at length in units 2 and 3 of this module. Please refer to these units as you practice developing monitoring plans.

Details of the Drug Therapy

Patients may require more frequent monitoring early in the course of therapy or while changing or titrating therapy. The more complex the regimen, the more monitoring may be required.

Biopsychosocial implications of the disease and drug therapy may affect the frequency and timing of monitoring. For example, with self-monitoring of blood glucose, patients who are highly motivated will probably monitor more than patients who are not motivated. A patient's occupation may have an influence on the self-monitoring schedule. Patients who work shift work may require changes in when they administer their medication during the day and, similarly, in their monitoring schedule.

Other issues affecting monitoring include the patient's support structure, family dynamics, and health beliefs. Patients who are encouraged to self-monitor blood glucose regularly, and who believe there is value in doing so, are more likely to monitor regularly.

Cost and Practicality of Monitoring

Many patients are surprised to learn about coupons and discounts on blood glucose monitors that enable patients to obtain a monitor at a very reasonable cost. The real cost of blood glucose monitoring, however, is purchasing the strips used by the monitors to collect the blood sample. Therefore, it is important that the patient have a good grasp of when he or she should be self-monitoring blood glucose and how the results will help guide his or her therapy. It is important that patients not test their blood glucose at times (or time intervals) that will not provide additional useful information.

An example of impractical monitoring would be a physician ordering monthly hemoglobin A_{1c} values for a patient who is stable but not controlled. Monthly hemoglobin A_{1c} values do not provide significantly useful information; plus, it is impractical to ask the patient to keep coming in for repeated laboratory assessments.

Designing a Monitoring Plan for Ambulatory Patients with Type 2 Diabetes

Case Study

You may want to refresh your memory of the American Diabetes Association–suggested monitoring parameters and frequency, as described in units 2

and 3. Following your review, let's consider the case of Mrs. Gonzalez and how we will monitor her progress toward pharmacotherapeutic and related health care goals. We will complete an APCP for Mrs. Gonzalez as well as develop an Ambulatory Monitoring Worksheet (AMW) to track selected monitoring parameters. Use the completed APCP and AMW in **Appendix A** to follow along.

Mrs. Gonzalez presented to the pharmacist after being diagnosed with type 2 diabetes, so the first pharmacotherapeutic and related health care goal is "improve diabetes control; prevent complications." The recommendation is to institute nonpharmacologic interventions (diet and exercise) and to monitor glycemic control indices. The physician has agreed with your goals, which are consistent with those recommended by the American Diabetes Association: fasting blood glucose <120 mg/dl; preprandial blood glucose <120 mg/dl; 2-hr postprandial blood glucose <140 mg/dl; and bedtime blood glucose between 100 and 140 mg/dl. The goal hemoglobin A_{1c} is <7%. The hemoglobin A_{1c} should be assessed quarterly for patients currently not under control and at least twice yearly for those with good control. Therefore, the pharmacist recommended obtaining a hemoglobin A_{1c} every 3 months until Mrs. Gonzalez's value is stable or her goal is achieved and then decreasing the monitoring to every 6 months. The pharmacist also recommended initial and follow-up laboratory and physical assessment monitoring as recommended by the American Diabetes Association. Mrs. Gonzalez was asymptomatic of diabetes, so she has no symptoms that we should monitor for resolution at this time; however, symptoms of hyperglycemia that she could experience are listed on the AMW and will be assessed at each visit to assure that she remains free of these complaints.

Mrs. Gonzalez's other pharmacotherapeutic and related health care goals were examined using this same process. The monitoring parameter for improved control of hypertension was blood pressure and absence of lisinopril-induced adverse effects. Based on the Joint National Committee on Prevention, Detection, Evaluation, and Treatment of High Blood Pressure (JNC VI) and American Diabetes Association guidelines, Mrs. Gonzalez's desired endpoint blood pressure was <130/85 mmHg unless specified otherwise by her physician; it should be monitored at each visit to the pharmacy. The visit frequency may be altered, however, depending on changes in her antihypertensive or other medications. The pharmacist will ask Mrs. Gonzalez about adverse effects caused by lisinopril therapy at each visit and request a potassium level to detect possible hyperkalemia every 6 months.

Lipid profile and total cholesterol were selected as monitoring parameters for improved cholesterol control. Based on recommendations established by American Diabetes Association, an LDL cholesterol value of <100 mg/dl and an HDL cholesterol value of >45 mg/dl were selected as desired endpoints, unless otherwise specified. The National Cholesterol Education Program (NCEP) recommendation for repeat blood work is 6–8 weeks after initiating drug therapy, with a second measurement in another 6 weeks. After the goal LDL cholesterol has been achieved, repeat assessments should occur every 8–12 weeks for a year, and then annually (assuming the patient is still at goal and no toxicities have been noted) with interim assessment of the total cholesterol (if no hypertriglyceridemia is present). The manufacturer of atorvastatin, on the other hand, recommends checking lipid levels 2–4 weeks after initiating therapy. The pharmacist recommended assessing the lipid panel 8 weeks after initiating atorvastatin therapy but assessing the total cholesterol as a measure of patient progress at each pharmacy visit. The manufacturer of atorvastatin also recommends checking liver enzymes prior to initiating therapy, 12 weeks after beginning therapy, and semiannually thereafter. The pharmacist will also ask Mrs. Gonzalez at each pharmacy visit about any subjective complaints suggestive of an adverse reaction to atorvastatin, including muscle pain, aches, tenderness, gastrointestinal upset, and headache.

As Mrs. Gonzalez begins therapy with conjugated estrogen/progestin, calcium carbonate, and enteric coated aspirin, the pharmacist will monitor for efficacy and subjective signs of adverse effects at every pharmacy visit. If the patient does not experience adverse effects on initiating therapy, frequency of questioning can be decreased to every 3 months.

To ensure the discontinuation of hydrochlorothiazide, monitor Mrs. Gonzalez's medication profile and interview her at every visit until she is no longer taking the drug.

Monitoring for adherence to an exercise plan and medical nutrition therapy can be accomplished by patient interview and weight measurement at every visit.

Mrs. Gonzalez's adherence to self-monitoring blood glucose and blood pressure can be evaluated through interviewing her, observing her technique, and reviewing her monitoring log books. The pharmacist will assess Mrs. Gonzalez's log books on every visit to the pharmacy. The goal is for Mrs. Gonzalez to monitor her blood glucose and blood pressure daily. Her adherence to self-monitoring will be reviewed at each pharmacy visit. Once Mrs. Gonzalez demonstrates adherence, you may confirm continued adherence through patient interview or review of her monitoring logs. Although demonstration is not needed at every visit, you may want to reassess her technique at least once a year to assure that no bad habits have been picked up.

Monitoring for follow-up with the ophthalmologist can be accomplished by patient interview at each visit until complete. Similarly, the pharmacist can ask Mrs. Gonzalez about completion of her annual home fecal blood test, her annual influenza vaccine, and whether she completes a monthly breast self-examination.

All the monitoring parameters have been transferred to the AMW, with frequencies noted. Having the parameters recorded on the AMW will enable the pharmacist to quickly identify which data needs to be collected at each visit.

Practice Example

Using the APCP for Mr. Jones in **Appendix B** completed through the "Recommendations for Therapy" column, complete the form as well as the blank AMW forms. When you have completed these forms, compare your responses to those in **Appendix C** and the following discussion.

The pharmacist strongly suspects that Mr. Jones has type 2 diabetes based on his risk factors, past medical history, chief complaint, and random blood glucose. The patient is referred to the primary care physician for confirmation of the diagnosis of diabetes, and the pharmacist makes a note to check with the physician every week until a diagnosis is obtained. When the diagnosis of type 2 diabetes is confirmed on 4/3/98, the pharmacist will add monitoring parameters to the APCP and AMW that are consistent with those recommended by the American Diabetes Association.

Mr. Jones also has hypertension. The monitoring parameter for improved control of hypertension is blood pressure and absence of lisinopril-induced adverse effects. Based on JNC VI guidelines, the general goal for a patient with hypertension is a systolic blood pressure <140 mmHg and a diastolic blood pressure <90 mmHg. The pharmacist in this case established a goal of <130/85 mmHg for two reasons. First, a blood pressure reading of <130/85 mmHg is considered normal. At the time the pharmacist established the blood pressure goal, Mr. Jones' diagnosis of type 2 diabetes had not been confirmed; however, the pharmacist felt comfortable listing <130/85 mmHg as the goal in this case. Similarly, the pharmacist recommended a switch from furosemide to lisinopril for improved blood pressure control, less effect on lipids and blood glucose, and potential protection of the kidneys. The pharmacist will ask Mr. Jones about adverse effects attributable to lisinopril therapy at each visit and request a potassium level to detect possible hyperkalemia every 6 months.

Mr. Jones has been instructed to talk with a dietitian about dietary interventions, and he is willing to start an exercise regimen. To monitor progress toward goals related to these interventions, the pharmacist will assess the patient's adherence, weight, body mass index (BMI), and blood pressure at every visit. The pharmacist will assess Mr. Jones' adherence to medication therapy and follow-up appointments at each encounter, through a review of his medication profile and by asking Mr. Jones questions about his regimen.

To ensure the discontinuation of furosemide, the pharmacist will monitor Mr. Jones' medication profile and interview him at every visit until he is no longer taking the drug.

Mr. Jones refuses to stop smoking or to stop drinking alcohol; therefore, asking him about tobacco and alcohol at each visit would not be useful. The pharmacist makes a note to bring this up each quarter with Mr. Jones.

Other monitoring parameters include Mr. Jones' adherence to therapy, his technique for peak flow monitoring, and eventually self-monitoring of blood glucose. These skills and behaviors can be evaluated through patient interview, observation of the patient's technique, and review of monitoring logs. The goal is for Mr. Jones to monitor his blood glucose and peak flow daily. His adherence to self-monitoring will be reviewed at each pharmacy visit. Once Mr. Jones demonstrates adherence, the pharmacist may confirm continued adherence through patient interview or review of his monitoring logs. Although demonstration is not needed at every visit, the pharmacist may want to reassess his technique at least once a year to ensure that no bad habits have been picked up.

For the annual prostate and rectal examination and the dilated eye examination, the pharmacist will inquire at every visit until done; then not again until the next year. The same will occur for twice-yearly activities such as a home fecal occult blood test and dental examination.

After Mr. Jones is officially diagnosed with type 2 diabetes, the pharmacist can add a goal to improve diabetes control and reduce the risk of complications. The treatment recommendation for Mr. Jones' diabetes was to continue dietary modification and exercise and begin oral repaglinide 0.5 mg before meals. Goals for Mr. Jones include fasting blood glucose <120 mg/dl, preprandial blood glucose <120 mg/dl, 2-hr postprandial <140 mg/dl, and bedtime blood glucose between 100 and 140 mg/dl. The goal hemoglobin A_{1c} is <7%. The pharmacist will assess Mr. Jones' blood glucose self-monitoring log at every visit, and the hemoglobin A_{1c} quarterly until at goal, then twice yearly. The pharmacist will also inquire about symptoms related to hyperglycemia, signs or symptoms of hypoglycemia attributable to repaglinide, and other drug-related adverse effects at every visit.

For treatment of Mr. Jones' fungal skin infection on his toe, the pharmacist recommended initiation of topical clotrimazole for 7–10 days with skin inspection monthly until resolution, then quarterly to monitor for recurrence.

Mr. Jones' APCP also lists poor control of cholesterol. At Mr. Jones' first presentation (3/3/98) the pharmacist confirmed the need for dietary intervention as a recommendation for therapy based on the patient's reported medical history. When the pharmacist received the laboratory results from 3/3/98, he recommended beginning pharmacotherapy (cholestyramine 4 g twice daily). As with Mrs. Gonzalez, the goal for LDL cholesterol is <100 mg/dl and that for HDL cholesterol is >45 mg/dl. Blood testing will be repeated 6–8 weeks after initiating drug therapy, with a second measurement in another 6 weeks. After the goal LDL cholesterol has been achieved, repeat assessments should occur every 8–12 weeks for a year, and then annually (assuming the patient is still at goal and no toxicities have been noted) with interim assessment of the total cholesterol (if no hypertriglyceridemia is present). The pharmacist recommends assessing the lipid panel 8 weeks after initiating drug therapy and assessing the total cholesterol as a measure of patient progress at each pharmacy visit. The pharmacist will monitor for adverse effects of therapy at every visit and then decrease to every 3 months. The pharmacist also made a note to check liver function tests every 3–6 months to monitor for worsening liver function.

Summary

Monitoring plans are designed to measure the achievement of pharmacotherapeutic and related health care goals established for a patient with type 2 diabetes. You should begin by determining what parameters should be assessed, what the target endpoints are, and how often these parameters should be assessed. You will only be able to say "We achieved the goal" if you clearly and prospectively define what constitutes the goal.

Reference

1. American Diabetes Association. Standards of medical care for patients with diabetes mellitus. *Diabetes Care* 1999;22 (*Suppl* 1):S32–41.

Self-Study Questions

Objective

State the customary monitoring parameters for medication regimens commonly prescribed for ambulatory patients with type 2 diabetes.

1. List customary monitoring parameters for medication regimens commonly prescribed in the ambulatory care setting for patients with type 2 diabetes.

Objective

Determine monitoring parameters that will measure achievement of pharmacotherapeutic goals for ambulatory patients with type 2 diabetes.

For questions 2–4, refer to the APCP completed through "Recommendations for Therapy" for Ms. McLucas in **Appendix D**.

2. Which of the following best describes a monitoring parameter that will measure achievement of Ms. McLucas' diabetes control?

   A. hemoglobin A_{1c}
   B. ALT
   C. LDL cholesterol
   D. BMI

3. Which of the following best describes a monitoring parameter that will measure achievement of Ms. McLucas' lipid control?

   A. fasting blood glucose
   B. blood pressure
   C. triglycerides
   D. complaint of foot pain

4. Which of the following best describes a monitoring parameter that will measure achievement of Ms. McLucas osteoarthritis control?

   A. bone scan
   B. patient's complaint of pain on a 10-point scale
   C. erythrocyte sedimentation rate
   D. appearance of reddened joints

Objective

Determine monitoring parameters that will measure achievement of related health care goals for ambulatory patients with type 2 diabetes.

For questions 5–7, refer to the APCP completed through "Recommendations for Therapy" for Ms. McLucas in Appendix D.

5. Which of the following best describes a monitoring parameter that will measure achievement of her self-monitoring of blood glucose?

   A. postprandial blood glucose
   B. proteinuria
   C. urine microalbuminuria
   D. hemoglobin A_{1c}

6. Which of the following best describes a monitoring parameter that will measure achievement of an annual dilated retinal examination?

   A. Patient shows you her appointment calendar, in which an appointment with an ophthalmologist was listed.
   B. Patient has made an appointment for next month with the ophthalmologist.
   C. You receive a consult report from an ophthalmologist.
   D. Patient cancelled her last appointment with the ophthalmologist but promises to reschedule soon.

7. Which of the following best describes a monitoring parameter that will measure achievement of adherence to a recommended meal plan?

   A. Patient talks knowledgeably about making better food choices.
   B. Patient's BMI has increased.
   C. Patient demonstrates a lack of understanding of the dietitian's instructions.
   D. Patient states that she no longer eats candy.

Objective

Determine desired endpoints for monitoring parameters in the treatment of ambulatory patients with type 2 diabetes.

8. Refer to Ms. McLucas in Appendix D. Determine measurable values for monitoring parameters in the treatment of patients with type 2 diabetes in the ambulatory care setting and complete the column for desired endpoints.

Objective

Describe factors that influence the frequency and timing of parameter measurement in monitoring plans for patients with type 2 diabetes.

9. Explain how cost would influence the frequency and timing of parameter measurement in monitoring plans for ambulatory patients with type 2 diabetes.

10. Explain how the specific needs of the patient would influence the frequency and timing of parameter measurement in monitoring plans for ambulatory patients with type 2 diabetes.

11. Explain how the biopsychosocial implications of type 2 diabetes would influence the frequency and timing of a parameter measurement in monitoring plans for ambulatory patients with type 2 diabetes.

Objective

Design a monitoring plan for a regimen for an ambulatory patient with type 2 diabetes that effectively evaluates achievement of pharmacotherapeutic and related health care goals.

12. Refer to Ms. McLucas in Appendix D. Design a monitoring plan for Mrs. McLucas, completing the APCP and the blank AMW forms.

Self-Study Answers

1. fasting blood glucose, results of SMBG, hemoglobin A_{1c}, signs and symptoms suggestive of drug toxicity, symptoms of disease progression or lack of resolution, adherence to recommended therapies, quality of life (patient satisfaction), adverse drug reactions, and drug interactions

2. A

3. C

4. B

5. A

6. C

7. A

8. Refer to the completed APCP for Ms. McLucas (**Appendix E**). Mrs. McLucas' physician has agreed with you on the following goals:

    fasting blood glucose <120 mg/dl

    hemoglobin A_{1c} <7%

    total cholesterol <200 mg/dl

    LDL cholesterol <130 mg/dl

    HDL cholesterol >45 mg/dl

    triglycerides <200 mg/dl

    blood pressure <130/85 mmHg

9. Type 2 diabetes is a relatively expensive disease to manage and monitor. Pharmacists need to be critical in selecting monitoring parameters that optimize ability to care for the patient but not waste health care dollars on monitoring tests that add little to the evaluation of the patient.

10. The patient's current metabolic control dictates frequency of monitoring, as does the glycemic goal (e.g., how tightly controlled). Patients who are prone to hypoglycemia should monitor more frequently.

11. Patient's motivational status will affect frequency of monitoring, as will the patient's work schedule (days or nights), support structure and family dynamics, as well as patient's health beliefs.

12. Refer to the completed APCP and AMW for Ms. McLucas (Appendix E).

AMBULATORY PHARMACIST'S CARE PLAN

Patient Rose Gonzalez   Pharmacist Jane Radcliffe   Date 2/20/98

Page 1 of 2

DATE IDENTIFIED	PROBLEM (TPL)	PHARMACOTHERAPEUTIC AND RELATED HEALTH CARE GOAL	RECOMMENDATIONS FOR THERAPY	MONITORING PARAMETER(S)	DESIRED ENDPOINT(S)	MONITORING FREQUENCY
2/20/98	poor control of diabetes	Improve diabetes control; prevent complications.	Institute non-pcol interventions (diet & exercise)	FBG SMBG HbA1c Pt. satisfac. SXs hypergly.	FBG<120 hsBG 100-140 HbA1c<7% ⊖ SXs HG	All q visit except HbA1c q 3 mo; ↓ to q 6 mo.
"	poor control of HTN	Improve BP control; prevent complications.	As above, plus rec. Δ to lisinopril 10 mg QD	BP AE lisinopril-cough, rash, K+	<130/85 K<5 ⊖ cough, rash	All q visit except WBC & K+ 2x q yr.
"	poor control of cholest.	Improve lipid control; prevent complications.	nonpcol interventions & Atorvastatin 10 mg	TC, CDL, HDL, TG LFT c/o muscle pain, GI upset, HA	LDL<100 HDL>45 TG<200 TC<200 ⊖ c/o AE	TC-q visit panel-q 8 wk x 2 SXs-q visit
"	not on daily ASA tx	↓ risk CV complic. of diabetes	Rec. EC ASA 325 mg QD	GI bleeding/upset; dark, tarry stools	⊖ bleeding or c/o	SX-q visit occult blood- 2x q yr.
"	post menopausal s̄ HRT	↓ risk post-men. SXs/↓ risks of post-menopause	Rec. conjugated estrogen/progestin	vasomotor SX c/o edema GI, breast pain, t'boembolic	⊖ SX or AE	q visit
"	not receiving calcium tx	↓ risk for osteoporosis	Rec calcium carbona 500 mg TID	AE GI upset constipation	⊖ height loss	quarterly
"	Potential of HCTZ to affect DM & chol.	Avoid worsened lipid control	D/C HCTZ	D/C → profile; pt. interview	D/C s̄ AE	q visit til D/C
"	no exercise plan	start & adhere to regular exercise program.	Begin regular walking program	report of regular walking prog	↓BMI, wt. ↓BP	q visit

AMBULATORY PHARMACIST'S CARE PLAN

Patient Rose Gonzalez   Pharmacist Jane Radcliffe   Date 2/20/98

Page 2 of 2

DATE IDENTIFIED	PROBLEM (TPL)	PHARMACOTHERAPEUTIC AND RELATED HEALTH CARE GOAL	RECOMMENDATIONS FOR THERAPY	MONITORING PARAMETER(S)	DESIRED ENDPOINT(S)	MONITORING FREQUENCY
2/20/98	no MNT plan	start & adhere to MNT plan.	refer to RD- follow meal plan	report of adherence to plan	↓ BMI, wt ↓ BP	q visit
"	no home BG monitoring	learn & regularly perform SMBG	select & explain use of BG monitor	-SMBG log -observe technique	-proper technique -adherence to use	observe 2x q yr. review log q visit
"	no home BP monitoring	learn & regularly perform BP measurements	select and explain use of BP cuff	-BP log -observe technique	-proper technique -adherence to use	observe 2x q yr.; review log every visit
"	no home fecal test	perform annual home fecal blood test	Provide home fecal blood test cards	cards returned	⊕ occult blood	2x q yr.
"	no influenza vaccine	receive annual influenza vaccine	Receive flu vaccine Fall 98	Pt. interview	flu shot received	q Fall
"	no monthly breast self-exam	learn & regularly perform exam	refer to primary physician for exam technique	pt. interview	monthly self-exam	q month

PHARMACIST'S CARE PLAN AMBULATORY MONITORING WORKSHEET (AMW)

Patient ___Rose Gonzalez___
Page 1

Pharmacist ___Jane Radcliffe___
Date ___2/20/98___

Pharmaco-therapeutic Goal	Monitoring Parameter	Desired Endpoint	Monitoring Frequency	Date										
1	FBG	<120	every visit											
1	SMBG-preprandial	<120												
1	SMBG-postprandial	<140												
1	SMBG-bedtime	100-140	→											
1	HbA1c	<7	q 3mo; ↓q 6mo											
1	dilated retinal exam	received	annual											
1	SCr	<1.2	q 6 month											
1	U/A	(1)	annual											
1	urine microalbumin	(1)	annual											
1	EKG	received	annual											
1	Foot screen	received	quarterly											
1	Skin screen	received	quarterly											
1	Dental exam	received	q 6 month											

PHARMACIST'S CARE PLAN AMBULATORY MONITORING WORKSHEET (AMW)

Patient Rose Gonzalez

Page 2 of 4

Pharmacist Jane Radcliffe

Date 2/20/98

Pharmaco-therapeutic Goal	Monitoring Parameter	Desired Endpoint	Monitoring Frequency	Date													
1	signs and symptoms of hyperglycemia	(−)	every visit													
1	(polyuria, polydipsia, polyphagia)	(−)	every visit													
2	BP	<130/85	every visit													
2	lisinopril AE− dizziness/headache	(−)	q visit; ↓ q 3 mo													
2	lisinopril AE− cough	(−)	→													
2	K+	<5	q 6 month													
3	Total cholesterol	<200	every visit													
3	LDL cholesterol	<100	q 8 wk x2; ↓													
3	HDL cholesterol	>45	→													
3	TG	<200	→													
4	ASA AE− GI upset	(−)	q visit; ↓ q 3 mo													
4	ASA AE− dark tarry stools	(−)	→													
4	ASA−efficacy prevent MI	(−)	every visit													

see additional items on page 4 —

PHARMACIST'S CARE PLAN AMBULATORY MONITORING WORKSHEET (AMW)

Patient Rose Gonzalez

Page 3 of 4

Pharmacist Jane Radcliffe

Date 2/20/98

Pharmaco-therapeutic Goal	Monitoring Parameter	Desired Endpoint	Monitoring Frequency	Date															
5	Vasomotor SXs	(-)	every visit															
5	Estrogen/progestin AE– breast pain, anorexia	(-)	2 visit, ↓ q 3 mo															
5	headache, edema	(-)	→															
5	thromboembolic c/o	(-)																
5	vaginal bleeding	(-)	↘															
6	height loss	(-)	quarterly															
6	calcium AE– GI upset, constipation	(-)	2 visit, ↓ q 3 mo															
7	patient interview and profile	(-)	every visit til D/C															
8	Pt. interview	adhere 4/5 days	every visit															
8	weight	<150 lb	→															
8	BMI	<27	↘															
9	Pt. interview	adhere 4/5 days	every visit															
10	correct technique	(+)	2x/yr															

PHARMACIST'S CARE PLAN AMBULATORY MONITORING WORKSHEET (AMW)

Patient __Rose Gonzalez__

Page __4 of 4__

Pharmacist __Jane Radcliffe__

Date __2/20/98__

Pharmaco-therapeutic Goal	Monitoring Parameter	Desired Endpoint	Monitoring Frequency	Date														
10	completing log	⊕	every visit														
11	correct technique	⊕	2x/yr														
11	completing log	⊕	every visit														
12	returned home fecal test cards	⊕	annual														
13	flu shot received	⊕	every fall														
14	patient interview	complete	every month														
3	AST	<35	baseline q 8 wks then q 6 mos														
3	ALT	<35	→														
3	AE of atorvastatin -GI upset	⊖	q visit														
3	-headache	⊖	→														
3	-muscle pain or tenderness	⊖	→														

see page 2

Ambulatory Pharmacist's Care Plan

Patient **George Jones**   Pharmacist **John O'Malley**   Date **3-3-98**

Page 1 of 3

DATE IDENTIFIED	PROBLEM (TPL)	PHARMACOTHERAPEUTIC AND RELATED HEALTH CARE GOAL	RECOMMENDATIONS FOR THERAPY	MONITORING PARAMETER(S)	DESIRED ENDPOINT(S)	MONITORING FREQUENCY
3/3/98	Sx and BG suggestive of DM. High risk of DM.	Rule in/out DM. Determine cause of high BG and nocturia	Refer to primary physician—await results			
	poor control of hypertension	Improve BP control; Prevent complications	D/C furosemide Begin lisinopril 10 mg q AM			
	nonadherence to diet	Start and adhere to prescribed meal plan	Referral to dietitian			
	h/o med schedule nonadherence	adherence to medication regimen	Provide written instructions			
	Furosemide may worsen lipids	Avoid worsened lipid profile	Rec d/c furosemide. Begin lisinopril			
	smoking history	Stop smoking	Nicotine replacement and counseling. Pt. refuses at this time			
	Alcohol use history	Stop alcohol use	↓ or stop alcohol use Pt. refuses at this time			

AMBULATORY PHARMACIST'S CARE PLAN

Patient ___George Jones___   Pharmacist ___John O'Malley___   Date ___3-3-98___

Page 2 of 3

DATE IDENTIFIED	PROBLEM (TPL)	PHARMACOTHERAPEUTIC AND RELATED HEALTH CARE GOAL	RECOMMENDATIONS FOR THERAPY	MONITORING PARAMETER(S)	DESIRED ENDPOINT(S)	MONITORING FREQUENCY
3/3/98	h/o nonadherence to f/u appts	Adherence to f/u appt. scheduling	Counsel pt.			
	nonadherence to exercise	start and adhere to exercise plan	Counsel pt.			
	Not doing peak flow monitoring	Learn and perform peak flow monitoring regularly	Instruct pt. on peak flow monitoring			
	No rectal/prostate exam	Annual rectal prostate exam	Refer to PCP. Pt. refuses at this time			
	No home Fecal test	Home fecal blood test q 6 months	Provide home fecal test cards. Pt. refuses at this time.			
	poor control of diabetes	Improve control; prevent complications	Rec. repaglinide 0.5 mg before meals			
4/3/98	Furosemide may ↑ BG	Avoid worsened BP control	Rec d/c furosemide Begin lisinopril			
	Fungal skin infection on toe	Eliminate fungal toe infection	Rec. Lotrimin cream to affected area BID for 7-10 days			

AMBULATORY PHARMACIST'S CARE PLAN

Patient ___George Jones___   Pharmacist ___John O'Malley___   Date ___3-3-98___

Page 3 of 3

DATE IDENTIFIED	PROBLEM (TPL)	PHARMACOTHERAPEUTIC AND RELATED HEALTH CARE GOAL	RECOMMENDATIONS FOR THERAPY	MONITORING PARAMETER(S)	DESIRED ENDPOINT(S)	MONITORING FREQUENCY
4/3	Insensate feet	Absence of infection trauma, ulcerations	Daily self-inspection Quarterly exam			
	Not on daily ASA tx	↓ risk CV complications 2° to diabetes	Rec EC ASA 325 mg QD			
	Poor control of cholesterol	Improve control, prevent complications	Refer for MNT Rec. cholestyramine 4 g BID			
	Not doing SMBG	Learn and perform regular SMBG	Instruct on SMBG			
	No dilated retinal exam	Annual dilated retinal exam	Refer to ophthalmologist			
	No recent dental exam	Dental exam q 6 months	Refer to dentist			
	liver dysfunction	monitor liver function	monitor LFTs			

PHARMACIST'S CARE PLAN AMBULATORY MONITORING WORKSHEET (AMW)

Patient _____

Pharmacist _____

Date _____

Pharmaco-therapeutic Goal	Monitoring Parameter	Desired Endpoint	Monitoring Frequency	Date											

PHARMACIST'S CARE PLAN AMBULATORY MONITORING WORKSHEET (AMW)

Patient _____

Pharmacist _____

Date _____

Pharmaco-therapeutic Goal	Monitoring Parameter	Desired Endpoint	Monitoring Frequency	Date											

PHARMACIST'S CARE PLAN AMBULATORY MONITORING WORKSHEET (AMW)

Patient _____

Pharmacist _____

Date _____

Pharmaco-therapeutic Goal	Monitoring Parameter	Desired Endpoint	Monitoring Frequency	Date													

PHARMACIST'S CARE PLAN AMBULATORY MONITORING WORKSHEET (AMW)

Patient _____

Pharmacist _____
Date _____

Pharmaco-therapeutic Goal	Monitoring Parameter	Desired Endpoint	Monitoring Frequency	Date												

PHARMACIST'S CARE PLAN AMBULATORY MONITORING WORKSHEET (AMW)

Patient _____

Pharmacist _____

Date _____

Pharmaco-therapeutic Goal	Monitoring Parameter	Desired Endpoint	Monitoring Frequency	Date											

AMBULATORY PHARMACIST'S CARE PLAN

Patient _George Jones_   Pharmacist _John O'Malley_   Date _3-3-98_

Page 1 of 3

DATE IDENTIFIED	PROBLEM (TPL)	PHARMACOTHERAPEUTIC AND RELATED HEALTH CARE GOAL	RECOMMENDATIONS FOR THERAPY	MONITORING PARAMETER(S)	DESIRED ENDPOINT(S)	MONITORING FREQUENCY
3/3/98	SX and BG suggestive of DM. High risk status	Rule in/out DM. Determine cause of high BG and nocturia	Refer to primary physician—await results	Consult report	Rule in/out diabetes	q week until resolved
	poor control of hypertension	Improve BP control; Prevent complications	D/C furosemide Begin lisinopril 10 mg q AM	BP; AE for lisinopril—cough rash, K+	<130/85 (-) SX AE	All q visit except K+— 2x/yr
	nonadherence to diet	start and adhere to prescribed meal plan	Referral to dietitian	pt. interview, wt, BMI	wt <160 BMI <27	q visit
	h/o med schedule nonadherence	Adherence to medication regimen	Provide written instructions	Pt. interview, review profile	proper medication use	q visit
	Furosemide may worsen lipids	Avoid worsened lipid profile	Rec d/c furosemide. Begin lisinopril	Profile and pt. interview	d/c w/o sequelae	q visit
	smoking history	Stop smoking	Nicotine replacement and counseling. Pt. refuses at this time	# cigs/day pt. interview	decreased or no smoking	discuss quarterly
	Alcohol use history	Stop alcohol use	↓ or stop alcohol use Pt. refuses at this time	Amt Etoh/wk Pt. interview	decreased or no Etoh use	discuss quarterly

AMBULATORY PHARMACIST'S CARE PLAN

Patient ___George Jones___   Page 2 of 3   Pharmacist ___John O'Malley___   Date ___3-3-98___

DATE IDENTIFIED	PROBLEM (TPL)	PHARMACOTHERAPEUTIC AND RELATED HEALTH CARE GOAL	RECOMMENDATIONS FOR THERAPY	MONITORING PARAMETER(S)	DESIRED ENDPOINT(S)	MONITORING FREQUENCY
3/3/98	h/o non-adherence to f/u appts	Adherence to f/u appt. scheduling	Counsel pt.	Pt. interview cc consult reports	Compliant c̄ other HCP	q visit
	nonadherence to exercise	start and adhere to exercise plan	Counsel pt.	Pt. interview, wt, BMI, BP	BMI<27, BP<130/85	q visit
	Not doing peak flow monitoring	Learn and perform peak flow monitoring regularly	Instruct pt. on peak flow monitoring	Observe technique, Review SM record	Proper technique use PFM w/o SX	Observe tech 2x then 2x/yr. Review log q visit
	No rectal/prostate exam	Annual rectal prostate exam	Refer to PCP. Pt. refuses at this time	Pt. interview consult report	complete exam	Discuss quarterly
	no home Fecal test	Home fecal blood test q 6 months	Provide home fecal test cards. Pt. refuses at this time.	Pt. interview	complete test	Discuss quarterly
4/3/98	poor control of diabetes	Improve control; prevent complications	Rec. repaglinide 0.5 mg before meals	FBG, SMBG, HBA1c, SX, AE, satisfaction	hs BG 100-14 FBG<120 HBA1c<7 ⊖SX and AE, ⊕satisfaction	FBG & SMBG q visit. HBA1c q 3 mo, q 6 mo
	Furosemide may ↑ BG	Avoid worsened BP control	Rec d/c furosemide Begin lisinopril	Profile and pt. interview	d/c w/o sequelae	q visit
	Fungal skin infection on toe	Eliminate fungal toe infection	Rec. Lotrimin cream to affected area BID for 7-10 days	Inspection of feet	No sign of infection	monthly x 3 then quarterly

Ambulatory Pharmacist's Care Plan

Patient __George Jones__   Pharmacist __John O'Malley__   Date __3-3-98__

Page 3 of 3

DATE IDENTIFIED	PROBLEM (TPL)	PHARMACOTHERAPEUTIC AND RELATED HEALTH CARE GOAL	RECOMMENDATIONS FOR THERAPY	MONITORING PARAMETER(S)	DESIRED ENDPOINT(S)	MONITORING FREQUENCY
4/3	Insensate feet	Absence of infection, trauma, ulcerations	Daily self-inspection. Quarterly exam	Foot exam, Pt. interview	No complications	Inspect quarterly. Interview q visit
	Not on daily ASA tx	↓ risk CV complications 2° to diabetes	Rec EC ASA 325 mg QD	GI upset, dark tarry stools, MI	-Sx - occult blood	Sx - q visit. Biannual fecal blood
	Poor control of cholesterol	Improve control, prevent complications	Refer for MNT. Rec. cholestyramine 4 g BID	TC, LDL, HDL, TG. c/o constipation. GI upset	TC<200 TG<200 LDL<100 HDL>45. - c/o AE	TC q visit. Panel q 8 wks x 2. Sxs - q visit
	Not doing SMBG	Learn and perform regular SMBG	Instruct on SMBG	Observation of technique, SMBG log	Proper tech. Use of BGM daily	Observe tech 2x/yr. Review log q visit
	No dilated retinal exam	Annual dilated retinal exam	Refer to ophthalmologist	-Pt. interview -copy of consult report	Compliant with annual exam	Annually
	No recent dental exam	Dental exam q 6 months	Refer to dentist	Pt. interview. Copy of consult report	Compliant with appts	q 6 mo
	liver dysfunction	monitor liver function	monitor LFTs	ALT, AST	<3S	q 3-6 mo

PHARMACIST'S CARE PLAN AMBULATORY MONITORING WORKSHEET (AMW)

Patient ___George Jones___ Page 1

Pharmacist ___John O'Malley___
Date ___3-3-98___

Pharmaco-therapeutic Goal	Monitoring Parameter	Desired Endpoint	Monitoring Frequency	Date													
1	Consult report	Rule in/out diabetes	q week until resolved														
2	BP	<130/85	q visit														
	lisinopril AE: dizziness	(-)	q visits ↓ q 3 mo														
	lisinopril AE: headache	(-)	→														
	lisinopril AE: cough	(-)															
	lisinopril AE: ↑K+	<5	2x year														
3	Pt. interview	Adhere 4/5 days	q visit														
	Weight	<160 lb	q visit														
	BMI	<27	q visit														
4	Profile and pt. interview	(+)	q visit														
5	Profile and pt. interview	d/c furosemide (-) symptoms	q visit														
6	# cigs/day Pt. currently refuses	⊘	revisit quarterly														
7	amt Etoh/wk pt. currently refuses	⊘	revisit quarterly														

PHARMACIST'S CARE PLAN AMBULATORY MONITORING WORKSHEET (AMW)

Patient: George Jones
Page 2

Pharmacist: John O'Malley
Date: 3-3-98

Pharmaco-therapeutic Goal	Monitoring Parameter	Desired Endpoint	Monitoring Frequency	Date									
8	Pt. interview w/ consult reports	(+)	q visit										
9	Pt. interview	adhere 4/5 days	q visit										
10	Observe technique	proper technique	2x; ↓ 2x/yr										
10	Review log	PFM w/o SX	q visit										
11	Pt. interview/ consult report Pt. currently refuses	annually complete exam	revisit quarterly										
12	Pt. interview Pt. currently refuses	complete test q 6 mos	revisit quarterly										
13	FBG	<120	every visit										
13	SMBG preprandial	<120											
13	SMBG postprandial	<140											
13	SMBG bedtime	100-140											
13	HbA1c	<7%	q 3 mo; ↓ q 6 mo										
13	SCr	<1.2	q 6 month										
13	U/A	(-)	annual										

PHARMACIST'S CARE PLAN AMBULATORY MONITORING WORKSHEET (AMW)

Patient _George Jones_

Page 3

Pharmacist _John O'Malley_

Date _3-3-98_

Pharmaco-therapeutic Goal	Monitoring Parameter	Desired Endpoint	Monitoring Frequency	Date																
13	urine microalbumin	<30	q 6 mo																	
13	urine culture	(-)	prn																	
13	EKG	received	annual																	
13	foot screen	received	quarterly																	
13	skin screen	received	quarterly																	
13	symptoms of hyperglycemia -nocturia	(-)	q visit																	
	-polyuria	(-)	q visit																	
	-polydypsia	(-)	q visit																	
	-polyphagia	(-)	q visit																	
13	dilated retinal exam	received	annual																	
13	dental exam- Pt. refuses at this time	received	revisit quarterly																	
13	Repaglinide AE- rash GI upset	(-)	q visit; ↓ q 3 mo																	
13	signs & symptoms of hypoglycemia	(-)	q visit																	

PHARMACIST'S CARE PLAN AMBULATORY MONITORING WORKSHEET (AMW)

Patient   George Jones

Page 4

Pharmacist   John O'Malley

Date   3-3-98

Pharmaco-therapeutic Goal	Monitoring Parameter	Desired Endpoint	Monitoring Frequency	Date													
14	Profile and pt. interview	d/c furosemide w/o symptoms	q visit													
15	Foot inspection	⊖ sign of infx	q month (×) 3													
16	Foot exam-sensation	10/10	quarterly													
16	Pt. interview	no complications	q visit													
17	ASA-AE GI upset	(−)	q visits ↓ q 3 mo													
17	ASA-AE dark, tarry stools	(−)	q visit; ↓ q 3 mo													
17	ASA-efficacy prevent MI	(−)	q visit													
18	Total cholesterol	<200	q visit													
18	LDL cholesterol	<100	q 8 wk (×2;) ↓ 2-3													
18	HDL cholesterol	>45	→													
18	TG	<200	↘													
18	Cholestyramine AE- constipation, GI upset	(−)	q visit; ↓ q 3 mo													

PHARMACIST'S CARE PLAN AMBULATORY MONITORING WORKSHEET (AMW)

Patient ___George Jones___

Page 5

Pharmacist ___John O'Malley___

Date ___3-3-98___

Pharmaco-therapeutic Goal	Monitoring Parameter	Desired Endpoint	Monitoring Frequency	Date												
19	Observe technique	proper technique	q 6 mo												
19	Review SMBG log	completes log	q visit												
20	Pt. interview, copy of report	receive exam	annual												
21	Pt. interview, copy of report	receive exam	q 6 month												
22	ALT	<35	q 3-6 mo												
22	AST	<35	q 3-6 mo												

AMBULATORY PHARMACIST'S CARE PLAN

Patient ___Sarah McLucas___   Pharmacist ___Alexa Sheffield___   Date ___4-23-98___

Page 1

DATE IDENTIFIED	PROBLEM (TPL)	PHARMACOTHERAPEUTIC AND RELATED HEALTH CARE GOAL	RECOMMENDATIONS FOR THERAPY	MONITORING PARAMETER(S)	DESIRED ENDPOINT(S)	MONITORING FREQUENCY
4/23/98	Poor control of diabetes	Improve control of diabetes; prevent complications	Refer to dietitian for meal planning			
"	Poor control of HTN	Improve control of HTN; prevent complications	Refer to dietitian for meal planning			
"	Poor control of lipids	Improve control of hypercholesterolemia; prevent complications	d/c cholestyramine Rec fluvastatin 20 mg q PM			
"	Postmenopausal w/o HRT	Eliminate post-menopausal Sxs and ↓ assoc risks (CV and osteoporosis)	Rec. conj. estrogen 0.625 mg QD and medroxyprogesterone 2.5 mg QD			
"	Not on ASA QD tx	Prevent cardiovascular complications	Rec Ec ASA 325 mg QD			
"	PPA in Tavist-D may worsen BP & BG	Avoid worsened BP and BG control	D/C Tavist-D Rec loratidine 10 mg QD w/ seasonal sym			
"	Nonadherence to diet	Adhere to prescribed diet	Refer to dietitian			
"	NSAID may ↑ BP	Avoid worsened BP control	D/C NSAIDS Rec acetaminophen up to 4 g QD			

AMBULATORY PHARMACIST'S CARE PLAN

Patient __Sarah McLucas__   Pharmacist __Alexa Sheffield__   Date __4-23-98__

Page 2

DATE IDENTIFIED	PROBLEM (TPL)	PHARMACOTHERAPEUTIC AND RELATED HEALTH CARE GOAL	RECOMMENDATIONS FOR THERAPY	MONITORING PARAMETER(S)	DESIRED ENDPOINT(S)	MONITORING FREQUENCY
4/23/98	Taking Tavist-D year-round	Control seasonal allergic rhinitis SXs	D/C Tavist-D take loratadine only w/seasonal SX			
"	Taking naprosyn and ibuprofen	Avoid duplicate tx	D/C naprosyn and ibuprofen			
"	Poor control of OA pain	Control pain Preserve/increase functional status	Rec. Acetaminophen up to 4 g QD and re-evaluate			
"	NSAID may ↑ SXs of GERD	Avoid SXs of GERD	D/C naprosyn			
"	Nonadherence to cholestyramine	Control hypercholest.	D/C cholestyramine Begin fluvastatin tx			
"	No SMBG	Regular SMBG	Instruct on self-monitoring			
"	No exercise plan	Adhere to exercise plan	Daily walk			

PHARMACIST'S CARE PLAN AMBULATORY MONITORING WORKSHEET (AMW)

Patient _____

Pharmacist _____

Date _____

Pharmaco-therapeutic Goal	Monitoring Parameter	Desired Endpoint	Monitoring Frequency	Date												

PHARMACIST'S CARE PLAN AMBULATORY MONITORING WORKSHEET (AMW)

Patient _____

Pharmacist _____

Date _____

Pharmaco-therapeutic Goal	Monitoring Parameter	Desired Endpoint	Monitoring Frequency	Date													

PHARMACIST'S CARE PLAN AMBULATORY MONITORING WORKSHEET (AMW)

Patient _____

Pharmacist _____

Date _____

Pharmaco-therapeutic Goal	Monitoring Parameter	Desired Endpoint	Monitoring Frequency	Date															

PHARMACIST'S CARE PLAN AMBULATORY MONITORING WORKSHEET (AMW)

Patient _____

Pharmacist _____

Date _____

Pharmaco-therapeutic Goal	Monitoring Parameter	Desired Endpoint	Monitoring Frequency	Date										

AMBULATORY PHARMACIST'S CARE PLAN

Patient Sarah McLucas   Pharmacist Alexa Sheffield   Date 4-23-98

Page 1 of 2

DATE IDENTIFIED	PROBLEM (TPL)	PHARMACOTHERAPEUTIC AND RELATED HEALTH CARE GOAL	RECOMMENDATIONS FOR THERAPY	MONITORING PARAMETER(S)	DESIRED ENDPOINT(S)	MONITORING FREQUENCY
4/23/98	Poor control of diabetes	Improve control of diabetes; prevent complications	Refer to dietitian for meal planning	FBG, SMBG, HbAlc Pt. symptoms SX of hypergly.	FBG<120 hsBG 100-140 HbAlc<7%	FBG and SMBG q visit HbAlc q 3 mo; then ↓ q 6 mo
"	Poor control of HTN	Improve control of HTN; prevent complications	Refer to dietitian for meal planning	BP	<130/85	q visit
"	Poor control of lipids	Improve control of hypercholesterolemia; prevent complications	d/c cholestyramine Rec fluvastatin 20 mg q PM	TC LDL, HDL, TG AE of fluvastatin	TC<200 LDL<100, HDL>45 TG <200 ⊖ AE	TC q visit; panel q 8 wks ⊗ AE q visit; LFTs baseline 8 wks, then q 6 mo
"	Postmenopausal w/o HRT	Eliminate post-menopausal SXs and ↓ assoc risks (CV and osteoporosis)	Rec. conj. estrogen 0.625 mg QD and medroxyprogesterone 2.5 mg QD	Vasomotor SX AE of HRT	⊖ symptoms and ⊖ AE	q visit
"	Not on ASA QD tx	Prevent cardiovascular complications	Rec EC ASA 325 mg QD	GI upset, bleeding, dark stools	⊖ SX or occult blood	SX q visit; occult blood 2x/yr.
"	PPA in Tavist-D may worsen BP & BG	Avoid worsened BP and BG control	D/C Tavist-D Rec loratidine 10 mg QD w/ seasonal symptoms	Pt. profile	D/C w/o ↑ SX	q visit until resolved
"	Nonadherence to diet	Adhere to prescribed diet	Refer to dietitian	report of adherence to meal plan	Pt. report ↓ wt, ↓BMI	q visit
"	NSAID may ↑ BP	Avoid worsened BP control	D/C NSAIDS Rec acetaminophen up to 4 g QD	Pt. profile	D/C w/o ↑ SX	q visit until resolved

AMBULATORY PHARMACIST'S CARE PLAN

Patient __Sarah McLucas__   Pharmacist __Alexa Sheffield__   Date __4-23-98__

Page 2 of 2

DATE IDENTIFIED	PROBLEM (TPL)	PHARMACOTHERAPEUTIC AND RELATED HEALTH CARE GOAL	RECOMMENDATIONS FOR THERAPY	MONITORING PARAMETER(S)	DESIRED ENDPOINT(S)	MONITORING FREQUENCY
4/23/98	Taking Tavist→D year-round	Control seasonal allergic rhinitis SXs	D/C Tavist-D take loratidine only w/seasonal SX	hayfever SX	⊖ SX ⊖ AE	q visit
"	Taking naprosyn and ibuprofen	Avoid duplicate tx	D/C naprosyn and ibuprofen	Pt. report and profile	no increased pain	q visit until resolved
"	Poor control of OA pain	Control pain Preserve/increase functional status	Rec. Acetaminophen up to 4 g QD and re-evaluate	OA pain	pain<2/10 (per pt. report)	q visit
"	NSAID may ↑ SXs of GERD	Avoid SXs of GERD	D/C naprosyn	Patient Profile	d/c w/o SX	q visit until resolved
"	Nonadherence to cholestyramine	Control hypercholest.	D/C cholestyramine Begin fluvastatin tx	Pt. report and profile	↑ compliance to tx	q visit until resolved.
"	No SMBG	Regular SMBG	Instruct on self-monitoring	Observation of technique -SMBG log	Proper technique Daily use of log	-Observe technique 2x/yr -Log → q visit
"	No exercise plan	Adhere to exercise plan	Daily walk	Report of adherence weight	Positive report ↓ wt and BMI	q visit

PHARMACIST'S CARE PLAN AMBULATORY MONITORING WORKSHEET (AMW)

Patient __Sarah McLucas__

Pharmacist __Alexa Sheffield__

Date __4/23/98__

Page 1

Pharmaco-therapeutic Goal	Monitoring Parameter	Desired Endpoint	Monitoring Frequency	Date										
1,6	FBG	<120	q visit											
1	SMBG preprandial	<120	q visit											
1	SMBG postprandial	<120	q visit											
1	SMBG Bedtime	100-140	q visit											
1	HBA1c	<7%	q 3 mo; ↓ q 6											
1	SX of hyperglycemia -polyuria	⊖	q visit											
1	-polydipsia	⊖	q visit											
1	-polyphagia	⊖	q visit											
1	Dilated retinal exam	received	annual											
1	Dental exam	received	2x/yr											
1	Skin screen/assess	received	quarterly											
1	Foot screen	received	quarterly											
1	SCr	<1.2	q 6 mo											

PHARMACIST'S CARE PLAN AMBULATORY MONITORING WORKSHEET (AMW)

Patient **Sarah McLucas**

Pharmacist **Alexa Sheffield**
Date **4/23/98**

Page 2

Pharmaco-therapeutic Goal	Monitoring Parameter	Desired Endpoint	Monitoring Frequency	Date													
1	U/A	(-)	annual													
1	Urine microalbumin	(-)	annual													
1	EKG	received WNL	annual													
2	BP	<130/85	q visit													
3	Total cholesterol	<200	q visit													
3	LDL cholesterol	<100	q 8 wk ⊗ 2													
3	HDL cholesterol	>45	→													
3	TG	<200	→													
3	AE of fluvastatin GI upset	(-)	q visit													
3	headache	(-)	q visit													
3	back or muscle pain or tenderness	(-)	q visit													
3	ALT	<35	Baseline; q 8 wk, q 6 mo													
3	AST	<35	→													

PHARMACIST'S CARE PLAN AMBULATORY MONITORING WORKSHEET (AMW)

Patient _Sarah McLucas_

Pharmacist _Alexa Sheffield_

Date _4/23/98_

Page 3

Pharmaco-therapeutic Goal	Monitoring Parameter	Desired Endpoint	Monitoring Frequency	Date											
4	Vasomotor SX	(–)	q visit												
4	AE of estrogen/progestin breast pain	(–)	q visit												
4	GI upset	(–)	q visit												
4	vaginal bleeding	(–)	q visit												
4	thromboembolic comp	(–)	q visit												
5	AE of ASA tx GI upset	(–)	q visit												
5	dark, tarry stools	(–)	q visit												
5	home fecal occult blood test	performed	2x/yr												
6	Patient profile	dc PPA	every visit until d/c												
7	Pt. interview	adhere 4/5 days	q visit												
7	Weight	<150	q visit												
7	BMI	<27	q visit												
8, 12	Patient profile	dc NSAIDs	every visit till d/c												

PHARMACIST'S CARE PLAN AMBULATORY MONITORING WORKSHEET (AMW)

Patient **Sarah McLucas**

Pharmacist **Alexa Sheffield**

Date **4-23-98**

Page 4

Pharmaco-therapeutic Goal	Monitoring Parameter	Desired Endpoint	Monitoring Frequency	Date										
9	SX of seasonal allergic rhinitis	(-)	q visit											
	AE of loratadine: dry mouth	(-)	q visit											
	sedation	(-)	q visit											
10	Pt. profile	d/c w/o SXs	q visit											
11	OA pain (knee)	pain <2/10	q visit											
13	Pt. profile	dc w/o SXs; ↑ compliance	q visit until resolved											
14	Correct technique	(+)	q 6 mo.											
14	Completing log	(+)	q visit											
15	Pt. interview	adhere 4/5 days	q visit											

Part III:

Managing an Ambulatory Pharmacist's Care Plan for Patients with Type 2 Diabetes

Implementing a Pharmacist's Care Plan for Patients with Type 2 Diabetes

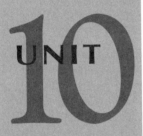

UNIT 10

So far in this module you have obtained data necessary to make therapeutic decisions, identified problems, defined goals of therapy, developed a therapeutic regimen, and designed a monitoring plan for an ambulatory patient with type 2 diabetes. But you're still not done! The next step is to implement your plan. As a pharmaceutical care provider, you cannot assure outcomes of drug therapy despite the best care plan in the world if you don't take steps to communicate and implement your plan.

Unit 17 of the *Ambulatory Care Clinical Skills Program: Core Module* addresses implementation issues, including how to communicate your plan to the patient as well as to other health care providers. Throughout this module you have seen examples of pharmacists working collaboratively with patients to develop plans. The same principle applies in implementing a plan of care; allow the patient to feel some sense of ownership in the plan.

In this unit, you will apply what you've already learned about sharing your plan with other health care providers.

Unit Objectives

After you successfully complete this unit, you will be able to:

- explain portions of the ambulatory diabetes patient's pharmacist's care plan that need to be communicated to the patient's pertinent health care providers, and
- explain methods of providing continuity of care to ambulatory diabetes patients.

Unit Organization

This unit begins by reviewing which portions of the ambulatory type 2 diabetes patient's pharmacist's care plan require the services of other health care providers. Then we consider how we can assure continuity of care by maintaining contact with patients. Last, you will be given an opportunity to practice these activities using Mr. Jones as an example.

Communicating the Plan to Pertinent Health Care Providers

In practice sites in which you do not have the ability to initiate or modify drug therapy, you need to communicate your plan to a health care provider who is responsible for making therapy changes. There's no guarantee the health care provider will agree with your plan, in which case you would need to negotiate a mutually acceptable plan of care for the patient that would lead to improved outcomes.

Case Study

Let's use Mrs. Gonzalez as an example. She was referred to the pharmacist by Dr. Thompson. Dr. Thompson was aware that the pharmacy routinely provides pharmaceutical care services for patients with type 2 diabetes, which makes the implementation of Pharmacist Radcliffe's recommendations somewhat easier, because pharmacists in this practice already have a working relationship with Dr. Thompson.

After collecting all relevant data, identifying pharmacotherapeutic and related health care problems, and developing a list of proposed interventions, Pharmacist Radcliffe prepares to contact Dr. Thompson. As discussed in the *Ambulatory Care Clinical Skills Program: Core Module*, the steps involved in communicating with other health care providers are to:
- present the plan,
- evaluate the provider's response,
- assess/identify issues,
- negotiate the plan, and
- make necessary changes to (fine tune) the original plan.

Let's listen in on a telephone conversation between Pharmacist Radcliffe and Dr. Thompson on February 25, 1998.

PHARMACIST:
"Hi, Dr. Thompson, this is Jane Radcliffe from Valley Pharmacy. Thanks for the referral of Mrs. Gonzalez; she was pretty upset when she first came in, but I met with her and got her started monitoring her blood glucose."

DR. THOMPSON:

"That's great, I knew you would. Do you have any suggestions now, or do you just want to follow her glucose for a while?"

PHARMACIST:

"Actually, I do have a few recommendations. I'm making a referral to Greta King, a dietitian in private practice; Mrs. Gonzalez is really looking forward to that. I think she has a good opportunity to make dietary changes to help her diabetes, hypertension, and hypercholesterolemia. She is also agreeable to joining a group of women in her neighborhood in a walking program. Mrs. Gonzalez told me that you had cleared her to start a walking program. Is this true?"

DR. THOMPSON:

"Yes, I encouraged her as well. Her EKG was normal, so there's no reason why she can't jump right in."

PHARMACIST:

"Great! Dr. Thompson, I also thought about recommending metformin therapy for Mrs. Gonzalez at this time, but she is extremely reluctant to start medication for her diabetes. She is convinced that she will be able to control her diabetes through diet alone. What do you think?"

DR. THOMPSON:

"I'm not sure if she'll be able to, but if she's that enthusiastic, let's give her 6–8 weeks and see how it goes. You'll keep an eye on how her glucose goes, won't you?"

PHARMACIST:

"Of course. I do think she should start therapy for her hyperlipidemia, though. I want to recommend atorvastatin."

DR. THOMPSON:

"Why don't we wait for the cholesterol as well, since we're waiting to see what the glucose does?"

PHARMACIST:

"Well, I'm concerned that her LDL cholesterol is already slightly over 200 mg/dl. I don't think her LDL cholesterol will come down more than 25 mg/dl, which leaves her quite a ways from goal. We can always back off if the diet proves to be more beneficial than I'm thinking."

DR. THOMPSON:

"All right, but start at a low dose, say 10 mg a day. Anything else?"

PHARMACIST:

"Yes, Mrs. Gonzalez and I talked about her setting up an appointment with her ophthalmologist; it's been two years since she was last seen. Also, I gave her some fecal occult blood test cards to use and return. I'll let you know how those turn out. I've also made a note in my records to remind Mrs. Gonzalez to get a flu vaccine this fall. We picked a blood glucose monitor, and I feel confident that she'll be able to check her glucose as I taught her. I did have a few drug therapy recommendations, though. I would like to discontinue the HCTZ, which can worsen her glucose and cholesterol, and start her on lisinopril 10 mg every day instead. As you know, lisinopril is a preferred agent in patients with diabetes; it doesn't alter the blood glucose or lipids and it protects the kidneys. Also, since Mrs. Gonzalez is postmenopausal, I think she should begin hormone replacement therapy. She should also receive calcium supplementation to prevent osteoporosis. Last, it's recommended that patients with diabetes who have cardiovascular risk factors such as hypertension and hypercholesterolemia be started on an aspirin a day, so I'd like to recommend one enteric-coated aspirin 325 mg a day for her."

DR. THOMPSON:

"Mrs. Gonzalez and I had already discussed initiating hormone replacement therapy to prevent osteoporosis. She seemed agreeable but wanted to think about it a bit more. In light of her new diagnosis and increased risk for cardiovascular disease, I think it would be good to start therapy now, as long as she is still agreeable. Why don't you discuss this further with her?"

PHARMACIST:

"Yes, I will. I'll also ask her to come back within a week so I can check her blood pressure. I'm seeing her in a few days to check her technique with blood glucose monitoring, so I can teach her about her new medications then. I set her goals per the American Diabetes Association recommendations—are you in agreement with that?"

Dr. Thompson:

"I agree, but I'm not sure that she'll hit the goals with just diet and exercise. Did you check her hemoglobin A_{1c}? She's not acutely symptomatic, so let's give the diet and exercise a couple of months and see how she does. I don't need to see her again for 2–3 months."

Pharmacist:

"Yes, I did check Mrs. Gonzalez' hemoglobin A_{1c}, and it was 10.2% on February 19. I can check it again by the first of May and have her make a follow-up appointment with you a week or so later, so you'll have the hemoglobin A_{1c} value for your visit. How does that sound?"

Dr. Thompson:

"That sounds great, Jane. Tell Mrs. Gonzalez to call me if she needs me, and you as well. Thanks for your help."

In this scenario, Dr. Thompson and Pharmacist Radcliffe had previously established a working relationship; therefore, the pharmacist's recommendations by telephone were appropriate and acceptable. For many practices, it would be more appropriate for the pharmacist to communicate with the physician in writing, sharing the plan of care as well as therapeutic recommendations. For example, the pharmacist may send the referring physician a SOAP (Subjective, Objective, Assessment, Plan) note summarizing a patient's recent upward trend in self-monitored blood glucose values, including a recommendation to increase the dose of the patient's antidiabetic medication. This would be an acceptable form of intervention, particularly if the pharmacist knew the patient had a follow-up appointment with the physician next week. Refer to unit 12 of the *Ambulatory Care Clinical Skills Program: Core Module* for a review of SOAP notes.

Pharmacist Radcliffe has now developed a care plan, and she and Dr. Thompson have agreed on interventions for Mrs. Gonzalez. She also sent a referral to the dietitian on the same day (see **Appendix A**). The pharmacist also needs to share this plan with the most important member of the team—Mrs. Gonzalez! The pharmacist should follow the same steps in communicating the plan to Mrs. Gonzalez as she did with Dr. Thompson:

- present the plan,
- evaluate the patient's response,
- assess/identify issues,
- negotiate the plan, and
- make necessary changes to (fine-tune) the original plan.

Pharmacist Radcliffe has a follow-up appointment with Mrs. Gonzalez for February 27, 1998 to review her blood glucose monitoring technique and to go over the care plan.

Pharmacist:

"Hello, Mrs. Gonzalez, how are you today?"

Mrs. Gonzalez (smiling):

"Well, a lot better than last week when I first met you, that's for sure."

Pharmacist:

"How has this week been for you? Any trouble with the blood glucose monitoring?"

Mrs. Gonzalez:

"Well, I can't say I'm crazy about sticking myself, but it wasn't as bad as I thought. I read all the booklets you gave me, and within a few days I got pretty good at it, if I say so myself! And I've been following the diet tips you gave me. When do I get to see the dietitian?"

Pharmacist:

"I sent the referral a few days ago; she should have it by now. I'll give you her name and telephone number, and you can make an appointment that suits your schedule. She's pretty good about seeing patients quickly. It sounds like you've really gotten off to a good start. How are you feeling about being diagnosed with diabetes, now that it's been a week?"

Mrs. Gonzalez:

"I'm still not crazy about that either, but I read the book you gave me all the way through, and I figure with you and Dr. Thompson I'll be OK. I plan on doing everything I'm supposed to do, so I can live a long time and not have any of those horrible complications of diabetes. I talked to the ladies in my neighborhood who walk every day, and they said I could join them. One of them has diabetes, too. She's had it for 5 years, and she said it was the wake-up call she needed. She's lost over 40 lb and she walks every day. She looks better now than she did 5 years ago!"

Pharmacist:

"That's wonderful! Since we last met, I've gone over all the information you gave me last week, and I'd like to talk to you about our plan for controlling your diabetes. How does that sound?"

MRS. GONZALEZ:

"Fine. I hope it's nothing too complicated, though."

PHARMACIST:

"No, a few medication changes, and things you've already started."

The pharmacist goes over the whole plan, including referrals to the dietitian and ophthalmologist. The pharmacist also provides fecal occult test cards for the patient to return at her convenience. The pharmacist watches the patient check her blood glucose and corrects any deficiencies she observes. Mrs. Gonzalez and Pharmacist Radcliffe discuss the issues surrounding hormone replacement therapy, and the patient is agreeable to starting therapy. The patient is instructed to discontinue the hydrochlorothiazide and given her new medications: lisinopril 10 mg by mouth daily; conjugated estrogen 0.625 mg daily; medroxyprogesterone 2.5 mg by mouth daily; enteric coated aspirin 325 mg by mouth daily; atorvastatin 10 mg by mouth daily; and calcium carbonate 500 mg TID. The pharmacist reviews all aspects of the new prescriptions with the patient and gives the patient opportunity to ask questions. She provides written information about each of Mrs. Gonzalez's new medications and works with her to establish a medication administration schedule.

PHARMACIST:

"I know it seems like a lot of changes, but I think we've come up with a good plan. Dr. Thompson is in full agreement as well. How will this plan work for you?"

MRS. GONZALEZ:

"I think it will be OK. I understand when I'm supposed to take all my medications and when to check my blood glucose. I'll keep up with my daily walk. When do I see you again?"

PHARMACIST:

"I would like to see you again next Friday so I can check your blood pressure. With luck, you will have seen the dietitian by then, and you can tell me all about it. Also, please try to line up your appointment with the ophthalmologist so I can make a note of when that is. Don't forget, though, you can call me anytime when you have a question; you don't have to wait until Friday. Do you have any other questions?"

MRS. GONZALEZ:

"No, I think I need to go home and go over all

this again. It's a lot to absorb. Thanks a lot, though. I'll see you next Friday."

Methods of Providing Continuity of Care

Unit 17 of the *Ambulatory Care Clinical Skills Program: Core Module* provides several excellent examples of how to maintain continuity of care with patients in an ambulatory care practice. In the case of Pharmacist Radcliffe and Mrs. Gonzalez, the pharmacist made a follow-up appointment with the patient before she left the pharmacy. The pharmacist maintains her own schedule and made a note of the time she would be seeing Mrs. Gonzalez next Friday. Also, the pharmacist made a note to call next Wednesday to remind Mrs. Gonzalez of their appointment and to see if she had any questions. If the ambulatory care pharmacist does not make these efforts, the tracking of patients and attention to their care can be jeopardized. The pharmacist needs to develop a tracking system to make sure patients keep appointments, that missed appointments are rescheduled, and a telephone call reminder system is in place. If this is not the case, more and more patients will be lost to follow-up, as the pharmacist's patient census increases. Patients who miss appointments cannot be followed and monitored per the care plan that was developed.

Another aspect of continuity of care is the need to document and communicate information between health care professionals as well as between practice settings. The following is an example that illustrates poor continuity of care. Mr. Kostkowski is a 64-year-old man with a 15-year history of type 2 diabetes. He is being treated with glyburide 10 mg by mouth daily and metformin 500 mg three times daily. He developed an ulcer on his left ankle and was hospitalized for debridement and treatment for osteomyelitis. He was discharged on intravenous antibiotics and sliding-scale (i.e., adjustable doses of) insulin provided through the hospital's home care program. Mrs. Kostkowski called the pharmacy asking for a refill of insulin, which was the first the ambulatory pharmacist had heard of Mr. Kostkowski's change in therapy. Pharmacists need to begin to work in an environment of seamless care and communicate with each other (hospital to ambulatory care pharmacist, and vice versa). Similarly, the home care pharmacist should be included in this loop. The ambulatory pharmacist must develop a mechanism to routinely communicate with the patient's other health care providers and foster a reciprocal arrangement.

Practice Example

Return to the case of Mr. Jones and determine how best to implement his care plan. What information should be communicated to the patient and other health care providers? What referrals should be made? Also, how could the pharmacist in this case maintain continuity of care with Mr. Jones? Write down your responses and, when you're done, compare them to what is written below.

Mr. Jones had approached the pharmacist initially with a complaint of nocturia on March 3, 1998. The pharmacist recognized that the patient had several risk factors for diabetes, did an assessment, and obtained a random blood glucose, which was 244 mg/dl. Suspecting a diagnosis of diabetes, the pharmacist completed his database and physical examination and referred the patient to Dr. Middleton for confirmation of the diagnosis of diabetes. The physician obtained another casual plasma glucose and fasting plasma glucose; both were diagnostic of diabetes. The patient had a lipid panel and liver function tests performed at a laboratory near his home on March 30, 1998, and returned to the pharmacy on April 3, 1998, for evaluation of hemoglobin A_{1c}, creatinine, and urinalysis. On April 6, 1998, the pharmacist discussed his proposed care plan by telephone with Dr. Middleton. The points the pharmacist covered included:

- the patient agreed to a dietary referral, and the pharmacist would send a letter to the dietitian;
- the patient was referred back to the physician for a rectal and prostate examination but refused to cooperate;
- the patient was referred to an ophthalmologist;
- the patient refused to see a dentist; the pharmacist made a note to discuss this with the patient every quarter;
- the pharmacist noted areas of sensation loss on foot examination and asked if the primary care provider wanted to perform a comprehensive foot examination or refer the patient to a podiatrist;

- the pharmacist would teach the patient how to use a peak flow meter and blood glucose monitor;
- the pharmacist recommended the following medication changes:
  - discontinue furosemide,
  - begin lisinopril 10 mg by mouth daily,
  - begin clotrimazole cream for early fungal infection in skin crease of toe,
  - begin repaglinide 0.5 mg by mouth before each meal,
  - begin enteric-coated aspirin 325 mg daily, and
  - begin cholestyramine 4 g twice daily;
- the pharmacist recommended nicotine replacement and smoking cessation when the patient agrees to stop smoking;
- the pharmacist asked the physician about an exercise program for the patient; and
- the pharmacist reviewed all desired endpoints for monitoring parameters with the physician.

The physician agreed with everything the pharmacist proposed, but he wanted to see the patient within a week of beginning repaglinide therapy, to follow up on the toe infection and to perform a comprehensive foot examination himself. The physician asked the pharmacist to check on the patient during the week to make sure his blood glucose didn't go too low during repaglinide therapy.

On April 8, 1998, the pharmacist met with Mr. Jones and reviewed the plan. Mr. Jones agreed with the plan (with exceptions noted above) and demonstrated good understanding of peak flow meter and blood glucose monitor use and medication changes. The pharmacist made a note to call Mr. Jones on April 10, 1998, to check his progress and had a follow-up appointment scheduled for April 22. Mr. Jones was also scheduled to see Dr. Middleton on April 15, 1998, as discussed above. The pharmacist sent a referral to the dietitian (**Appendix B**).

Summary

Once you have designed a therapeutic regimen, you must implement it. There are several techniques you can use to facilitate this process, including sending a letter or making direct telephone contact. Be sure to document all conversations with other health care providers, as well as patient progress.

Self-Study Questions

Objective

Explain which portions of the ambulatory diabetes patient's pharmacist's care plan need to be communicated to the patient's pertinent health care providers.

1. Name and explain which portions of the diabetes patient's pharmacist's care plan need to be communicated to the patient's pertinent health care providers.

2. Explain why medication changes need to be communicated to the patient's primary care provider.

3. Explain why dietary nonadherence needs to be communicated to the dietitian.

Objective

Explain methods of providing continuity of care to ambulatory diabetes patients.

4. Explain special concerns in providing continuity of care to ambulatory patients with diabetes.

5. Explain why ensuring follow-up appointments is a concern in providing continuity of care to ambulatory patients with diabetes.

6. Explain why remembering to contact patients by telephone between appointments is important in providing continuity of care to ambulatory patients with diabetes.

Self-Study Answers

1. In many practice settings, recommendations to initiate or modify drug therapy must be communicated to the patient's primary care physician. Other portions of the care plan that require communication include referrals to a dietitian, exercise physiologist, dentist, podiatrist, and ophthalmologist.

2. Unless the pharmacist has authority to initiate drug therapy, the pharmacist must speak to the prescriber to obtain a prescription for recommended medication changes.

3. The dietitian is best suited to work one-on-one with the patient to amend dietary habits.

4. The biggest concern with continuity of care in ambulatory practice is maintaining the pharmacist-patient relationship. The pharmacist needs to develop a tracking system to make sure patients keep appointments, that missed appointments are rescheduled, and that a telephone call reminder system is in place. Documentation and communication between health care professionals are important elements in providing this continuity of care.

5. If the patient misses an appointment with the pharmacist, the patient may not be appropriately monitored according to the specifications of the plan of care.

6. The pharmacist needs to have a system to remind him- or herself to make these telephone calls. Once the pharmacist's patient census increases, the telephone contact will not be maintained if these reminders are not documented.

Appendix A. Referral Letter to Dietitian for Mrs. Gonzalez

VALLEY PHARMACY

654 Main Street
Annapolis, MD 21401

February 25, 1999

Greta King, RD, CDE
Dietary Consultants, Inc.
553 Water Street
Annapolis, MD 21401

Dear Ms. King:

Mrs. Rose Gonzalez is a 55-year-old obese Hispanic woman with a history of hypertension for 4 years who has been newly diagnosed with type 2 diabetes and hypercholesterolemia. She also has occasional gastroesophageal reflux disease and constipation. Her laboratory values (all obtained this month) are:

Fasting plasma glucose 184 mg/dl
Casual plasma glucose 242 mg/dl
HbA_{1c} 10.2%
Total cholesterol 290 mg/dl
LDL cholesterol 204 mg/dl
HDL cholesterol 30 mg/dl
Triglycerides 280 mg/dl
Serum creatinine 1.1 mg/dl
Proteinuria—negative

She is 5'5" and on February 20, 1998, weighed 228 lb. Her blood pressure on that day was 152/100 mmHg, pulse 92 bpm and regular.

Her metabolic goals have been set as follows, on discussion with Dr. Thompson:

Fasting plasma glucose and preprandial glucose <120 mg/dl
Postprandial blood glucose <140 mg/dl
Bedtime blood glucose 100–140 mg/dl
HbA_{1c} <7%
Blood pressure <130/85 mmHg
Total cholesterol <200 mg/dl
LDL cholesterol <130 mg/dl
HDL cholesterol >45 mg/dl
Triglycerides <200 mg/dl
Weight <150 lb
BMI <27

Appendix A. Referral Letter to Dietitian for Mrs. Gonzalez (cont.)

Her medication regimen is:

Lisinopril 10 mg PO qd
Conjugated estrogen 0.625 mg PO qd
Medroxyprogesterone 2.5 mg PO qd
Enteric-coated aspirin 325 mg PO qd
Calcium carbonate 500 mg PO tid
Docusate 100 mg PO prn
Nonprescription famotidine PO prn
Acetaminophen PO prn

Mrs. Gonzalez is eager to meet with you to design a meal plan that will optimize control of her diabetes, hypertension, and hypercholesterolemia. Please work with Mrs. Gonzalez in meal planning for a low-fat, low-calorie, low-salt diet. She is very motivated to improve her health.

If you disagree with any of the goals or have any feedback on this plan, please contact me as soon as you are able. My work number is 555-5693, or you may page me at 555-9853. I'd appreciate if you could send a copy of your consult to me as well as to Dr. Thompson.

Sincerely,

Jane Radcliffe

Jane Radcliffe, R.Ph.

Appendix B. Referral Letter to Dietitian for Mr. Jones

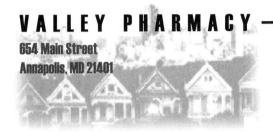

VALLEY PHARMACY

654 Main Street
Annapolis, MD 21401

April 3, 1998

Anthony Rosella, RD, CDE
Dietary Consultants, Inc.
553 Water Street
Annapolis, MD 21401

Dear Mr. Rosella:

Mr. George Jones is a 66-year-old obese African American man with a history of asthma for 5 years, hypertension for 4 years, angina for 3 years, and hypercholesterolemia for 1 year. He has been newly diagnosed with type 2 diabetes. His laboratory values (all obtained this month) are:

Fasting plasma glucose 190 mg/dl
Casual plasma glucose 244 mg/dl (on 3/13/98); 258 mg/dl (on 3/14/98)
HbA$_{1c}$ 11.6%
Total cholesterol 290 mg/dl
LDL cholesterol 229 mg/dl
HDL cholesterol 45 mg/dl
Triglycerides 80 mg/dl
Serum creatinine 1.8 mg/dl
Proteinuria—positive

He is 5'8' and on March 3, 1998, weighed 240 lb. His blood pressure on that day was 152/98 mmHg seated and 140/90 mmHg standing. His pulse was 84 bpm seated and 92 bpm standing; and regular.

His metabolic goals have been set as follows, on discussion with Dr. Middleton:

Fasting plasma glucose and preprandial glucose <120 mg/dl
Postprandial blood glucose <140 mg/dl
Bedtime blood glucose 100–140 mg/dl
HbA$_{1c}$ <7%
Blood pressure <130/85 mmHg
Total cholesterol <200 mg/dl
LDL cholesterol <130 mg/dl
HDL cholesterol >45 mg/dl
Triglycerides <200 mg/dl
Weight <160 lb
BMI <27

Appendix B. Referral Letter to Dietitian for Mr. Jones (cont.)

His medication regimen is:

Lisinopril 10 mg PO qd
Repaglinide 0.5 mg PO tid with meals
Enteric-coated aspirin 325 mg PO qd
Cholestyramine 4 g PO bid
Multivitamin 1 tablet PO qd
Albuterol inhalation prn
Acetaminophen PO prn
Sublingual nitroglycerin 0.4 mg SL prn

Mr. Jones is eager to meet with you to design a meal plan that will optimize control of his diabetes, hypertension, and hypercholesterolemia. Please work with Mr. Jones in meal planning for a low-fat, low-calorie, low-salt diet. He understand the importance of dietary modifications in improving his health but is reluctant to change his dietary habits.

If you disagree with any of the goals or have any feedback on this plan, please contact me as soon as you are able. My work number is 555-7948, or you may page me at 555-7949. I'd appreciate if you could send a copy of your consult to me as well as to Dr. Middleton.

Sincerely,

John O'Malley

John O'Malley, Pharm.D.

Evaluating Outcomes for Patients with Type 2 Diabetes

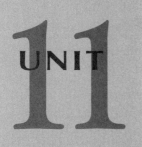

UNIT 11

In unit 9 we discussed which monitoring parameters to follow as part of the pharmaceutical care plan. Next we will discuss how to track the monitoring parameters to determine if the desired endpoints have been met, thus accomplishing the pharmacotherapeutic and related health care goals for the patient. Because diabetes is largely a self-managed disease, it is imperative to also assess the effectiveness of the patient-specific education programs you have instituted for your type 2 diabetes patients.

Unit Objectives

After you successfully complete this unit, you will be able to:

- interpret data unique to ambulatory patients with type 2 diabetes that are gathered as specified in a monitoring plan,
- assess data to determine achievement of or state of progress toward an ambulatory type 2 diabetes patient's pharmacotherapeutic and related health care goals,
- determine reasons for an ambulatory patient's progress or lack of progress toward stated health care goals,
- explain the importance of the analysis of trends that are unique to the monitoring parameter measurements for ambulatory patients with type 2 diabetes, and
- assess the effectiveness of patient-specific education programs for ambulatory patients with type 2 diabetes.

Unit Organization

In this unit we will discuss and practice the approach to evaluating outcomes. This approach begins with an assessment of patient status, condition, and therapy changes; we then discuss assessing the need for missing or additional data. We will use Mrs. Gonzalez as an example to illustrate the process of evaluating patient outcomes by assessing available data. Then you will have an opportunity to practice with the case of Mr. Jones.

Assessing Goal Achievement

As discussed in unit 20 of the *Ambulatory Care Clinical Skills Program: Core Module*, there are four sequential steps in assessing whether desired endpoints have been achieved:

1. Consider changes in patient status, condition, drug therapy, or nondrug therapy since developing the monitoring plan.
2. Assess if required data are missing.
3. Assess the need for additional data.
4. Assess the achievement of the desired endpoint for each parameter in the monitoring plan and judge whether that pharmacotherapeutic goal was met.

Case Study

Assessing Patient Status, Condition, and Therapy Changes

Refer to Mrs. Gonzalez's APCP and AMW in **Appendix A**. During her visit today, May 4, 1998, with Mrs. Gonzalez, Pharmacist Radcliffe inquires if the patient has experienced any change in her condition or drug therapy since her last visit. She has no new complaints and has had no changes in her drug therapy since the lisinopril dose was last increased in April. She has continued with her diet (adhering to her regimen 3 out of every 5 days) and an exercise plan. Mrs. Gonzalez has not experienced any change in status, condition, or therapy and no change is required in her APCP or AMW.

Assessing Whether Missing Data Are Still Required

As you can see from Mrs. Gonzalez's AMW, the pharmacist does not have all the needed data. The pharmacist does not have a baseline potassium level, needed to monitor for possible drug-induced hyperkalemia from the lisinopril therapy, and a lipid panel is overdue. In addition to obtaining a total cholesterol at every visit, the pharmacist also planned to assess the entire fasting lipid panel every 8 weeks for the first 4 months. Pharmacist Radcliffe will need to make arrangements for Mrs. Gonzalez to stop by a local laboratory for a potassium level and fasting lipid profile.

The monitoring frequency specified for the hemoglobin A_{1c} is every 3 months until stable and then every 6 months. The hemoglobin A_{1c} is repeated at this visit, a little sooner than 3 months since her diagnosis, so the physician would also have the value for his next visit with Mrs. Gonzalez.

All other required data have been obtained, including the presence/absence of subjective complaints that the pharmacist asked the patient about directly, a fasting blood glucose that the pharmacist obtained directly, weight, blood pressure, adherence to nonpharmacologic therapies, and analysis of the average values of self-monitoring of blood glucose. On interviewing the patient, the pharmacist learned that Mrs. Gonzalez received a dilated retinal examination on April 28; the pharmacist marked this as complete on the AMW. According to Mrs. Gonzalez, her eye examination was unremarkable, and the ophthalmologist instructed her to make another appointment in a year. No consult report was received from the ophthalmologist.

As a reminder, Pharmacist Radcliffe will make a note that aspartate aminotransferase (AST) and alanine aminotransferase (ALT) values, height measurement, foot screening, and skin examination should all be obtained within the next 4–6 weeks.

Assessing Need for Additional Data

In Mrs. Gonzalez's case, the pharmacist obtained the majority of the data needed or analyzed data provided by the patient (e.g., self-monitoring of blood glucose). No additional data are needed at this time.

Assessing Achievement of Desired Endpoints

Once you have assessed the patient's AMW for new problems or changes, missing data, and additional data requirements, you need to assess achievement of or state of progress toward desired endpoints for each parameter in the monitoring plan. This is your last assessment and should not be attempted until you have considered possible changes in the patient's condition or status.

You now need to match your monitoring parameter measurements with your desired endpoints. Have you achieved your goals? If not, why not? Are you making progress toward the goal? If so, is the rate of progress acceptable? If not, why not?

For example, Mrs. Gonzalez has not achieved her glycemic goals, although she is making progress. The pharmacist can observe the downward trends in fasting blood glucose, self-monitoring results, and hemoglobin A_{1c} (from 10.2% to 9.5%). The importance of evaluating trends is discussed later in this unit.

Mrs. Gonzalez's second goal is to improve her blood pressure control and prevent complications. Her blood pressure is coming down in response to the lisinopril dosage increase.

Her third goal is to improve her lipid control and prevent complications. Mrs. Gonzalez's total cholesterol has dropped from 290 to 164 mg/dl over 2.5 months, since beginning atorvastatin therapy. Her total cholesterol is <200, which is the goal, but a lipid panel should be drawn to assess the remaining cholesterol values. The LDL cholesterol is the best indicator of the achievement of lipid goals.

Another goal for Mrs. Gonzalez is to eliminate postmenopausal symptoms and reduce cardiovascular risks. She was not symptomatic of her postmenopausal state initially; not surprisingly, there has been no change in her complaint of vasomotor symptoms. She did complain of mild nausea the first week after beginning conjugated estrogen, progestin, enteric-coated aspirin and lisinopril therapy, which resolved by the time of her appointment 2 weeks later.

Mrs. Gonzalez's adherence to nonpharmacologic therapies has been declining since inception. On interview, she states it is very difficult to plan her meals. She and her husband like to eat at restaurants, and this is not always conducive to following her prescribed meal plan. However, she is making progress toward her weight loss goal.

Mrs. Gonzalez is achieving her goal of regular self-monitoring of blood pressure and blood glucose. The pharmacist reassessed her technique on February 27 and March 6, 1998, respectively, with good results. Mrs. Gonzalez also returned the fecal occult blood test cards on March 6, 1998.

Evaluating Reasons for Failure to Achieve Endpoints

You have completed your assessment of the monitoring data and, by examining the attainment of each of the desired endpoints, have determined whether the patient reached each of the pharmacotherapeutic goals. In areas where the patient did not attain the desired endpoint, you should explore why the therapy failed. Four possible causes for failure to achieve desired therapeutic endpoints follow. For a complete discussion of these causes, refer to unit 20 of the *Ambulatory Care Clinical Skills Program: Core Module*.

Failure to Receive Therapy
The first reason for therapy failure is that patients may not receive therapy; this is a common occurrence among outpatients. There are a variety of reasons why patients do not adhere to therapies, including inappropriate use of a delivery system, difficulty adhering to a prescribed diet or exercise regimen, or a conscious choice not to adhere

because of inconvenience or an adverse effect. Mrs. Gonzalez is having difficulty adhering to her diet and exercise regimen, although she is very compliant with her medication regimen, as shown by her refill record.

Change in Patient Status or Condition

The second reason for therapy failure is change in the patient's status or condition, in which case you need to modify your monitoring plan. Mrs. Gonzalez has not experienced any noticeable disease progression, complications, or adverse effects from her medication regimen.

Change in Patient Therapy

The third reason for therapy failure is change in the patient's therapy, such as change resulting from drug interactions or changes made by other health care providers. If such were the case with Mrs. Gonzalez, you would need to make sure the APCP was communicated to the provider that made the change; and alter it to monitor the new therapy.

Therapeutic Failure

Unfortunately, not all interventions will be successful in all patients. Despite making the most appropriate drug recommendations and appropriately monitoring outcomes, the therapy you prescribe for a patient may still fail.

As discussed above, Mrs. Gonzalez is not at the desired endpoint for several of her goals. This may be because she has not been fully adherent to her nonpharmacologic interventions, and also because of the need for pharmacologic interventions for glucose control.

Analyzing Trends

When evaluating achievement of outcomes, it is important to evaluate not only the latest measurements but also trends. By looking at data obtained at subsequent visits, you can determine if a patient is making progress toward glycemic control goals, a blood pressure goal, freedom from adverse medication effects, adherence to nonpharmacologic therapies, a total cholesterol goal, and adherence to other recommendations such as health maintenance and referrals to other health care providers. Even if the patient is not at the goal for a given parameter, it is important to appreciate trends toward achieving the goal. The pharmacist may also choose to establish short- and intermediate-term goals.

With Mrs. Gonzalez, for example, her blood glucose, blood pressure, and total cholesterol are not at goal, but they are on a favorable trend. If her blood glucose, blood pressure, and lipid values were unchanged, the pharmacist would suspect lack of adherence to recommended therapies.

When evaluating a patient's results from self-monitoring of blood glucose, it is important to look for trends. Despite the accuracy of the home blood glucose monitors, you should rarely respond to one value. Instead, look at averages and trends and try to identify patterns. For example, consider a patient receiving isophane (NPH) and regular insulin twice daily. If over the past 3–5 days the patient experiences a trend toward an increased pre-lunch blood glucose reading, the pharmacist may recommend increasing the regular insulin before breakfast, after ruling out the influence of a variable such as an unusually large breakfast for the past 5 days. This is referred to as pattern assessment and is part of observing trends.

Practice Example

Now turn to the case of Mr. Jones in **Appendix B**. Review his APCP and AMW and interpret the data provided as of his visit on June 17, 1998. Has he achieved his pharmacotherapeutic and related health care goals? Is he making progress toward these goals? What types of questions could you ask Mr. Jones to assess the effectiveness of the patient education provided to him? When you have completed this exercise, compare your answers to those given below.

The first step in assessment is to ascertain if there have been any changes in patient status, condition, drug therapy, or nondrug therapy since you developed the monitoring plan. Mr. Jones told you on April 22 that Dr. Middleton said his fungal toe infection had resolved. You inspected the toe and concurred with Dr. Middleton's prognosis. On May 6, the physician increased the Questran Light to 8 g twice daily. The physician also increased his repaglinide from 0.5 to 1 mg by mouth before meals on May 18, 1998. The patient does complain of recent constipation.

Next, assess if data are missing. You do not have a potassium level for Mr. Jones or confirmation that he has received a dilated retinal examination. The pharmacist will need to make arrangements for Mr. Jones to stop by a local laboratory for testing of his potassium level. The remaining data the pharmacist can personally collect or get from the patient (e.g., self-monitoring of blood glucose and peak flow meter use). As a reminder, the pharmacist should make a note to obtain liver function test results and perform a skin and foot examination to assess sensation within the next 6 weeks. No additional data are needed at this time.

The next step is to assess and evaluate the achievement of desired endpoints. Mr. Jones' second health care goal is control of his hypertension. Again, his blood pressure is coming down but is not at goal yet. He denies having symptoms of toxicity from lisinopril therapy.

Mr. Jones has been adherent to medication administration (as evidenced by refill history) and keeping appointments. He still refuses to give up smoking or drinking beer, but otherwise he has been compliant with diet and exercise. His weight has decreased to 218 lb, but he is still over 50 lb above goal.

He has demonstrated good technique with both the peak flow meter and the blood glucose monitor. Mr. Jones still refuses to undergo a prostate/rectal examination or to accept a referral to the dentist. He agreed to a home fecal occult blood test and an ophthalmologist referral.

Another health care goal for Mr. Jones is to improve control of his diabetes. After 6 weeks of therapy with repaglinide 0.5 mg before each meal, his fasting blood glucose was still ≥ 180 mg/dl. Subsequent to increasing the repaglinide dose, his fasting plasma glucose dropped an additional 20–30 mg/dl but still remains above the goal of <120 mg/dl.

Mr. Jones' final health care goal is to improve control of cholesterol; his total cholesterol has decreased since beginning Questran Light therapy. After the physician increased the dose to 8 g twice daily on May 6, Mr. Jones showed additional improvement, as indicated by the results of the lipid profile on June 17, 1998. However, the LDL cholesterol is still above goal. It is important to remember that not every patient will achieve the goal you have established. In Mr. Jones' case, it is unlikely that we can gain any significant benefit from increasing the Questran Light again. Even though Mr. Jones may not achieve an LDL cholesterol of 100, the closer he gets to goal, the more favorable. Mr. Jones has been fairly compliant with the recommended meal plan, which was tailored to meet his busy schedule, but he emphasizes it is unlikely he can reduce his fat intake further.

Assessing Patient-Specific Education

As discussed in unit 8, you should assess the effectiveness of patient-specific education at the time

each objective is taught and provide reinforcement at subsequent visits. The patient education program form in unit 8 is an excellent tool for documenting and assessing the effectiveness of patient education.

Case Study

Refer to the completed patient education program form for Mrs. Gonzalez in Appendix A. The pharmacist questioned Mrs. Gonzalez each time they met about the content taught at the previous session regarding diabetes education. Mrs. Gonzalez had good recall and did not require additional explanation of previously covered material. On March 6, 1998, the pharmacist reviewed Mrs. Gonzalez's understanding of self-monitoring of blood glucose monitoring and observed her technique.

Practice Example

Refer to the completed patient education program form for Mr. Jones in Appendix B to assess the effectiveness of the education provided. Determine areas where additional education is required and then compare your answers to those described below.

Mr. Jones requires additional education about the role of diet and exercise in controlling diabetes, hypertension, and hypercholesterolemia. Follow-up education is also required about preventive measures and the risks of alcohol and tobacco use.

Summary

Assessing the achievement of each of the desired endpoints for the parameters selected in the monitoring plan enables the pharmacist to determine whether the patient's pharmacotherapeutic goals have been achieved. Because judgment is frequently complicated by conflicting and missing data, it is imperative that pharmacists use a systematic approach in evaluation.

Self-Study Questions

Objective

Interpret data unique to ambulatory patients with type 2 diabetes that are gathered as specified in a monitoring plan.

For questions 1–3, refer to the APCP and AMW for Ms. McLucas in **Appendix C**.

1. Which data would you assess to determine whether Ms. McLucas' health care goal to "improve control of diabetes and prevent complications" was achieved?

2. Which data would you assess to determine whether Ms. McLucas' health care goal to "improve control of hypertension and prevent complications" was achieved?

3. Which data would you assess to determine whether Ms. McLucas' health care goal to "improve control of hypercholesterolemia and prevent complications" was achieved?

Objective

Assess data to determine achievement of or state of progress toward an ambulatory type 2 diabetes patient's pharmacotherapeutic and related health care goals.

For questions 4–6, refer to the APCP and AMW for Ms. McLucas in Appendix C.

4. What do the parameters used to assess diabetes control indicate about Ms. McLucas' progress toward her goals?

5. What does the parameter used to assess hypertension control indicate about Ms. McLucas' progress toward her goals?

6. What do the parameters used to assess hypercholesterolemia indicate about Ms. McLucas' progress toward her goals?

Objective

Determine reasons for an ambulatory type 2 diabetes patient's progress or lack of progress toward stated health care goals.

For questions 7–9, refer to the APCP and AMW for Ms. McLucas in Appendix C.

7. Give a possible reason why Ms. McLucas has not achieved her goal weight.

8. Give a possible reason why Ms. McLucas has not achieved her glycemic goals.

9. Determine if Ms. McLucas has achieved her LDL cholesterol goal.

Objective

Explain the importance of the analysis of trends that are unique to the monitoring parameter measurements for ambulatory patients with type 2 diabetes.

10. Explain the importance of the analysis of self-monitoring of blood glucose trends for ambulatory patients with type 2 diabetes.

Objective

Assess the effectiveness of patient-specific education programs for ambulatory patients with type 2 diabetes.

For question 11, refer to the APCP, AMW, and patient education program for Ms. McLucas in Appendix C.

11. How would you assess the effectiveness of patient-specific education for this patient?

Self-Study Answers

1. To assess diabetes control, the following monitoring parameters should be assessed: fasting blood glucose, self-monitoring glucose results, hemoglobin A$_{1c}$, and complaints related to hyperglycemia, such as polyuria, polydipsia, and polyphagia. To assess prevention of complications monitoring parameters include dilated retinal and dental exams, foot and skin screening, serum creatinine measurement, and urinalysis.

2. blood pressure

3. Total cholesterol, LDL cholesterol, HDL cholesterol, and triglycerides should be monitored to assess efficacy of therapy. Monitoring parameters to detect adverse effects of fluvastatin therapy (e.g., gastrointestinal upset, headache, muscle pain, and increased liver enzymes) should be assessed to detect complications.

4. Ms. McLucas is not at goal, although she had made some progress. Clearly her predominant abnormality is postprandial hyperglycemia.

5. Ms. McLucas has met her goal for blood pressure control.

6. The total cholesterol is at goal (<200); however, we need a whole lipid panel to determine whether she has reached her LDL cholesterol goal (considered to be a better predictor of risk status than total cholesterol).

7. Ms. McLucas is steadily losing weight and is near her goal; the fact that she is not yet at goal does not indicate she will not reach it.

8. Ms. McLucas has made some progress toward this goal. Perhaps with continued weight loss and exercise she will achieve the goal.

9. Ms. McLucas may have achieved her LDL cholesterol goal; we do not have the data at this time. Based on her total cholesterol, she is going in the right direction.

10. Some patients require adjustments to their insulin regimen based on trends in self-monitoring of blood glucose. This adjustment is referred to as pattern assessment.

11. Ms. McLucas shows good understanding of all educational objectives except for the role of hormone replacement therapy and the importance of diet and exercise in managing her disease. These topics require reinforcement. All educational objectives require follow-up as described in the AMW.

APPENDIX A

Patient Education Program for Mrs. Gonzalez

Goals:

1. To educate Mrs. Gonazlez about diabetes mellitus and the importance of blood glucose control.
2. To educate Mrs. Gonzalez about uncontrolled hypertension and hypercholesterolemia and potential complications.
3. To educate Mrs. Gonzalez on the importance of health maintenance.

Educational Objective	Date Taught	Outcome	Follow-up Required?
1. Mrs. Gonzalez will understand what diabetes	2/20/98	1	yes
mellitus is, including:	2/27/98	1	yes
-basic pathophysiology	3/6/98	1	yes
-the role of blood glucose control	3/20/98	1	yes
-potential complications of diabetes	4/3/98	1	yes
-signs and symptoms of hyperglycemia	5/4/98	1	yes
2. Mrs. Gonzalez will understand the role of hypertension and hypercholesterolemia and complications of each, which may interact with and worsen complications of diabetes.	3/6/98	1	yes
3. Mrs. Gonzalez will understand the role of hormone replacement therapy and daily aspirin therapy as part of her therapeutic regimen.	2/27/98	1	no
4. Mrs. Gonzalez will understand how to properly	2/27/98	1	yes
evaluate blood glucose and will monitor	3/6/98	1	yes
blood glucose as recommended.	5/4/98	1	yes
5. Mrs. Gonzalez will understand how to properly	2/27/98	1	yes
monitor blood pressure and will monitor	3/6/98	1	yes
blood pressure as recommended.			
6. Mrs. Gonzalez will understand the importance	2/27/98	2	yes
of adherence to dietary recommendations for	3/20/98	1	yes
control of diabetes, hypertension, and	5/4/98	2	yes
hypercholesterolemia.			
7. Mrs. Gonzalez will understand the importance	2/27/98	2	yes
of adherence to an exercise program for control	3/20/98	1	yes
of diabetes, hypertension, and hyper-	5/4/98	1	yes
cholesterolemia.			
8. Mrs. Gonzalez will understand the importance	2/27/98	1	yes
of performing annual home fecal occult blood	3/20/98	1	yes
tests and monthly breast self-examinations.	5/4/98	1	yes

Educational Objective	Date Taught	Outcome	Follow-up Required?
9. Mrs. Gonzalez will understand the importance of follow-up with health care providers, including the ophthalmologist, dentist, pharmacist, and primary care provider.	2/19/98	1	yes
10. Mrs. Gonzalez will understand the importance of taking her medications as prescribed and at the recommended times.	2/27/98 3/6/98 4/3/98	1 1 1	yes yes yes
11. Mrs. Gonzalez will recognize adverse effects of her medications and what action to take should they occur.	2/27/98 3/6/98 4/3/98	1 1 1	yes yes yes
12. Mrs. Gonzalez will understand the importance of and demonstrate good technique for foot and skin inspection.	3/20/98 4/3/98	2 1	yes yes

Outcome:

1. Patient restated content correctly/performed task acceptably well.
2. Patient needs reinforcement of content or performance of task.
3. Patient cannot or will not restate content correctly or perform task.

Content:

Content will depend on Mrs. Gonzalez' current understanding of the above issues. Educational content will fill in gaps in her knowledge base.

Delivery Methods:

Method is verbal for all objectives. Provided video on introduction to diabetes mellitus. Provided book, *Right from the Start*, on type 2 diabetes. Demonstrated blood glucose and blood pressure monitoring.

Evaluation of Effectiveness:

1. Patient interview for health beliefs, restate content when requested, adherence to recommended follow-up
2. Demonstrate use of blood glucose monitoring; demonstrate foot and skin inspection
3. Refill records for medications and metabolic control

Ambulatory Pharmacist's Care Plan

Patient __Rose Gonzalez__   Pharmacist __Jane Radcliffe__   Date __2/20/98__

Page 1 of 2

DATE IDENTIFIED	PROBLEM (TPL)	PHARMACOTHERAPEUTIC AND RELATED HEALTH CARE GOAL	RECOMMENDATIONS FOR THERAPY	MONITORING PARAMETER(S)	DESIRED ENDPOINT(S)	MONITORING FREQUENCY
2/20/98	poor control of diabetes	Improve diabetes control; prevent complications.	Institute non-pharmacol interventions (diet & exercise)	FBG SMBG, HbA1c, Pt. satisfac., SXs hypergly.	FBG<120, hsBG 100-140, HbA1c<7%, ⊖ SXs HG	All q visit except HbA1c q 3 mo; ↓ to q 6 mo.
"	poor control of HTN	Improve BP control; prevent complications.	As above, plus rec. Δ to ^{abc} lisinopril 10 mg QD	BP, AE lisinopril- cough, rash, K⁺	<130/85, K<5, ⊖ cough, rash	All q visit except WBC & K⁺ 2x q yr.
"	poor control of cholest.	Improve lipid control; prevent complications.	nonpharmacol interventions & Atorvastatin 10 mg*	TC, LDL, HDL, TG, LFT, c/o muscle pain, GI upset, HA	LDL<100 HDL>45, TG<200 TC<200, ⊖ c/o AE	TC-q visit panel-q 8 wk x 2, SXs-q visit
"	Not on daily ASA tx	↓ risk CV complic. of diabetes	Rec. EC ASA 325 mg QD*	GI bleeding/upset; dark, tarry stools	⊖ bleeding or c/o	SX-q visit occult blood- 2x q yr.
"	post menopausal c̄ HRT	↓ risk post-men. SXs/↓ risks of post-menopause	Rec. conjugated estrogen/progestin*	vasomotor SX c/o edema GI, breast pain t'boembolic	⊖ SX or AE	q visit
"	not receiving calcium tx	↓ risk for osteoporosis	Rec calcium carbonate 500 mg TID*	AE GI upset constipation	⊖ height loss	quarterly
"	Potential of HCTZ to affect DM & chol.	Avoid worsened BG & lipid control	D/C HCTZ	D/C → profile; pt. interview	D/C c̄ AE	q visit til D/C
"	no exercise plan	start & adhere to regular exercise program.	Begin regular walking program	report of regular walking prog	↓ BMI, wt. ↓BP	q visit

*Treatment began 2/7/98.   b 3/6 Lisinopril ↑ to 15 mg qd.   c 4/3 Lisinopril ↑ to 20 mg qd.

AMBULATORY PHARMACIST'S CARE PLAN

Patient Rose Gonzalez   Pharmacist Jane Radcliffe   Date 2/20/98

Page 2 of 2

DATE IDENTIFIED	PROBLEM (TPL)	PHARMACOTHERAPEUTIC AND RELATED HEALTH CARE GOAL	RECOMMENDATIONS FOR THERAPY	MONITORING PARAMETER(S)	DESIRED ENDPOINT(S)	MONITORING FREQUENCY
2/20/98	no MNT plan	start & adhere to MNT plan.	refer to RD- follow meal plan	report of adherence to plan	↓ BMI, wt ↓ BP	q visit
"	no home BG monitoring	learn & regularly perform SMBG	select & explain use of BG monitor	-SMBG log -observe technique	-proper technique -adherence to use	observe 2x q yr. review log q visit
"	no home BP monitoring	learn & regularly perform BP measurements	select and explain use of BP cuff	-BP log -observe technique	-proper technique -adherence to use	Observe 2x q yr.; review log every visit
"	no home fecal test	perform annual home fecal blood test	Provide home fecal blood test cards	cards returned	⊖ occult blood	2x q yr.
"	no influenza vaccine	receive annual influenza vaccine	Receive flu vaccine Fall 98	Pt. interview	flu shot received	q Fall
"	no monthly breast self-exam	learn & regularly perform exam	refer to primary physician for exam technique	pt. interview	monthly self-exam	q month

PHARMACIST'S CARE PLAN AMBULATORY MONITORING WORKSHEET (AMW)

Patient: Rose Gonzalez

Pharmacist: Jane Radcliffe

Date: 2/20/98

Pharmaco-therapeutic Goal	Monitoring Parameter	Desired Endpoint	Monitoring Frequency	2/9	2/18	2/19	2/27	3/6	3/20	4/3	5/4			
—	FBG	<120	every visit		184		AVG 170	AVG 160	AVG 165	AVG 155	AVG 152			
—	SMBG-preprandial	<120	→				AVG 174	AVG 170	AVG 170	AVG 160	AVG 160			
—	SMBG-postprandial	<140	→	random 242			AVG 200	190	192	184	→180			
—	SMBG-bedtime	100-140					AVG 180	176	170	160	→148			
—	HbA1c	<7	q 3mo; ↓ q 6mo			10.2					9.5			
—	dilated retinal exam	received	annual			①	①	made appt	①	①	✓			
—	SCr	<1.2	q 6 month	0.9										
—	U/A	①	annual			⊕ glucose / 0 protein / 0 ketone								
—	urine microalbumin	⓪	annual			①								
—	EKG	received	annual	WNL										
—	Foot screen	received	quarterly	✓										
—	Skin screen	received	quarterly	✓										
—	Dental exam	received	q 6 month	✓ 1/98										

PHARMACIST'S CARE PLAN AMBULATORY MONITORING WORKSHEET (AMW)

Patient ___Rose Gonzalez___
Page 2

Pharmacist ___Jane Radcliffe___
Date ___2/20/98___

Pharmaco-therapeutic Goal	Monitoring Parameter	Desired Endpoint	Monitoring Frequency	2/9	2/18	2/19	2/27	3/6	3/20	4/3	5/4
1	signs and symptoms of hyperglycemia	(-)	every visit			(-)	(-)	(-)	(-)	(-)	(-)
1	(polyuria, polydipsia, polyphagia)	(-)	every visit			(-)	(-)	(-)	(-)	(-)	(-)
2	BP	<130/85	every visit			152/100	142/90	140/90	134/82	136/84	130/80
2	lisinopril AE- dizziness/headache	(-)	q visit; ↓ q 3 mo				(-)	(+)	(-)	(-)	(-)
2	lisinopril AE- cough	(-)	→				(-)	(-)	(-)	(-)	(-)
2	K+	<5	q 6 month								
3	Total cholesterol	<200	every visit	286	290			205	184	172	164
3	LDL cholesterol	<100	q 8 wk x2; ↓		204						
3	HDL cholesterol	>45	→		30						
3	TG	<200	→		280						
4	ASA AE- GI upset	(-)	q visit; ↓ q 3 mo					(+)	(-)	(-)	(-)
4	ASA AE- dark tarry stools	(-)	→					(-)	(-)	(-)	(-)
4	ASA-efficacy prevent MI	(-)	every visit					(-)	(-)	(-)	(-)

see page 4 for additional items _____

PHARMACIST'S CARE PLAN AMBULATORY MONITORING WORKSHEET (AMW)

Patient __Rose Gonzalez__
Page **3**

Pharmacist __Jane Radcliffe__
Date _____

Pharmaco-therapeutic Goal	Monitoring Parameter	Desired Endpoint	Monitoring Frequency	2/9	2/18	2/19	2/27	3/6	3/20	4/3	5/4		
5	Vasomotor Sxs	(↓)	every visit			(↓)	(↓)	(↓)	(↓)	(↓)	(↓)		
5	Estrogen/progestin AE- breast pain, anorexia	(↓)	q visit, ↓ q 3 mo					(+)	(↓)	(↓)	(↓)		
5	headache, edema	(↓)	→					(↓)	(↓)	(↓)	(↓)		
5	thromboembolic c/o	(↓)	→					(↓)	(↓)	(↓)	(↓)		
5	vaginal bleeding	(↓)	→					(↓)	(↓)	(↓)	(↓)		
6	height loss	(↓)	quarterly				5'5"						
6	calcium AE- GI upset, constipation	(↓)	q visit, ↓ q 3 mo					(↓)	(↓)	(↓)	(↓)		
7	patient interview and profile	(↓)	every visit til D/C				(↓)	(↓)					
8	Pt. interview	adhere 4/5 days	every visit					(+)	(+)	3/5	3/5 1-2/5		
8	weight	<150 lb	→				228	223	220	216	210		
8	BMI	<27	→				38	37	37	36	36	35	
9	Pt. interview	adhere 4/5 days	every visit					(+)	(+)	3/5	3/5 2-3/5		
10	correct technique	(+)	2x/yr					(+)					

PHARMACIST'S CARE PLAN AMBULATORY MONITORING WORKSHEET (AMW)

Patient __Rose Gonzalez__

Page 4

Pharmacist __Jane Radcliffe__

Date _____

Pharmaco-therapeutic Goal	Monitoring Parameter	Desired Endpoint	Monitoring Frequency	Date 2/9	2/18	2/19	2/27	3/6	3/20	4/3	5/4		
10	completing log	(+)	every visit					(+)	(+)	(+)	(+)		
11	correct technique	(+)	2x/yr			(+)							
11	completing log	(+)	every visit				(+)	(+)	(+)	(+)	(+)		
12	returned home fecal test cards	(+)	annual					(+)					
13	flu shot received	(+)	every fall										
14	patient interview	complete	every month						✓	✓	✓		
3	AST	<35	baseline g 8 wks then g 6 mos			8			12				
3	ALT	<35	→			11			20				
3	AE of atorvastatin -GI upset	(-)	g visit					(-)	(-)	(-)	(-)		
3	-headache	(-)	→					(-)	(-)	(-)	(-)		
3	-muscle pain or tenderness	(-)	→					(-)	(-)	(-)	(-)		

see page 1

APPENDIX B

Patient Education Program for Mr. George Jones

Goals:

1. To educate Mr. Jones about diabetes mellitus and the importance of blood glucose control.
2. To educate Mr. Jones about uncontrolled hypertension and hypercholesterolemia and potential complications.
3. To educate Mr. Jones on monitoring and management of asthma.
4. To educate Mr. Jones on importance of health maintenance.
5. To educate Mr. Jones on importance of and techniques to improve health care compliance.

Educational Objective	*Date Taught*	*Outcome*	*Follow-up Required?*

1. Mr. Jones will understand what diabetes mellitus is, including:
   -basic pathophysiology
   -the role of blood glucose control
   -potential complications of diabetes
   -signs and symptoms of hyperglycemia
	4/3/98
	4/8/98
	5/6/98
	5/20/98
	6/17/98
		1
		1
		1
		1
		1
			yes
			yes
			yes
			yes
			yes

2. Mr. Jones will understand the role of hypertension and hypercholesterolemia and complications of each, which may interact with and worsen complications of diabetes.	5/6/98 6/17/98	2 2	yes yes
3. Mr. Jones will understand how to properly perform peak flow monitoring and administer albuterol at appropriate times.	4/3/98 4/8/98	1 1	yes yes
4. Mr. Jones will understand how to properly evaluate blood glucose and will monitor blood glucose as recommended.	4/22/98 5/20/98 6/17/98	1 1 1	yes yes yes
5. Mr. Jones will understand the importance of adherence to dietary recommendations for control of diabetes, hypertension, and hypercholesterolemia.	4/22/98 5/20/98 6/17/98	2 2 2	yes yes yes
6. Mr. Jones will understand the importance of adherence to an exercise program for control of diabetes, hypertension, and hypercholesterolemia.	4/3/98 4/22/98 5/20/98 6/17/98	2 2 2 2	yes yes yes yes
7. Mr. Jones will understand the importance of performing annual home fecal occult blood test.	3/3/98 6/17/98	3 3	yes yes
8. Mr. Jones will understand the importance of follow-up with health care providers, including the ophthalmologist, dentist, pharmacist, and primary care provider.	3/3/98 5/10/98	2 2	yes yes

Educational Objective	Date Taught	Outcome	Follow-up Required?
9. Mr. Jones will understand the importance of taking his medications as prescribed and at the recommended times.	4/8/98 5/18/98	1 1	yes yes
10. Mr. Jones will recognize adverse effects of his medications, particularly hypoglycemia, and what action to take should they occur.	4/8/98 5/18/98	1 1	yes yes
11. Mr. Jones will understand the importance of and demonstrate appropriate foot and skin inspection.	5/6/98	1	yes

Outcome:

1. Patient restated content correctly/performed task acceptably well.
2. Patient needs reinforcement of content or performance of task.
3. Patient cannot or will not restate content correctly or perform task.

Content:

Content will depend on Mr. Jones' current understanding of the above issues. Educational content will fill in gaps in his knowledge base.

Delivery Methods:

Methods are verbal for all objectives. Provided video on introduction to diabetes mellitus. Provided book, *Right from the Start*, on type 2 diabetes. Provided written materials on repaglinide. Demonstrated blood glucose and peak flow monitoring.

Evaluation of Effectiveness:

1. Patient interview for health beliefs, restate content when requested, adherence to recommended follow-up
2. Demonstrated use of peak flow and blood glucose monitoring; demonstrated foot and skin inspection
3. Refill records for repaglinide and metabolic control

AMBULATORY PHARMACIST'S CARE PLAN

Patient __George Jones__   Pharmacist __John O'Malley__   Date __3-3-98__

Page 1 of 3

DATE IDENTIFIED	PROBLEM (TPL)	PHARMACOTHERAPEUTIC AND RELATED HEALTH CARE GOAL	RECOMMENDATIONS FOR THERAPY	MONITORING PARAMETER(S)	DESIRED ENDPOINT(S)	MONITORING FREQUENCY
3/3/98	SX and BG suggestive of DM. High risk status	Rule in/out DM. Determine cause of high BG and nocturia	Refer to primary physician—await results	Consult report	Rule in/out diabetes	q week until resolved
	poor control of hypertension	Improve BP control; Prevent complications	D/C furosemide Begin lisinopril 10 mg q AM*	BP, AE for lisinopril—cough rash, ↑K+	<130/85 ⊖ SX AE	All q visit except K+- 2x/yr
	nonadherence to diet	start and adhere to prescribed meal plan	Referral to dietitian	pt. interview, wt, BMI	wt<160 BMI<27	q visit
	h/o med schedule nonadherence	adherence to medication regimen	Provide written instructions	Pt. interview, review profile	proper medication use	q visit
	Furosemide may worsen lipids	Avoid worsened lipid profile	Rec d/c furosemide. Begin lisinopril	Profile and pt. interview	d/c w/o sequelae	q visit
	smoking history	Stop smoking	Nicotine replacement and counseling. Pt. refuses at this time	# cigs/day pt. interview	decreased or no smoking	discuss quarterly
	Alcohol use history	Stop Alcohol use	↓ or stop alcohol use Pt. refuses at this time	amt Etoh/wk Pt. interview	decreased or no Etoh use	discuss quarterly

*Treatment began 4/8

AMBULATORY PHARMACIST'S CARE PLAN

Patient George Jones Pharmacist John O'Malley Date 3-3-98

Page 2 of 3

DATE IDENTIFIED	PROBLEM (TPL)	PHARMACOTHERAPEUTIC AND RELATED HEALTH CARE GOAL	RECOMMENDATIONS FOR THERAPY	MONITORING PARAMETER(S)	DESIRED ENDPOINT(S)	MONITORING FREQUENCY
3/3/98	h/o non-adherence to flu appts	Adherence to flu appt. scheduling	Counsel pt.	Pt. interview cc consult reports	Compliant c̄ other HCP	q visit
	nonadherence to exercise	start and adhere to exercise plan	Counsel pt.	Pt. interview, wt, BMI, BP	BMI<27 BP<130/85	q visit
	Not doing peak flow monitoring	Learn and perform peak flow monitoring regularly	Instruct pt. on peak flow monitoring	Observe technique, Review SM record	Proper technique use PFM w/o SX	Observe tech 2x then 2x/yr Review log q visit
	No rectal/prostate exam	Annual rectal prostate exam	Refer to PCP. Pt. refuses at this time	Pt. interview consult report	complete exam	Discuss quarterly
	No home fecal test	Home fecal blood test q 6 months	Provide home fecal test cards. Pt. refuses at this time.	Pt. interview	complete test	Discuss quarterly
4/3/98	poor control of diabetes	Improve control; prevent complications	Rec. repaglinide 0.5 mg a.c. before meals	FBG, SMBG, HBA1c, SX AE, satisfaction	FBG<120 hs BG 100-140 HBA1c <7 ⊖ SX and AE, ⊕ satisfaction	FBG & SMBG q visit HBA1c q 3 mo, ↓ q 6 mo satisfaction
	Furosemide may ↑ BG	Avoid worsened BP control	Rec d/c furosemide Begin lisinopril	Profile and pt. interview	d/c w/o sequelae	q visit
	Fungal skin infection on toe	Eliminate fungal toe infection	Rec. Lotrimin cream to affected area BID* for 7-10 days	Inspection of feet	No sign of infection	monthly x 3 then quarterly

*Treatment began 4/8.   °5/18 repaglinide ↑ to 1 mg with meals.

AMBULATORY PHARMACIST'S CARE PLAN

Patient George Jones   Pharmacist John O'Malley   Date 3-3-98

Page 3 of 3

DATE IDENTIFIED	PROBLEM (TPL)	PHARMACOTHERAPEUTIC AND RELATED HEALTH CARE GOAL	RECOMMENDATIONS FOR THERAPY	MONITORING PARAMETER(S)	DESIRED ENDPOINT(S)	MONITORING FREQUENCY
4/3	Insensate feet	Absence of infection trauma, ulcerations	Daily self-inspection Quarterly exam	Foot exam, Pt. interview	No complications	Inspect quarterly Interview q visit q visit
	Not on daily ASA tx	↓ risk CV complications 2° to diabetes	Rec EC ASA 325 mg QD*	GI upset, dark tarry stools, MI	⊖SX ⊖ occult blood	SX – q visit Biannual fecal blood
	Poor control of cholesterol	Improve control, prevent complications	Refer for MNT Rec. cholestyramine 4 g BIDᵇ	TC, CDL, HDL, TG c/o constipation GI upset	TC<200 TG<200 CDL<100 HDL>45, ⊖ c/o AE	TC q visit Panel q 8 wks x2 Sxs – q visit
	Not doing SMBG	Learn and perform regular SMBG	Instruct on SMBG	Observation of technique, SMBG log	Proper tech. Use of BGM daily	Observe tech 2x/yr Review log q visit
	No dilated retinal exam	Annual dilated retinal exam	Refer to ophthalmologist	–Pt. interview –copy of consult report	Compliant with annual exam	Annually
	No recent dental exam	Dental exam q 6 months	Refer to dentist	Pt. interview Copy of consult report	Compliant with appts	q 6 mo
	liver dysfunction	monitor liver function	monitor LFTs	ALT, AST	<3S	q 3-6 mo

ᵃTreatment began 4/8.   ᵇS/b cholestyramine ↑ to 8 g BID.   *Treatment began 4/8.

PHARMACIST'S CARE PLAN AMBULATORY MONITORING WORKSHEET (AMW)

Patient ___George Jones___
Page 1

Pharmacist ___John O'Malley___
Date ___3-3-98___

Pharmaco-therapeutic Goal	Monitoring Parameter	Desired Endpoint	Monitoring Frequency	3/3	3/18	3/23	3/30	4/3	4/8	4/10	4/22	5/6	5/20	6/17
1	Consult report	Rule in/out diabetes	q week until resolved					✓						
2	BP	<130/85	q visit	152/98 40/90				140/84	140/85	138/85	138/85	136/82	140/86	136/82
	lisinopril AE: dizziness	(−)	q visit						⊖	⊖	⊖	⊖	⊖	⊖
	lisinopril AE: headache	(−)	q visits ↓ q 3 mo						⊖	⊖	⊖	⊖	⊖	⊖
	lisinopril AE: cough	(−)	→						⊖	⊖	⊖	⊖	⊖	⊖
	lisinopril AE: ↑ K+	<5	2x year											
3	Pt. interview	adhere 4/5 days	q visit	⊖				⊕	⊕	⊖	⊕	⊕	⊕	⊕
	Weight	<160 lb	q visit	240				235	235	235	230	225	218	210
	BMI	<27	q visit	37				36	36	36	35	34	33	32
4	Profile and pt. interview	⊕	q visit	+/−				⊕	⊕	⊕	⊕	⊕	⊕	⊕
5	Profile and pt. interview	d/c furosemide ⊖ symptoms	q visit					✓	⊖	⊖	⊖	⊖		
6	# cigs/day	Pt. currently refuses	revisit quarterly	1 ppd				− ppd						
7	Amt Etoh/wk	pt. currently refuses	revisit quarterly	4 beers								4 beers		

PHARMACIST'S CARE PLAN AMBULATORY MONITORING WORKSHEET (AMW)

Patient: George Jones   Page 2

Pharmacist: John O'Malley

Date: 3-3-98

Pharmaco-therapeutic Goal	Monitoring Parameter	Desired Endpoint	Monitoring Frequency	3/3	3/18	3/23	3/30	4/3	4/8	4/10	4/22	5/6	5/20	6/17
8	Pt. interview w/ consult reports	(+)	q visit	+(+)				(+)	(+)	(+)	(+)	(+)	(+)	(+)
9	Pt. interview	adhere 4/5 days	q visit	(−)				(+)	(+)	(+)	(+)	(+)	(+)	(+)
10	Observe technique	proper technique	2x; ↓2x/yr					✓	✓					
10	Review log	PFM w/o SX	q visit					✓	✓	✓	✓	✓	✓	✓
11	Pt. interview/consult report — Pt. currently refuses	Annually complete exam	revisit quarterly					(−)						
12	Pt. interview w/ — Pt. currently refuses	complete test q 6 mos	revisit quarterly	(−)				(−)						(−)
13	FBG	<120	every visit		190						avg 190 180	avg 190 180	avg 160 160	avg 160 150
13	SMBG preprandial	<120		Random 244	Random 258						avg 190 180	avg 190 180	avg 162	avg 162 152
13	SMBG postprandial	<140	↓								avg 240 230	avg 240 230	avg 200 200	avg 200 200
13	SMBG bedtime	100-140	↓								avg 180 170	avg 180 170	avg 160 160	avg 160 160
13	HbA1c	<7%	q 3 mo; ↓q 6 mo					11.6						
13	SCr	<1.2	q 6 month				1.8							
13	U/A	(−)	annual				+prot +glue -ket							

PHARMACIST'S CARE PLAN AMBULATORY MONITORING WORKSHEET (AMW)

Patient George Jones
Page 3

Pharmacist John O'Malley
Date 3-3-98

Pharmaco-therapeutic Goal	Monitoring Parameter	Desired Endpoint	Monitoring Frequency	3/3	3/18	3/23	3/30	4/3	4/8	4/10	4/22	5/6	5/20	6/17
13	urine microalbumin	<30	q 6 mo					35						
13	urine culture	(-)	prn			(-)								
13	EKG	received	annual					isch oldMI						
13	Foot screen	received	quarterly					✓	✓	✓	✓	✓	✓	✓
13	skin screen	received	quarterly					✓						
13	symptoms hyperglycemia -nocturia	(-)	q visit	(+)				(+)	(+)	(+)	(+)	+/-	(-)	(-)
	-polyuria	(-)	q visit	(-)				(-)	(-)	(-)	(-)	(-)	(-)	(-)
	-polydypsia	(-)	q visit	(-)				(-)	(-)	(-)	(-)	(-)	(-)	(-)
	-polyphagia	(-)	q visit	(-)				(-)	(-)	(-)	(-)	(-)	(-)	
13	dilated retinal exam	received	annual					to schedule						
13	dental exam- Pt. refuses at this time	received	revisit quarterly					(-)						
13	Repaglinide AE- rash GI upset	(-)	q visit; ↓ q 3 mo							(-)	(-)	(-)	(-)	(-)
13	signs & symptoms of hypoglycemia	(-)	q visit							(-)	(-)	(-)	(-)	(-)

PHARMACIST'S CARE PLAN AMBULATORY MONITORING WORKSHEET (AMW)

Patient George Jones

Page 4

Pharmacist John O'Malley

Date 3-3-98

Pharmaco-therapeutic Goal	Monitoring Parameter	Desired Endpoint	Monitoring Frequency	3/3	3/18	3/23	3/30	4/3	4/8	4/10	4/22	5/6	5/20	6/17
14	Profile and pt. interview	d/c furosemide w/o symptoms	q visit					✓	①	①	①	①		
15	Foot inspection	⊖ sign of infx	q month ⊗3						①			①		①
16	Foot exam-sensation	10/10	quarterly					7/10						
16	Pt. interview	no complications	q visit					①	①			①	①	①
17	ASA-AE GI upset	⊖	2 visits ↓ q 3 mo							①	①	①	①	①
17	ASA-AE dark, tarry stools	⊖	q visit; → q 3 mo							①	①	①	①	①
17	ASA-efficacy prevent MI	⊖	q visit							①	①	①	①	①
18	Total cholesterol	<200	q visit				290				215	220	210	198
18	LDL cholesterol	<100	q 8 wk ⊗2; ↓ 2-3 mo				229							135
18	HDL cholesterol	>45	→				45							46
18	TG	<200	↓				80							84
18	Cholestyramine AE-constipation, GI upset	⊖	q visit; ↓ q 3 mo							(-)	(+)	(+)(+)	(+)(+)(+)	(+)(+)

PHARMACIST'S CARE PLAN AMBULATORY MONITORING WORKSHEET (AMW)

Patient ___George Jones___

___Page 5___

Pharmacist ___John O'Malley___

Date ___3-3-98___

Pharmaco-therapeutic Goal	Monitoring Parameter	Desired Endpoint	Monitoring Frequency	Date 3/3	3/18	3/23	3/30	4/3	4/8	4/10	4/22	5/6	5/20	6/17
19	Observe technique	proper technique	q 6 mo						✓		✓			
19	Review SMBG log	completes log	q visit								✓	✓	✓	✓
20	Pt. interview, copy of report	receive exam	annual	⊖				⊖						⊕ 5/13
21	Pt. interview, copy of report	receive exam	q 6 month	⊖				⊖						⊖
22	ALT	<35	q 3-6 mo				56							
22	AST	<35	q 3-6 mo				98							

APPENDIX C

Patient Education Program for Ms. McLucas

Goals:

1. To educate Ms. McLucas about diabetes mellitus and the importance of blood glucose control.
2. To educate Ms. McLucas about uncontrolled hypertension and hypercholesterolemia and potential complications.
3. To educate Ms. McLucas on importance of health maintenance.

Educational Objective	*Date Taught*	*Outcome*	*Follow-up Required?*
1. Ms. McLucas will understand what diabetes mellitus is, including: -basic pathophysiology -the role of blood glucose control -potential complications of diabetes -signs and symptoms of hyperglycemia	4/23/98 5/7/98 6/18/98 7/30/98	1 1 1 1	yes yes yes yes
2. Ms. McLucas will understand the role of hypertension and hypercholesterolemia and complications of each, which may interact with and worsen complications of diabetes.	5/7/98 6/18/98	1 1	yes yes
3. Ms. McLucas will understand the role of hormone replacement therapy (HRT) and daily aspirin therapy as part of her therapeutic regimen.	4/23/98 5/7/98	2, HRT not accepted 2, HRT not accepted	yes yes
4. Ms. McLucas will understand how to properly evaluate blood glucose and will monitor blood glucose as recommended.	5/7/98	1	yes
5. Ms. McLucas will understand the importance of adherence to dietary recommendations for control of diabetes, hypertension, and hyper-cholesterolemia.	4/23/98 5/7/98 6/18/98 7/30/98	2 2 1 1	yes yes yes yes
6. Ms. McLucas will understand the importance of adherence to an exercise program for control of diabetes, hypertension, and hypercholesterolemia.	4/23/98 5/7/98 7/30/98	2 2 1	yes yes yes
7. Ms. McLucas will understand the importance of performing annual home fecal occult blood test.	4/20/98	1	yes
8. Ms. McLucas will understand the importance of follow-up with health care providers, including the ophthalmologist, dentist, pharmacist, and primary care provider.	4/3/98	2	yes
9. Ms. McLucas will understand the importance of taking her medications as prescribed and at the recommended times (including as-needed seasonal allergy medications).	4/23/98 6/18/98	1 1	yes yes

Educational Objective	Date Taught	Outcome	Follow-up Required?
10. Ms. McLucas will recognize adverse effects of her medications and what action to take should they occur.	4/23/98 5/7/98	1 1	yes yes
11. Ms. McLucas will understand the importance of and demonstrate good technique for foot and skin inspection.	4/23/98 6/18/98	2 1	yes yes

Outcome:

1. Patient restated content correctly/performed task acceptably well.
2. Patient needs reinforcement of content or performance of task.
3. Patient cannot or will not restate content correctly or perform task.

Content:

Content will depend on Ms. McLucas' current understanding of the above issues. Educational content will fill in gaps in her knowledge base.

Delivery Methods:

Method is verbal for all objectives. Provided video on introduction to diabetes mellitus. Provided book, *Right from the Start*, on type 2 diabetes. Demonstrated blood glucose monitoring.

Evaluation of Effectiveness:

1. Patient interview for health beliefs, restate content when requested, adherence to recommended follow-up
2. Demonstrated use of blood glucose monitoring; demonstrated foot and skin inspection
3. Refill records for medications and metabolic control

AMBULATORY PHARMACIST'S CARE PLAN

Patient **Sarah McLucas**   Pharmacist **Alexa Sheffield**   Date **4-23-98**

DATE IDENTIFIED	PROBLEM (TPL)	PHARMACOTHERAPEUTIC AND RELATED HEALTH CARE GOAL	RECOMMENDATIONS FOR THERAPY	MONITORING PARAMETER(S)	DESIRED ENDPOINT(S)	MONITORING FREQUENCY
4/23/98	Poor control of diabetes	Improve control of diabetes; prevent complications	Refer to dietitian for meal planning	FBG, SMBG, HbA1c, Pt. symptoms SX of hypergly.	FBG<120 hsBG 100-140 HbA1c<7%	FBG and SMBG q visit HbA1c q 3 mo; then ↓ q 6 mo
"	Poor control of HTN	Improve control of HTN; prevent complications	Refer to dietitian for meal planning†	BP	<130/85	q visit
"	Poor control of lipids	Improve control of hypercholesterolemia; prevent complications	d/c cholestyramine Rec fluvastatin 20 mg q PM	TC, LDL, HDL, TG AE of fluvastatin	TC<200 LDL<100, HDL>45 TG <200 ⊖ AE	TC q visit; panel q 8 wks x2 AE q visit; LFTs baseline, 8 wks, then q 6 mo
"	Postmenopausal w/o HRT	Eliminate post-menopausal SXs and ↓ assoc risks (CV and osteoporosis)	Rec. conj. estrogen 0.625 mg QD and medroxyprogesterone 2.5 mg QD	Vasomotor SX AE of HRT	⊖ symptoms and ⊖ AE	q visit
"	Not on ASA QD tx	Prevent cardiovascular complications	Rec Ec ASA 325 mg QD*	GI upset, bleeding, dark stools	⊖ SX or occult blood	SX q visit; occult blood 2x/yr.
"	PPA in Tavist-D may worsen BP & BG	Avoid worsened BP and BG control	D/C Tavist-D Rec loratadine* 10 mg QD w/ seasonal symptoms	Pt. profile	D/C w/o ↑ SX	q visit until resolved
"	Nonadherence to diet	Adhere to prescribed diet	Refer to dietitian	report of adherence to meal plan	Pt. report ↓ wt, ↓BMI	q visit
"	NSAID may ↑ BP	Avoid worsened BP control	D/C NSAIDS Rec acetaminophen up to 4 g QD*	Pt. profile	D/C w/o ↑ SX	q visit until resolved

†Treatment began 4/23/98.

AMBULATORY PHARMACIST'S CARE PLAN

Patient **Sarah McLucas**   Pharmacist **Alexa Sheffield**   Date **4-23-98**

Page **2 of 2**

DATE IDENTIFIED	PROBLEM (TPL)	PHARMACOTHERAPEUTIC AND RELATED HEALTH CARE GOAL	RECOMMENDATIONS FOR THERAPY	MONITORING PARAMETER(S)	DESIRED ENDPOINT(S)	MONITORING FREQUENCY
4/23/98	Taking Tavist-D year-round	Control seasonal allergic rhinitis SXs	D/C Tavist-D take loratidine only w/seasonal SX	hayfever SX	⊝ SX ⊝ AE	q visit
"	Taking Naprosyn and ibuprofen	Avoid duplicate tx	D/C Naprosyn and ibuprofen	Pt. report and profile	no increased pain	q visit until resolved
"	Poor control of OA pain	Control pain Preserve/increase functional status	Rec. Acetaminophen up to 4 g QD and re-evaluate	OA pain	pain<2/10 (per pt. report)	q visit
"	NSAID may ↑ SXs of GERD	Avoid SXs of GERD	D/C Naprosyn	Patient Profile	d/c w/o SX	q visit until resolved
"	Nonadherence to cholestyramine	Control hypercholest.	D/C cholestyramine Begin fluvastatin tx	Pt. report and profile	↑ compliance to tx	q visit until resolved.
"	No SMBG	Regular SMBG	Instruct on self-monitoring	Observation of technique -SMBG log	Proper technique Daily use of log	-Observe technique 2x/yr -Log → q visit
"	No exercise plan	Adhere to exercise plan	Daily walk	Report of adherence weight	Positive report Wt and BMI	q visit

PHARMACIST'S CARE PLAN AMBULATORY MONITORING WORKSHEET (AMW)

Patient Sarah McLucas

Page 1

Pharmacist Alexa Sheffield

Date 4/23/98

Pharmaco-therapeutic Goal	Monitoring Parameter	Desired Endpoint	Monitoring Frequency	4/14	4/20	4/23	5/7	6/18	7/30					
1,6	FBG	<120	q visit	142	138		140	136	130					
1	SMBG preprandial	<120	q visit				140	135	130					
1	SMBG postprandial	<120	q visit				200	180	180					
1	SMBG Bedtime	100-140	q visit				160	150	150					
1	HBAlc	<7%	q 3 mo; ↓ q 6		9.4				8.8					
1	SX of hyperglycemia –polyuria	(-)	q visit				(-)	(-)	(-)					
1	–polydipsia	(-)	q visit				(-)	(-)	(-)					
1	–polyphagia	(-)	q visit				(-)	(-)	(-)					
1	Dialated retinal exam	received	annual					(+)						
1	Dental exam	received	2x/yr			(+)								
1	Skin screen/assess	received	quarterly			(+)								
1	Foot screen	received	quarterly			(+)								
1	SCr	<1.2	q 6 mo		0.8									

PHARMACIST'S CARE PLAN AMBULATORY MONITORING WORKSHEET (AMW)

Patient __Sarah McLucas__

Page 2

Pharmacist __Alexa Sheffield__

Date __4/23/98__

Pharmaco-therapeutic Goal	Monitoring Parameter	Desired Endpoint	Monitoring Frequency	Date 4/14	4/20	4/23	5/7	6/18	7/30					
1	U/A	⊖	annual		⊖									
1	Urine microalbumin	⊖	annual		⊖									
1	EKG	received WNL	annual	WNL										
2	BP	<130/85	q visit			134/ 86	132/ 88	130/ 82	128/ 80					
3	Total cholesterol	<200	q visit		232		230	220	200					
3	LDL cholesterol	<100	q 8 wk ⊗2		145									
3	HDL cholesterol	>45	→		30									
3	TG	<200	→		284									
3	AE of fluvastatin GI upset	⊖	q visit				⊖	⊖	⊖					
3	headache	⊖	q visit				⊖	⊖	⊖					
3	back or muscle pain or tenderness	⊖	q visit				⊖	⊖	⊖					
3	ALT	<35	Baseline; q 8 wk, q 6 mo		10			=						
3	AST	<35	→		9			9	9					

PHARMACIST'S CARE PLAN AMBULATORY MONITORING WORKSHEET (AMW)

Patient Sarah McLucas

Pharmacist Alexa Sheffield

Date 4/23/98

Page 3

Pharmaco-therapeutic Goal	Monitoring Parameter	Desired Endpoint	Monitoring Frequency	Date 4/14	4/20	4/23	5/7	6/18	7/30
4	Vasomotor SX	(-)	q visit				(-)	(-)	(-)
4	AE of estrogen/progestin breast pain	(-)	q visit				refuses tx		
4	GI upset	(-)	q visit				→		
4	vaginal bleeding	(-)	q visit				→		
4	thromboembolic comp	(-)	q visit				→		
5	AE of ASA tx GI upset	(-)	q visit				(-)	(-)	(-)
5	dark, tarry stools	(-)	q visit				(-)	(-)	(-)
5	home fecal occult blood test	performed	2x/yr			✓			
6	Patient profile	dc PPA	every visit until d/c				d/c		
7	Pt. interview	adhere 4/5 days	q visit				(+)	(+)	(+)
7	Weight	<150	q visit			162	160	154	152
7	BMI	<27	q visit			27	27	26	26
8, 12	Patient profile	dc NSAIDs	every visit till d/c				d/c		

PHARMACIST'S CARE PLAN AMBULATORY MONITORING WORKSHEET (AMW)

Patient **Sarah McLucas**

Page 4

Pharmacist **Alexa Sheffield**

Date **4-23-98**

Pharmaco-therapeutic Goal	Monitoring Parameter	Desired Endpoint	Monitoring Frequency	4/14	4/20	4/23	5/7	6/18	7/30
9	SX of seasonal allergic rhinitis	(-)	q visit				(-)	(-)	(-)
	AE of loratadine: dry mouth	(-)	q visit				(-)	(-)	(-)
	sedation	(-)	q visit				(-)	(-)	(-)
10	Pt. profile	d/c w/o SXs	q visit				dc		
11	OA pain (knee)	pain <2/10	q visit				3/10	2/10	3/10
13	Pt. profile	dc w/o SXs; ↑ compliance	q visit until resolved				dc		
14	Correct technique	(+)	q 6 mo.				(+)	(+)	(+)
14	Completing log	(+)	q visit				(+)	(+)	(+)
15	Pt. interview	adhere 4/5 days	q visit				(+)	(+)	(+)

Redesigning the Pharmacist's Care Plan for Patients with Type 2 Diabetes

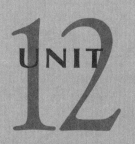

In unit 21 of the *Ambulatory Care Clinical Skills Program: Core Module*, you learned to redesign a pharmacist's ambulatory care plan. Throughout this module you have followed along and worked through several cases of patients with type 2 diabetes. Now you are ready to take the last step and complete the circle of pharmaceutical care by redesigning your care plans.

Unit Objectives

After you successfully complete this unit, you will be able to:

- determine if a change in pharmacotherapeutic and related health care goals, regimen, or monitoring plan is required in the treatment of ambulatory patients with type 2 diabetes, and
- modify a pharmacist's care plan for ambulatory patients with type 2 diabetes as necessary based on the achievement of pharmacotherapeutic and related health care goals.

Unit Organization

This unit begins with a discussion of how the need for changes in the goals, regimen, or monitoring plan of a patient with type 2 diabetes is determined. Once the need to change is decided, you will then learn to modify the care plan to reflect these changes. You will see an example of redesigning a care plan for an ambulatory patient with type 2

diabetes. You will then redesign a care plan using a practice case.

Adjusting the APCP

There are several elements in a care plan that may require adjustment. The most obvious is a change in the therapy regimen (to add, delete, or modify therapy). A change to the therapy regimen or other precipitating variables may necessitate a change in the educational goals or plans or in the monitoring plan. You may want to review unit 21 of the *Ambulatory Care Clinical Skills Program: Core Module*, particularly the discussion on considerations to make prior to changing a care plan.

Changes to Pharmacotherapeutic and Related Health Care Goals

As discussed in unit 21 of the *Ambulatory Care Clinical Skills Program: Core Module*, three factors that can help you identify whether you need to change your pharmacotherapeutic and health care related goals are:

- the patient's quality of life,
- change in the patient's status, and
- the receipt of updated or more complete patient information.

Patient's Quality of Life

The first question to ask is: Will the patient's quality of life be improved if you change the goal? This can be interpreted two ways. Will the patient's quality of life be improved if we make the goal more stringent? Or, will the patient's quality of life be improved if we relax this goal? For example, a patient has a goal hemoglobin A_{1c} of <7%. The patient's quality of life may be comfortable with an easily achieved hemoglobin A_{1c} of 7.5–8%, but trying to get it down that extra bit causes a disproportionate increase in stress for the patient. Conversely, if the patient feels better as the hemoglobin A_{1c} decreases (which is generally the case), it might be prudent to aim for the most reasonable hemoglobin A_{1c} possible, keeping patient-specific variables in mind. Remember: Treat the patient, not the number!

Change in Patient Status

If a diabetes patient develops a propensity toward more frequent episodes of hypoglycemia, you may consider setting less ambitious glycemic control goals. It is better that the patient have a little higher blood glucose and have less risk of developing hypoglycemic episodes.

Receipt of Updated or More Complete Patient Information

You may decide to change pharmacotherapeutic and related health care goals based on receipt of updated or more complete patient information. For example, you are following a patient with type 2 diabetes who is not currently controlled by behavioral interventions alone. After you review the patient's self-monitored blood glucose results, it is clear that postprandial hyperglycemia is the patient's predominant abnormality. Based on this information, you may be more inclined to recommend therapy with an α-glucosidase inhibitor, instead of other potential monotherapeutic options.

Changes to the Therapy Recommendations

There are three changes you can make to a patient's therapy regimen:

- add a new therapy,
- delete a current therapy, or
- modify a current therapy.

Modifications to the therapy regimen for any of these reasons requires altering the APCP, monitoring parameters, and monitoring frequency.

Adding a New Therapy

Patients with type 2 diabetes who do not meet their blood glucose goals frequently require the addition of a pharmacologic agent to their nonpharmacologic therapy. Also, patients on one pharmacologic agent to treat type 2 diabetes may require the addition of a second drug to meet their goals. For example, Mr. Clifford has been receiving metformin and is at the maximum dose per day, without achieving goal glycemic control. In this case, you will most likely recommend combination oral therapy. New drug entities available to treat type 2 diabetes allow many possible combinations of two and even three drugs at a time. Research is ongoing to evaluate each of these potential combinations.

Deleting a Current Therapy

There are several reasons why you might delete a drug from the current regimen of a patient with type 2 diabetes. First, the patient might have achieved the goal for which the therapy was prescribed. For example, a patient with a vaginal yeast infection has successfully completed a course of therapy. The patient has achieved the goal of therapy, so you will no longer need to monitor the parameters you had defined.

You may also delete a drug from therapy as the result of changing a pharmacotherapeutic goal for a patient. For example, a patient with type 2 diabetes who develops cancer may have a declining oral intake, thus lowering his or her need for medications that lower blood glucose. You will certainly relax your glycemic control goals and may be able to discontinue one or more medications. This in turn affects your monitoring parameters, some of which you may discontinue.

You may recommend discontinuing a medication due to the occurrence of adverse drug reactions, drug interactions, or patient adherence issues. For example, a patient with type 2 diabetes receiving hydrochlorothiazide (HCTZ) may have increased blood glucose or experience an adverse effect on his or her lipid profile. You may decide to recommend discontinuing the HCTZ for these reasons.

Another reason for deleting drug therapy is a change in the patient's status. Mrs. Riggins has been taking metformin for a little over a year with good response; however, her most recent serum creatinine was >1.4 mg/dl. Variables that could falsely elevate the serum creatinine have been ruled out, and a subsequent serum creatinine value is 1.5 mg/dl. It would be appropriate at this time to remove metformin from Mrs. Riggins' therapy, as elevated serum creatinine is a risk factor for the development of lactic acidosis. After an alternative agent has been selected, the pharmacist would modify the monitoring and education plans.

Finally, you may have to delete a therapy because of therapeutic failure. For example, you have recommended glipizide for a patient with type 2 diabetes. If the patient experiences primary failure, you may have to discontinue therapy and select an alternate approach to treating the patient's diabetes. This will require a modification to your monitoring plan as well.

Modifying a Current Therapy

As discussed in unit 21 of the *Ambulatory Care Clinical Skills Program: Core Module*, there are several reasons why you may need to modify a patient's therapy regimen.

Drug Dosage Not Maximized

A major reason for modifying a current drug regimen could be that the drug dosage has not been maximized. For example, you have been following Mr. Montgomery, who is taking glyburide 10 mg orally every day. Glyburide is an appropriate choice for this patient, but he has not achieved his glycemic goals; therefore, it would be reasonable to increase the dose to 15 or even 20 mg every day. This would probably be preferred to adding a second and possibly more expensive medication to his regimen.

Patient Nonadherence

There are many reasons why a patient may be nonadherent to a medication regimen, some of which may be remedied by altering the therapeutic regimen. For example, Mr. Brookins was started on repaglinide, and he has had only a fair response to therapy. On questioning, the patient admitted that he cannot afford the medication and sometimes has to go without it. Despite the convenience of dosing prior to each meal and the flexibility inherent in this regimen, the pharmacist recommended switching to a sulfonylurea, which is less expensive. The patient agreed, and the pharmacist modified the monitoring and education plan accordingly.

Bioavailability/Pharmacokinetic Issues

Another reason for modifying the drug regimen concerns bioavailability and pharmacokinetic issues. Suppose for some reason a prescriber wants to switch a patient from the Micronase brand of glyburide to the Glynase brand. The Glynase brand of glyburide is more bioavailable due to drug particle micronization; therefore, the equivalent glycemic effect is accomplished with a lower dose. The dose of Glynase required to bring the patient to the goal value would have to be determined.

Another issue with pharmacokinetics relates to the half-life of a given drug. For example, chlorpro-

pamide is not used as frequently as it has been in the past for several reasons, one is the duration that hypoglycemia lasts, should it occur. Chlorpropamide has a half-life of 30–42 hours and as high as 200 hours in patients with end-stage renal disease. For this reason, chlorpropamide dosing for patients experiencing declining renal function or frequent episodes of hypoglycemia may require adjustments.

Changes in Educational Goals and Plans

Several factors might contribute to your decision to change your education plan for a patient with type 2 diabetes. These factors include:

- a change in therapy,
- a change in the patient's status, or
- stabilization of the patient on current therapy.

Change in Therapy

Any time a patient's therapy is changed, the patient needs to be educated to ensure the intended changes are carried out. New medications, discontinued medications, and increased or decreased dosages are all changes to therapy that require thorough patient education.

Change in Patient Status

Using the example again of the patient with type 2 diabetes who develops a life-limiting illness, you may decide to recommend discontinuing hypoglycemic therapy. The patient will require education about this decision, and the decision will have implications for monitoring (e.g., increased or decreased blood glucose monitoring) as well.

Stabilization of the Patient on Current Therapy

Once a patient has reached and maintains your desired endpoints, decrease the frequency of your patient education. For example, you may change your patient education schedule from every quarter to once every 6 months for a patient who is well-educated and repeatedly shows good understanding of diabetes self-management.

Changes in the Monitoring Plan

As you learned in unit 21 of the *Ambulatory Care Clinical Skills Program: Core Module*, there are four factors that may lead to changing your monitoring plan:

- change in the pharmacotherapeutic and related health care goal,
- change in therapy,

- change in the patient's setting or acuity level, or
- stabilization of the patient on current therapy.

For example, it was recently reported that troglitazone can cause liver toxicity. As a result, it is recommended patients prescribed troglitazone have liver function tests according to a prescribed plan. This new recommendation will directly affect the frequency that you monitor liver enzymes for a patient receiving troglitazone. Review unit 21 of the *Ambulatory Care Clinical Skills Program: Core Module* for additional details on monitoring plan changes.

Modifying a Pharmacist's Care Plan for Patients with Type 2 Diabetes

At this point, let's practice making and recording decisions concerning your APCP, monitoring parameters, and therapy. We will use the case of Mrs. Gonzalez as an example, then you will practice with the case of Mr. Jones.

Case Study

Let's review each of Mrs. Gonzalez's pharmacotherapeutic and related health care goals and monitoring parameters from the APCP and AMW (**Appendix A**). Based on these documents, we will determine which modifications, if any, are needed.

Pharmacotherapeutic and Related Health Care Goal #1

Her APCP shows that Mrs. Gonzalez's first goal was to improve her diabetes control and prevent complications. The therapeutic interventions used up to this point are medical nutrition therapy and exercise. Monitoring parameters for diabetes control include assessment of fasting blood glucose, review of self-monitoring of blood glucose results that the patient provides, and hemoglobin A_{1c}. At this time there is no need to modify the frequency of monitoring for these parameters. When Mrs. Gonzalez does reach her goal hemoglobin A_{1c} the frequency for this parameter can be decreased to every 6 months. The monitoring parameters for diabetes complications do not require changes at this time.

Mrs. Gonzalez has made some progress toward her goals, but not much between April 3 and May 4. Her weight has decreased 18 lb in nearly 3 months, but she admits that her adherence to her meal and exercise plans is waning.

Refer to the Diabetes Treatment Satisfaction Questionnaire (DTSQ) that Mrs. Gonzalez completed during her May 4, 1998, visit to the pharmacy. She is not satisfied with her current treatment and thinks her blood glucose is too high. When questioned further, she states that the diet and exercise treatment plan is not convenient, allows for no flexibility, and, most importantly, is not giving her the desired results. Mrs. Gonzalez is more than willing to consider drug therapy if it means her blood glucose control will improve.

Pharmacist Radcliffe agrees with Mrs. Gonzalez. While the pharmacist can encourage improved adherence to diet and exercise, Mrs. Gonzalez's diabetes is not currently under control, and it would be appropriate at this point to add additional therapy. The monotherapeutic options available include an insulin secretagogue (sulfonylurea or repaglinide), metformin, a thiazolidinedione (rosiglitazone), an α-glucosidase inhibitor (acarbose or miglitol), or insulin. She is not very symptomatic of diabetes, so insulin is probably not required at this point. She has both pre- and postprandial hyperglycemia, and her hemoglobin A_{1c} is still >1% above goal, so acarbose would be of limited usefulness. Mrs. Gonzalez is obese, with excess central adiposity. Insulin secretagogues are used more in patients who are within 120% of ideal body weight.

Either metformin or rosiglitazone would be reasonable for Mrs. Gonzalez, as she is probably insulin resistant. She has concomitant hypercholesterolemia, her serum creatinine is not above the cutoff for using metformin, and she does not have any other risk factors for lactic acidosis as a result of metformin therapy. Patients in the United Kingdom Prospective Diabetes Study (UKPDS) who received metformin had excellent treatment outcomes, so this seems a reasonable choice for Mrs. Gonzalez. The pharmacist recommends beginning metformin therapy at 500 mg by mouth, twice daily (with the morning and evening meal). The physician agrees to this recommendation and Pharmacist Radcliffe adds the new therapy to Mrs. Gonzalez's APCP. Monitoring parameters for metformin must be added to the AMW, and the patient needs to be educated about this new medication. The pharmacist should reassess Mrs. Gonzalez's level of satisfaction with her diabetes treatment again in 2–3 months to see if better blood glucose control has had a positive impact.

Pharmacotherapeutic and Related Health Care Goal #2

Mrs. Gonzalez's second goal was to improve hypertension control. HCTZ was discontinued, and she was started on lisinopril 10 mg by mouth, every day. The pharmacist discussed this with Dr. Thompson, and he agreed with recommendations to increase the lisinopril to 15 mg by mouth, every day, on March 6 and to 20 mg by mouth, every day, on April 3. The pharmacist educated Mrs. Gonzalez on the increased doses, and as of May 4 she achieved her blood pressure goal. The patient has not experienced adverse effects of dizziness, headache, or cough; however, no potassium level has been drawn. The patient has no risk factors for developing hyperkalemia, such as renal dysfunction or concomitant therapy with medications that increase serum potassium. Blood pressure monitoring should continue to be performed at every visit. If Pharmacist Radcliffe believes that Mrs. Gonzalez is able to recognize possible adverse effects of her therapy, questioning her about these effects may be decreased to every 3 months.

Pharmacotherapeutic and Related Health Care Goal #3

Mrs. Gonzalez's next goal was to improve control of her hypercholesterolemia. Judging by the total cholesterol, some progress has been made toward this goal. Mrs. Gonzalez has avowed that she will be more conscientious with her diet. On further discussion with Dr. Thompson, it is agreed to continue managing Mrs. Gonzalez's hypercholesterolemia with the current therapy regimen and to draw a total lipid profile to determine if this goal is being met.

Pharmacotherapeutic and Related Health Care Goals #4 and #12

Per the American Diabetes Association standards, all diabetes patients at risk for cardiovascular complications should receive one aspirin per day. Mrs. Gonzalez has been adherent to this recommendation and denies adverse effects such as gastrointestinal upset or dark stools. The pharmacist gave Mrs. Gonzalez stool cards to assess for occult blood (goal #12), which was negative. The pharmacist will continue to ask about dark stools and will check stool cards twice yearly. This goal is currently being met. On the AMW, the frequency for questioning the patient about adverse drug affects related to aspirin therapy can be decreased to every 3 months.

Pharmacotherapeutic and Related Health Care Goal #5

Because Mrs. Gonzalez is postmenopausal, the next goal was to institute hormone replacement therapy. She was slightly nauseated at the beginning of therapy, but this has passed. She denied vasomotor symptoms and other adverse effects, as well as cardiovascular complications. This goal is being met. No change in the AMW should be made at this time; monitoring of adverse effects should continue at every visit.

Pharmacotherapeutic and Related Health Care Goal #6

The sixth goal for Mrs. Gonzalez was to initiate calcium therapy to decrease risk of developing osteoporosis. Although we do not yet have evidence that this goal is being achieved, the patient is not experiencing adverse drug effects and no changes are required at this time.

Pharmacotherapeutic and Related Health Care Goal #7

The seventh goal was to discontinue HCTZ and institute lisinopril therapy. This was accomplished; therefore, the goal was achieved. The goal, recommendation, and its monitoring plan can be deleted.

Pharmacotherapeutic and Related Health Care Goals #8 and #9

Goals #8 and #9 are adherence to a recommended meal and exercise plan. Mrs. Gonzalez has had some success with these goals, but lately has not been as adherent to the plans as the pharmacist would like her to be. Mrs. Gonzalez expressed her intention to try harder in these areas; the pharmacist will continue to monitor parameters such as adherence, weight, and body mass index (BMI). The pharmacist will reinforce patient education and determine if the patient's insurance will permit additional visits to the dietitian or a referral to an exercise physiologist.

Pharmacotherapeutic and Related Health Care Goals #10 and #11

Mrs. Gonzalez was instructed to institute regular self-monitoring of blood glucose and blood pressure monitoring, which she has done. The monitoring parameters include correct technique and completion of blood glucose and blood pressure logs, which are being met. The pharmacist will continue to monitor these parameters, as described in the AMW.

Pharmacotherapeutic and Related Health Care Goals #13 and #14

The patient has not yet had the influenza vaccine; the pharmacist has made a note to remind the patient for fall of 1998. Meanwhile, she did have a dilated retinal eye examination in April 1998. The pharmacist will leave this on the AMW as a reminder to make an appointment for next year. Mrs. Gonzalez also reports completing monthly breast self-examinations.

Now turn to **Appendix A** to see how the pharmacist amended the APCP and AMW in response to these recommendations.

Practice Example

Turn to the APCP and AMW for Mr. Jones in **Appendix B**. Assess the achievement of each pharmacotherapeutic and related health care goal based on the available data and determine any necessary changes to the care plan following the same thought processes as those just used for Mrs. Gonzalez. Record these changes on the AMW and APCP, then compare your changes with those recorded in **Appendix C**.

Pharmacotherapeutic and Related Health Care Goal #1

The first goal for Mr. Jones was to determine if he had diabetes. This goal was achieved when the patient was diagnosed with type 2 diabetes; the APCP and AMW should be changed to indicate that this goal is achieved.

Pharmacotherapeutic and Related Health Care Goal #2

The next goal was to improve blood pressure control and prevent complications. Mr. Jones' blood pressure has decreased somewhat over the past 3 months. He is currently taking lisinopril 10 mg by mouth, once daily; the pharmacist recommends increasing it to 15 mg by mouth, once daily. If Mr. Jones continues to lose weight and his blood pressure falls as a result of weight loss, the lisinopril dose can be reduced. The dosage increase is added to the APCP after the increase is approved by the physician; no change is needed to the monitoring plan. The pharmacist needs to educate Mr. Jones about the dosage increase.

Pharmacotherapeutic and Related Health Care Goals #3 and #9

Mr. Jones has followed the care plan in regard to adherence to diet and exercise therapy. He is making progress toward his goal weight and BMI. No modification is needed in the goal, therapy, or monitoring plan for these goals. The pharmacist will reinforce the need to maintain this adherence through patient education.

Pharmacotherapeutic and Related Health Care Goals #4 and #8

Mr. Jones has reported adhering to his medication regimen and has kept all scheduled appointments. The pharmacist will leave these goals on the APCP and AMW as a reminder to revisit them occasionally.

Pharmacotherapeutic and Related Health Care Goals #5 and #14

These goals recommended discontinuing the furosemide to avoid adverse effects on the lipid profile and blood glucose control. This was accomplished without adversely affecting the patient's blood pressure control. Therefore, the goal was achieved and the goal, recommendation, and monitoring plan can be marked as resolved.

Pharmacotherapeutic and Related Health Care Goals #6 and #7

At this time, Mr. Jones refuses to follow recommendations to decrease or stop smoking and alcohol use. The pharmacist will leave the goals as they are and revisit them quarterly.

Pharmacotherapeutic and Related Health Care Goal #10

Mr. Jones is performing his peak flow monitoring and maintaining a log book. No change in goal, therapy, or monitoring plan is needed.

Pharmacotherapeutic and Related Health Care Goals #11 and #12

Mr. Jones still refuses to perform home fecal occult blood testing or to have a rectal/prostate examination. The pharmacist has discussed these interventions with the patient more often than specified in the monitoring plan and is likely making progress in convincing the patient of the importance of these interventions. The pharmacist will leave the plan as it is and revisit these issues occasionally.

Pharmacotherapeutic and Related Health Care Goal #13

Following his diagnosis of type 2 diabetes, Mr. Jones began therapy with repaglinide 0.5 mg before each meal, in addition to nonpharmacologic interventions. The pharmacist and physician agreed that it was unlikely this dose would control Mr. Jones' blood glucose; therefore, the physician agreed to increase the dose to 1 mg by mouth before meals. Following this modification, Mr. Jones' blood glucose has decreased for all parameters. The patient has not experienced any signs or symptoms of hypoglycemia or other toxicities from repaglinide, and the complaint of nocturia has resolved. The pharmacist will monitor for improvement before recommending additional changes in the therapy or monitoring plan.

Follow-up parameters to monitor for the development of diabetes complications indicate that the patient's condition has not worsened, but the pharmacist will need to monitor the serum creatinine closely because of the increase in the value obtained on March 30.

Pharmacotherapeutic and Related Health Care Goal #15

The goal to eliminate the fungal skin infection on Mr. Jones' toe has been met. The goal, recommendation, and monitoring plan can be marked as resolved.

Pharmacotherapeutic and Related Health Care Goal #16

Mr. Jones has met this goal (with the clearing of the fungal infection). The pharmacist will continue quarterly foot inspections for the absence of foot infection, trauma, and ulceration. Completion of daily foot examinations by the patient will continue to be assessed at every visit and reinforced in patient education. No change to the APCP or AMW is needed.

Pharmacotherapeutic and Related Health Care Goal #17

Mr. Jones adheres to the recommendation to take a daily aspirin tablet and is free from toxicity. He continues to deny dark stools or gastrointestinal upset. No change to the APCP or AMW is needed.

Pharmacotherapeutic and Related Health Care Goal #18

Mr. Jones has made significant progress toward his goal of improving lipid control; his total cholesterol has decreased by over 90 mg/dl in 3 months, and his LDL cholesterol is at 135 mg/dl (goal <100 mg/dl) following the increase in the dosage of Questran Light to 8 grams bid on May 6. It is unlikely that the patient will gain any additional benefit from increasing the dose of cholestyramine again. Adding additional drug therapy is not feasible for Mr. Jones:

Niacin is not a good choice as it increases blood glucose, and the HMG-CoA reductase inhibitors are not a good first choice because Mr. Jones has elevated liver enzymes baseline. The pharmacist recommends that he maintain diet and exercise interventions, which may continue to show a beneficial trend. The pharmacist will also revisit the need to stop smoking, which would also improve the situation. Some patients may not hit their ideal goal, but an LDL cholesterol of 135 mg/dl is considerably better than 229 mg/dl. No change in the goal, therapy, or monitoring plan is required at this time.

Mr. Jones' Questran Light therapy is probably the culprit in the new problem of constipation. The pharmacist recommended Metamucil therapy (which may actually help Mr. Jones' lipids as well!) and will monitor therapy accordingly. This problem is noted on the APCP and AMW as "Pharmacotherapeutic and Related Health Care Goal #23." The pharmacist will educate the patient about increasing fluid intake and monitoring for adverse effects while receiving this therapy.

Pharmacotherapeutic and Related Health Care Goal #19

The goal to learn and perform regular self-monitoring of blood glucose (SMBG) has been met and the pharmacist will continue to reassess technique every 6 months and evaluate the patient's blood glucose log at every visit. No changes are required to the care plan at this time.

Pharmacotherapeutic and Related Health Care Goal #20

Mr. Jones has not yet received his annual dilated retinal examination. The pharmacist will encourage Mr. Jones to schedule this examination promptly.

Pharmacotherapeutic and Related Health Care Goal #21

Mr. Jones continues to refuse a dental examination every 6 months. The pharmacist will leave the plan as it is, and revisit this issue occasionally.

Pharmacotherapeutic and Related Health Care Goal #22

The final goal for Mr. Jones is to monitor for worsening liver function. The monitoring plan indicated that liver function would be assessed every 3–6 months. It has not been 3 months since the last assessment and no new information is available to indicate worsening liver function. No change to the APCP or AMW should be made for this goal.

Summary

When evaluating the carefully assessed results of an implemented APCP, the pharmacist must make decisions using a systematic approach. The APCP can be altered by changing the patient's pharmaco-therapeutic and related health care goals, regimen, monitoring plan, education plan, or any combination of these elements. The pharmacist should expect that a change in one aspect will precipitate a change in the others.

Self-Study Questions

Objective

Determine if a change in pharmacotherapeutic and related health care goals, regimen, or monitoring plan is required in the treatment of ambulatory patients with type 2 diabetes.

Refer to the APCP and AMW for Ms. McLucas in **Appendix D**.

1. Is a change needed in Ms. McLucas' goal to improve control of hypertension and prevent complications?

2. Is a change needed in Ms. McLucas' goal to improve control of diabetes and prevent complications?

3. Is a change needed in Ms. McLucas' goal to improve control of hypercholesterolemia and prevent complications?

Objective

Modify a pharmacist's care plan for patients with type 2 diabetes as necessary based on the achievement of pharmacotherapeutic and related health care goals.

Refer to the APCP and AMW for Ms. McLucas (**Appendix D**).

4. Modify Ms. McLucas' care plan as necessary based on the achievement of her pharmacotherapeutic and related health care goals.

Self-Study Answers

1. Yes, she has achieved the goal of improving control of hypertension. The goal should be modified to read, "maintain control of hypertension and prevent complications."

2. No, she has not achieved the goal, so the goal remains unchanged. Addition of pharmacologic therapy may be considered at this time.

3. Yes, she has probably achieved the goal of improving control of hyperlipidemia based on the total cholesterol. Once a fasting lipid panel is drawn, if the LDL cholesterol is <100 mg/dl the goal can be changed to read, "maintain control of hypercholesterolemia and prevent complications."

4. See **Appendix E**. Ms. McLucas has met her goals for improving control of hypertension; therefore, the goal was changed to "maintain control." Once a fasting lipid panel is drawn, the goal for hypercholesterolemia may also need to be changed to "maintain control."

   Ms. McLucas has not met the goals for glycemic control and pharmacologic therapy could be initiated to improve control. Her predominant abnormality is postprandial hyperglycemia, and her hemoglobin A_{1c} is within 1% of goal.

Therefore, acarbose is a good choice for Ms. McLucas and the pharmacist made this recommendation to the physician. The physician agreed and the pharmacist added adverse effects of acarbose to the AMW (e.g., abdominal pain, flatulence, and diarrhea) and will educate the patient about use of this drug.

Goals that have been met and should be marked as resolved are Pharmacotherapeutic and Related Health Care Goals #6, #8, #10, #12, and #13.

A goal that has not been met but that she is making progress toward is Pharmacotherapeutic and Related Health Care Goal #11. No changes are required in the goals, therapy, or monitoring plan at this time.

Goals that have been met but do not require a change in the APCP or AMW are Pharmacotherapeutic and Related Health Care Goals #5, #7, #9, #14, and #15.

For Pharmacotherapeutic and Related Health Care Goal #4, the patient still does not wish to begin hormone replacement therapy. The pharmacist should make a note to revisit this issue.

APPENDIX A

Mrs. Gonzalez
5/4/98

The Diabetes Treatment Satisfaction Questionnaire: DTSQ

The following questions concern your diabetes treatment (including insulin, tablets, and/or diet) and your experience over the past few weeks. Please answer each question by circling a number on each of the scales.

1. How satisfied are you with your current treatment?

| *very satisfied* | 6 | 5 | 4 | 3 | (2) | 1 | 0 | *very dissatisfied* |

2. How often have you felt that your blood sugars have been unacceptably high recently?

| *most of the time* | 6 | 5 | (4) | 3 | 2 | 1 | 0 | *none of the time* |

3. How often have you felt that your blood sugars have been unacceptably low recently?

| *most of the time* | 6 | 5 | 4 | 3 | 2 | 1 | (0) | *none of the time* |

4. How convenient have you been finding your treatment to be recently?

| *very convenient* | 6 | 5 | 4 | 3 | (2) | 1 | 0 | *very inconvenient* |

5. How flexible have you been finding your treatment to be recently?

| *very flexible* | 6 | 5 | 4 | 3 | 2 | (1) | 0 | *very inflexible* |

6. How satisfied are you with your understanding of your diabetes?

| *very satisfied* | (6) | 5 | 4 | 3 | 2 | 1 | 0 | *very dissatisfied* |

7. Would you recommend this form of treatment to someone else with your kind of diabetes?

| *Yes, I would definitely recommend the treatment* | 6 | 5 | 4 | 3 | 2 | (1) | 0 | *No, I would definitely not recommend the treatment* |

8. How satisfied would you be to continue with your present form of treatment?

| *very satisfied* | 6 | 5 | 4 | 3 | 2 | 1 | (0) | *very dissatisfied* |

Please make sure that you have circled one number on each of the scales.

AMBULATORY PHARMACIST'S CARE PLAN

Patient __Rose Gonzalez__   Pharmacist __Jane Radcliffe__   Date __2/20/98__

Page 1 of 2

DATE IDENTIFIED	PROBLEM (TPL)	PHARMACOTHERAPEUTIC AND RELATED HEALTH CARE GOAL	RECOMMENDATIONS FOR THERAPY	MONITORING PARAMETER(S)	DESIRED ENDPOINT(S)	MONITORING FREQUENCY
2/20/98	poor control of diabetes	Improve diabetes control; prevent complications.	Institute non-pcal interventions (diet & exercise)	FBG SMBG HbA1c Pt. satisfac. SXs hypergly.	FBG<120 hsBG 100-140 HbA1c<7% ⊖SXs HG	All q visit except HbA1c q 3 mo; ↓ to q 6 mo. _(REVISED 5/4/98)_
"	poor control of HTN	Improve BP control; prevent complications.	As above, plus rec. Δ to abc lisinopril 10 mg QD	BP AE lisinopril- cough, rash, K+	<130/85 K<S ⊖ cough, rash	All q visit except WBC & K+ 2x q yr.
"	poor control of cholest.	Improve lipid control; prevent complications.	nonpcal interventions & Atorvastatin 10 mg*	TC, CDL, HDL, TG LFT c/o muscle pain, GI upset, HA	CDL<100 HDL>4S TG<200 TC<200 ⊖ c/o AE	TC-q visit panel-q @ 8 wk x 2 SXs-q visit
"	not on daily ASA tx	↓ risk CV compli. of diabetes	Rec. EC ASA 325 mg QD*	GI bleeding/ upset; dark, tarry stools	⊖ bleeding or c/o	SX-q visit occult blood- 2x q yr.
"	post-menopausal s̄ HRT	↓ risk post-men. SXs/↓ risks of post-menopause	Rec. conjugated estrogen/progestin"	vasomotor SX c/o edema GI, breast pain t'boembolic,	⊖ SX or AE	q visit
"	not receiving calcium tx	↓ risk for osteoporosis	Rec calcium carbonate 500 mg TID	AE GI upset constipation	⊖ height loss	quarterly
"	Potential of HCTZ to affect DM & chol.	Avoid worsened BG & lipid control	D/C HCTZ	D/C → profile; pt. interview	D/C s̄ AE	q visit D/C RESOLVED
"	no exercise plan	start & adhere to regular exercise program.	Begin regular walking program	report of regular walking prog	↓ BMI, wt. ↓BP	q visit

*Treatment began 2/7/98.   b3/6 Lisinopril ↑ to 15 mg qd.   4/3 Lisinopril ↑ to 20 mg qd.

AMBULATORY PHARMACIST'S CARE PLAN

Patient __Rose Gonzalez__   Pharmacist __Jane Radcliffe__   Date __2/20/98__

Page 2 of 2

DATE IDENTIFIED	PROBLEM (TPL)	PHARMACOTHERAPEUTIC AND RELATED HEALTH CARE GOAL	RECOMMENDATIONS FOR THERAPY	MONITORING PARAMETER(S)	DESIRED ENDPOINT(S)	MONITORING FREQUENCY
2/20/98	no MNT plan	start & adhere to MNT plan.	refer to RD- follow meal plan	report of adherence to plan	↓ BMI, wt. ↓ BP	q visit
"	no home BG monitoring	learn & regularly perform SMBG	select & explain use of BG monitor	-SMBG log -observe technique	-proper technique -adherence to use	observe 2x q yr. review log q visit
"	no home BP monitoring	learn & regularly perform BP measurements	select and explain use of BP cuff	-BP log -observe technique	-proper technique -adherence to use	Observe 2x q yr review log every visit
=	no home fecal test	perform annual home fecal blood test	Provide home fecal blood test cards	cards returned	⊕ occult blood	2x q yr.
=	no influenza vaccine	receive annual influenza vaccine	Receive flu vaccine Fall 98	Pt. interview	flu shot received	q Fall
=	no monthly breast self-exam	learn & regularly perform exam	refer to primary physician for exam technique	pt. interview	monthly self-exam	q month
5/4/98	not meeting goals for control of DM	Improve diabetes control; prevent complications	metformin 500mg po bid	FBG/SMBG HbA1c, sx of hypoglycemia, Hct/Hb, SCr, GI	FBG <120, hsBG 100-140, HBA1c <7 ⊖ sx of hypoglycemia, ⊖ decrease in Hct/Hb, SCr <1.2, ⊖ adverse effects	All q visit except HbA1c q 3 months then to q ↓ 6 mo Hct/Hb, SCr q 6 mo
				upset, rash, malaise, myalgia, somnolence, pt satisfaction		

PHARMACIST'S CARE PLAN AMBULATORY MONITORING WORKSHEET (AMW)

Patient Rose Gonzalez
Page 1

Pharmacist Jane Radcliffe
Date 2/20/98

Pharmaco-therapeutic Goal	Monitoring Parameter	Desired Endpoint	Monitoring Frequency	2/9	2/18	2/19	2/27	3/6	3/20	4/3	5/4
1	FBG	<120	every visit		184		avg 170	avg 160	avg 165	avg 155	avg 152
1	SMBG–preprandial	<120	→				avg 174	avg 170	avg 170	avg 160	avg 160
1	SMBG–postprandial	<140	→	random 242			avg 200	190	192	184	→ 180
1	SMBG–bedtime	100–140	→				avg 180	176	170	160	→ 148
1	HbA1c	<7	q 3mo; ↓ q 6mo			10.2					9.5
1	dilated retinal exam	received	annual			⊝	⊝	made appt	⊕	⊕	✓
1	SCr	<1.2	q 6 month	0.9							
1	U/A	⊝	annual	WNL		⊕ glucose / ⊝ protein / ⊝ ketone					
1	urine microalbumin	⊝	annual			⊕					
1	EKG	received	annual								
1	Foot screen	received	quarterly			✓					
1	Skin screen	received	quarterly			✓					
1	Dental exam	received	q 6 month	1/98		✓					

PHARMACIST'S CARE PLAN AMBULATORY MONITORING WORKSHEET (AMW)

Patient Rose Gonzalez
Page 2

Pharmacist Jane Radcliffe
Date 2/20/98

Pharmaco-therapeutic Goal	Monitoring Parameter	Desired Endpoint	Monitoring Frequency	2/9	2/18	2/19	2/27	3/6	3/20	4/3	5/4			
1	signs and symptoms of hyperglycemia	(−)	every visit			(−)	(−)	(−)	(−)	(−)	(−)			
1	(polyuria, polydipsia, polyphagia)	(−)	→			(−)	(−)	(−)	(−)	(−)	(−)			
2	BP	<130/85	every visit			152/100	142/90	140/90	134/82	136/84	130/80			
2	lisinopril AE-dizziness/headache	(−)	q visit; ↓ q 3 mo					(+)		(−)				
2	lisinopril AE-cough	(−)	→					(−)		(−)				
2	K+	<5	q 6 month											
3	Total cholesterol	<200	every visit	286	290			205	184	172	164			
3	LDL cholesterol	<100	q 8 wk x2; ↓		204									
3	HDL cholesterol	>45	→		30									
3	TG	<200	→		280									
4	ASA AE-GI upset	(−)	q visit; ↓ q 3 mo					(+)		(−)	(−)			
4	ASA AE-dark tarry stools	(−)	→					(−)		(−)	(−)			
4	ASA-efficacy prevent MI	(−)	every visit					(−)		(−)	(−)			

see also page ↑

PHARMACIST'S CARE PLAN AMBULATORY MONITORING WORKSHEET (AMW)

Patient _____ Rose Gonzalez _____ Page 3

Pharmacist _____ Jane Radcliffe _____

Date _____

Pharmaco-therapeutic Goal	Monitoring Parameter	Desired Endpoint	Monitoring Frequency	2/9	2/18	2/19	2/27	3/6	3/20	4/3	5/4
5	Vasomotor SXs	(−)	every visit		(−)	(−)	(−)	(−)	(−)	(−)	(−)
5	Estrogen/progestin AE- breast pain, anorexia	(−)	q visit, ↓ q 3 mo					(+)	(−)	(−)	(−)
5	headache, edema	(−)	→					(−)	(−)	(−)	(−)
5	thromboembolic c/o	(−)	→					(−)	(−)	(−)	(−)
5	vaginal bleeding	(−)	→					(−)	(−)	(−)	(−)
6	height loss	(−)	quarterly				5'5"				
6	calcium AE- GI upset, constipation	(−)	q visit, ↓ q 3 mo					(−)	(−)		(−)
7	patient interview and profile	(−)	every visit til D/C				(−)	(−)	Resolved		
8	Pt. interview	adhere 4/5 days	every visit					(+)	(+)	3/5	3/5 1-2/5
8	weight	<150 lb	→				228	223	220	216	210
8	BMI	<27	→				38	37	37	36	35
9	Pt. interview	adhere 4/5 days	every visit					(+)	(+)	3/5	3/5 2-3/5
10	correct technique	(+)	2x/yr					(+)			

PHARMACIST'S CARE PLAN AMBULATORY MONITORING WORKSHEET (AMW)

Patient ___Rose Gonzalez___

Page 4

Pharmacist ___Jane Radcliffe___

Date _____

Pharmaco-therapeutic Goal	Monitoring Parameter	Desired Endpoint	Monitoring Frequency	2/9	2/18	2/19	2/27	3/6	3/20	4/3	5/4			
10	completing log	(+)	every visit					(+)	(+)	(+)	(+)			
11	correct technique	(+)	2x/yr				(+)							
11	completing log	(+)	every visit					(+)	(+)	(+)	(+)			
12	returned home fecal test cards	(+)	annual					(+)						
13	flu shot received	(+)	every fall											
14	patient interview	complete	every month						✓		✓			
3	AST	<35	baseline q 8 wks then q 6 mos				8		12					
3	ALT	<35	→				11		20					
3	AE of atorvastatin -GI upset	(−)	q visit					(−)	(−)	(−)	(−)			
3	-headache	(−)	→					(−)	(−)	(−)	(−)			
3	-muscle pain or tenderness	(−)	→					(−)	(−)	(−)	(−)			
15	Hematocrit	36-44	q 6 mo											
15	hemoglobin	12-15	→											

PHARMACIST'S CARE PLAN AMBULATORY MONITORING WORKSHEET (AMW)

Patient ___Rose Gonzalez___

Page 5

Pharmacist ___Jane Radcliffe___

Date ___2/20/98___

Pharmaco-therapeutic Goal	Monitoring Parameter	Desired Endpoint		Date 2/9	2/18	2/19	2/27	3/6	3/20	4/3	5/4			
IS	GI upset	(-)	q visit											
IS	rash	(-)	→→											
IS	malaise/somnolence	(-)												
IS	myalgia	(-)												

Ambulatory Pharmacist's Care Plan

Patient ___George Jones___   Pharmacist ___John O'Malley___   Date ___3-3-98___

Page 1 of 3

DATE IDENTIFIED	PROBLEM (TPL)	PHARMACOTHERAPEUTIC AND RELATED HEALTH CARE GOAL	RECOMMENDATIONS FOR THERAPY	MONITORING PARAMETER(S)	DESIRED ENDPOINT(S)	MONITORING FREQUENCY
3/3/98	SX and BG suggestive of DM. High risk status	Rule in/out DM. Determine cause of high BG and nocturia	Refer to primary physician—await results	Consult report	Rule in/out diabetes	q week until resolved
	poor control of hypertension	Improve BP control; Prevent complications	D/C furosemide Begin lisinopril 10 mg q AM	BP; AE for lisinopril—cough rash, ↑K+	<130/85 ⊖ SX AE	All q visit except K+ 2x/yr
	nonadherence to diet	start and adhere to prescribed meal plan	Referral to dietitian	pt. interview, wt, BMI	wt <160 BMI <27	q visit
	h/o med schedule nonadherence	adherence to medication regimen	Provide written instructions	Pt. interview, review profile	proper medication use	q visit
	Furosemide may worsen lipids	Avoid worsened lipid profile	Rec d/c furosemide. Begin lisinopril	Profile and pt. interview	d/c w/o sequelae	q visit
	smoking history	Stop smoking	Nicotine replacement and counseling. Pt. refuses at this time	# cigs/day pt. interview	decreased or no smoking	discuss quarterly
	Alcohol use history	Stop alcohol use	↓ or stop alcohol use Pt. refuses at this time	amt Etoh/wk Pt. interview	decreased or no Etoh use	discuss quarterly

*Treatment began 4/8

AMBULATORY PHARMACIST'S CARE PLAN

Patient ___George Jones___ Pharmacist ___John O'Malley___ Date ___3-3-98___

Page 2 of 3

DATE IDENTIFIED	PROBLEM (TPL)	PHARMACOTHERAPEUTIC AND RELATED HEALTH CARE GOAL	RECOMMENDATIONS FOR THERAPY	MONITORING PARAMETER(S)	DESIRED ENDPOINT(S)	MONITORING FREQUENCY
3/3/98	h/o non-adherence to flu appts	Adherence to flu appt. scheduling	Counsel pt.	Pt. interview c̄ consult reports	Compliant c̄ other HCP	q visit
	nonadherence to exercise	start and adhere to exercise plan	Counsel pt.	Pt. interview, wt, BMI, BP	BMI<27 BP<130/85	q visit
	Not doing peak flow monitoring	Learn and perform peak flow monitoring regularly	Instruct pt. w/ peak flow monitoring	Observe technique, Review SM record	Proper technique use PFM w/o SX	Observe tech 2x then 2x/yr Review log q visit
	No rectal/prostate exam	Annual rectal prostate exam	Refer to PCP. Pt. refuses at this time	Pt. interview consult report	complete exam	Discuss quarterly
	no home fecal test	Home fecal blood test q 6 months	Provide home fecal test cards. Pt. refuses at this time.	Pt. interview	complete test	Discuss quarterly
4/3/98	poor control of diabetes	Improve control; prevent complications	Rec. repaglinide 0.5 mg^ac before meals	FBG, SMBG, HBA1c, SX AE, satisfaction	FBG<120 hs BG 100-140 HBA1c <7 ⊕ SX and AE, ⊕ satisfaction	FBG & SMBG q visit HBA1c q 3 mo, ↓ 6 mo
	Furosemide may ↑ BG	Avoid worsened BP control	Rec d/c furosemide Begin lisinopril	Profile and pt. interview	d/c w/o sequelae	q visit
	Fungal skin infection w toe	Eliminate fungal toe infection	Rec. Lotrimin cream to affected area BID^+ for 7-10 days	Inspection of feet	No sign of infection	monthly x 3 then quarterly

^Treatment began 4/8 ^S/18 repaglinide ↑ to 1 mg with meals

Ambulatory Pharmacist's Care Plan

Patient ___George Jones___   Pharmacist ___John O'Malley___   Date ___3-3-98___

Page 3 of 3

DATE IDENTIFIED	PROBLEM (TPL)	PHARMACOTHERAPEUTIC AND RELATED HEALTH CARE GOAL	RECOMMENDATIONS FOR THERAPY	MONITORING PARAMETER(S)	DESIRED ENDPOINT(S)	MONITORING FREQUENCY
4/3	Insensate feet	Absence of infection trauma, ulcerations	Daily self-inspection Quarterly exam	Foot exam, Pt. interview	No complications	Inspect quarterly Interview q visit
	Not on daily ASA tx	↓ risk CV complications 2° to diabetes	Rec EC ASA 325 mg QD^a	GI upset, dark tarry stools, MI	⊖SX ⊖ occult blood	SX - q visit Biannual fecal blood
	Poor control of cholesterol	Improve control, prevent complications	Refer for MNT Rec. cholestyramine 4 g BID^b	TC, LDL, HDL, TG c/o constipation GI upset	TC<200 TG<200 LDL<100 HDL>45, ⊖ c/o AE	TC q visit Panel q 8 wks ⊗2 Sxs - q visit
	Not doing SMBG	Learn and perform regular SMBG	Instruct on SMBG	Observation of technique, SMBG log	Proper tech. Use of BGM daily	Observe tech 2x/yr Review log q visit
	No dilated retinal exam	Annual dilated retinal exam	Refer to ophthalmologist	-Pt. interview -copy of consult report	Compliant with annual exam	Annually
	No recent dental exam	Dental exam q 6 months	Refer to dentist	Pt. interview Copy of consult report	Compliant with appts	q 6 mo
	liver dysfunction	monitor liver function	monitor LFTs	ALT, AST	<35	q 3-6 mo

^a Treatment began 4/8   ^b S/b cholestyramine ↑ to 8 g BID

PHARMACIST'S CARE PLAN AMBULATORY MONITORING WORKSHEET (AMW)

Patient __George Jones__ Page 1

Pharmacist __John O'Malley__

Date __3-3-98__

Pharmaco-therapeutic Goal	Monitoring Parameter	Desired Endpoint	Monitoring Frequency	3/3	3/18	3/23	3/30	4/3	4/8	4/10	4/22	5/6	5/20	6/17
1	Consult report	Rule in/out diabetes	q week until resolved				✓							
2	BP	<130/85	q visit	152/98 140/90				140/84	140/85	138/85	138/85	136/84	140/86	136/82
	lisinopril AE: dizziness	⊖	q visits ↓ q 3 mo						⊖	⊖	⊖	⊖	⊖	⊖
	lisinopril AE: headache	⊖	→						⊖	⊖	⊖	⊖	⊖	⊖
	lisinopril AE: cough	⊖							⊖	⊖	⊖	⊖	⊖	⊖
	lisinopril AE: ↑ K+	<5	2x year											
3	Pt. interview	⊕	q visit	⊖				⊕	⊕	⊕	⊕	⊕	⊕	⊕
	Weight	<160 lb	q visit	240				235	235	235	230	225	218	210
	BMI	<27	q visit	37				36	36	36	35	34	33	32
4	Profile and pt. interview	⊕	q visit	+/-				⊕	⊕	⊕	⊕	⊕	⊕	⊕
5	Profile and pt. interview	d/c furosemide ⊖ symptoms ∅	q visit	1				✓	⊖	⊖	⊖	⊖		
6	# cigs/day Pt. currently refuses	∅	revisit quarterly ppd	1 quarterly ppd				1 ppd						
7	Amt EtoH/wk Pt. currently refuses	∅	revisit quarterly beers	4 quarterly beers								4 beers		

PHARMACIST'S CARE PLAN AMBULATORY MONITORING WORKSHEET (AMW)

Patient __George Jones__
Page 2

Pharmacist __John O'Malley__
Date __3-3-98__

Pharmaco-therapeutic Goal	Monitoring Parameter	Desired Endpoint	Monitoring Frequency	3/3	3/18	3/23	3/30	4/3	4/8	4/10	4/22	5/6	5/20	6/17
8	Pt. interview w/ consult reports	(+)	q visit	+/-				⊕	⊕	⊕	⊕	⊕	⊕	⊕
9	Pt. interview	adhere 4/5 days	q visit	(-)				⊕	⊕	⊕	⊕	⊕	⊕	⊕
10	Observe technique	proper technique	2x; ↓2x/yr					✓	✓					
10	Review log	PFM w/o Sx	q visit					✓	✓	✓	✓	✓	✓	✓
11	Pt. interview/ consult report Pt. currently refuses	annually complete exam	revisit quarterly	(-)				(-)						
12	Pt. interview Pt. currently refuses	complete test q 6 mos	revisit quarterly	(-)				(-)						(-)
13	FBG	<120	every visit		190					AVG 190	AVG 190	AVG 180	AVG 160	AVG 150
13	SMBG preprandial	<120	→	Random 244	Random 258					AVG 190	AVG 190	AVG 180	AVG 162	AVG 152
13	SMBG postprandial	<140	↓							AVG 240 230	AVG 240 230	AVG 200 200	AVG 200	AVG 200
13	SMBG bedtime	100-140	↓							AVG 180	AVG 180	AVG 170	AVG 160	AVG 160
13	HbA1c	<7%	q 3 mo; ↓q 6 mo					11.6						
13	SCr	<1.2	q 6 month				1.8							
13	U/A	(-)	annual					+prot +glu -ket						

PHARMACIST'S CARE PLAN AMBULATORY MONITORING WORKSHEET (AMW)

Patient: George Jones
Page 3

Pharmacist: John O'Malley
Date: 3-3-98

Pharmaco-therapeutic Goal	Monitoring Parameter	Desired Endpoint	Monitoring Frequency	3/3	3/18	3/23	3/30	4/3	4/8	4/10	4/22	5/6	5/20	6/17
13	urine microalbumin	<30	q 6 mo					35						
13	urine culture	(-)	prn			(-)								
13	EKG	received	annual					isch old MI ✓	✓	✓	✓	✓	✓	✓
13	foot screen	received	quarterly					✓	✓	✓	✓	✓	✓	✓
13	skin screen	received	quarterly					✓						
13	symptoms of hyperglycemia -nocturia	(-)	q visit	(+)				(+)	(+)	(+)	(+)	+/-	(-)	(-)
	-polyuria	(-)	q visit	(-)				(-)	(-)	(-)	(-)	(-)	(-)	(-)
	-polydipsia	(-)	q visit	(-)				(-)	(-)	(-)	(-)	(-)	(-)	(-)
	-polyphagia	(-)	q visit	(-)				(-)	(-)	(-)	(-)	(-)	(-)	(-)
13	dilated retinal exam	received	annual					to schedule						
13	dental exam - Pt. refuses at this time	received	revisit quarterly					(-)						
13	Repaglinide AE- rash GI upset	(-)	q visit; ↓, q 3 mo							(-)	(-)	(-)	(-)	(-)
13	signs & symptoms of hypoglycemia	(-)	q visit					(-)	(-)	(-)	(-)	(-)	(-)	(-)

PHARMACIST'S CARE PLAN AMBULATORY MONITORING WORKSHEET (AMW)

Patient: George Jones — Page 4

Pharmacist: John O'Malley

Date: 3-3-98

Pharmaco-therapeutic Goal	Monitoring Parameter	Desired Endpoint	Monitoring Frequency	3/3	3/18	3/23	3/30	4/3	4/8	4/10	4/22	5/6	5/20	6/17
14	Profile and pt. interview	d/c furosemide w/o symptoms	q visit					✓	⊖	⊖	⊖	⊖		
15	Foot inspection	sign of infx ⊖	q month ×3											⊖
16	Foot exam–sensation	10/10	quarterly					7/10						
16	Pt. interview	no complications	q visit					⊖	⊖	⊖	⊖	⊖	⊖	⊖
17	ASA–AE GI upset	⊖	q visits ↓q 3 mo						⊖	⊖	⊖	⊖	⊖	⊖
17	ASA–AE dark, tarry stools	⊖	q visit; ↓q 3 mo						⊖	⊖	⊖	⊖	⊖	⊖
17	ASA–efficacy prevent MI	⊖	q visit						⊖	⊖	⊖	⊖	⊖	⊖
18	Total cholesterol	<200	q visit				290				215	220	210	198
18	LDL cholesterol	<100	q 8 wk ×2; ↓q 2–3 mo				229							135
18	HDL cholesterol	>45	→				45							46
18	TG	<200	→				80							84
18	Cholestyramine AE– constipation, GI upset	⊖	q visit; ↓q 3 mo						⊖/⊖/⊕		⊖/⊕	⊖/⊕		⊖/⊕

PHARMACIST'S CARE PLAN AMBULATORY MONITORING WORKSHEET (AMW)

Patient _____ George Jones _____   Pharmacist _____ John O'Malley _____

Page 5   Date _____ 3-3-98 _____

Pharmaco-therapeutic Goal	Monitoring Parameter	Desired Endpoint	Monitoring Frequency	3/3	3/18	3/23	3/30	4/3	4/8 4/10	4/22	5/6	5/20	6/17
19	Observe technique	proper technique	q 6 mo						✓	✓	✓	✓	✓
19	Review SMBG log	completes log	q visit							✓	✓	✓	✓
20	Pt. interview, copy of report	receive exam	annual	(−)				(−)					(+) 5/13
21	Pt. interview, copy of report	receive exam	q 6 month	(−)				(−)					(−)
22	ALT	<35	q 3-6 mo				56						
22	AST	<35	q 3-6 mo				98						

AMBULATORY PHARMACIST'S CARE PLAN

Patient George Jones   Page 1 of 3   Pharmacist John O'Malley   Date 3-3-98

DATE IDENTIFIED	PROBLEM (TPL)	PHARMACOTHERAPEUTIC AND RELATED HEALTH CARE GOAL	RECOMMENDATIONS FOR THERAPY	MONITORING PARAMETER(S)	DESIRED ENDPOINT(S)	MONITORING FREQUENCY
3/3/98	SX and BG suggestive of DM. High risk status	Rule in/out DM. Determine cause of high BG and nocturia	Refer to primary physician—await results	Consult report	Rule in/out diabetes	q week until resolved — resolved
	poor control of hypertension	Improve BP control; Prevent complications	D/C furosemide; Begin lisinopril 10 mg q AM[a]	BP; AE for lisinopril—cough rash, ↑K+	<130/85, ⊖ SX AE	All q visit except K+ 2x/yr
	nonadherence to diet	start and adhere to prescribed meal plan	Referral to dietitian	pt. interview, wt, BMI	wt<160, BMI<27	q visit
	h/o med schedule nonadherence	adherence to medication regimen	Provide written instructions	Pt. interview, review profile	proper medication use	q visit
	Furosemide worsened lipids	Avoid worsened lipid profile	Rec d/c furosemide. Begin lisinopril	Profile and pt. interview	d/c w/o sequelae	q visit — resolved
	smoking history	Stop smoking	Nicotine replacement and counseling. Pt. refuses at this time	# cigs/day pt. interview	decreased or no smoking	discuss quarterly
	Alcohol use history	Stop alcohol use	↓ or stop alcohol use. Pt. refuses at this time	amt Etoh/wk Pt. interview	decreased or no Etoh use	discuss quarterly

[a] Treatment began 4/8.

6/17 ↑ lisinopril to 15 mg qd.

AMBULATORY PHARMACIST'S CARE PLAN

Patient __George Jones__   Pharmacist __John O'Malley__   Date __3-3-98__

Page 2 of 3

DATE IDENTIFIED	PROBLEM (TPL)	PHARMACOTHERAPEUTIC AND RELATED HEALTH CARE GOAL	RECOMMENDATIONS FOR THERAPY	MONITORING PARAMETER(S)	DESIRED ENDPOINT(S)	MONITORING FREQUENCY
3/3/98	h/o non-adherence to flu appts	Adherence to flu appt. scheduling	Counsel pt.	Pt. interview c̄ consult reports	Compliant c̄ other HCP	q̄ visit
	Nonadherence to exercise	start and adhere to exercise plan	Counsel pt.	Pt. interview, wt, BMI, BP	BMI<27 BP<130/85	q̄ visit
	Not doing peak flow monitoring	Learn and perform peak flow monitoring regularly	Instruct pt. on peak flow monitoring	Observe technique, Review SM record	Proper technique use PFM w/o SX	Observe tech 2x then 2x/yr Review log q̄ visit
	No rectal/prostate exam	Annual rectal prostate exam	Refer to PCP. Pt. refuses at this time	Pt. interview consult report	complete exam	Discuss quarterly
	no home Fecal test	Home fecal blood test q̄ 6 months	Provide home fecal test cards. Pt. refuses at this time.	Pt. interview	complete test	Discuss quarterly
4/3/98	poor control of diabetes	Improve control; prevent complications	Rec. repaglinide 0.5 mg⁴ᶜ before meals	FBG, SMBG, HBAlc, SX AE, satisfaction	FBG<120 ↓s BG 100-140 HBAlc <7 ⊖ SX and AE, ⊕ satisfaction	FBG & SMBG q̄ visit HBAlc q̄ 3 mo, ↓6 mo ⊕ satisfaction
	Furosemide may ↑ BG	Avoid worsened BP control	Rec d/c furosemide Begin lisinopril	Profile and pt. interview	d/c w/o sequelae	q̄ visit → resolved
	Fungal skin infection on toe	Eliminate fungal toe infection	Rec. Lotrimin cream to affected area BID for 7-10 days	Inspection of feet	No sign of infection	monthly x 3 then quarterly → resolved

*Treatment began 4/8.   °5/18 repaglinide ↑ to 1 mg with meals.

AMBULATORY PHARMACIST'S CARE PLAN

Patient George Jones   Pharmacist John O'Malley   Date 3-3-98

Page 3 of 3

DATE IDENTIFIED	PROBLEM (TPL)	PHARMACOTHERAPEUTIC AND RELATED HEALTH CARE GOAL	RECOMMENDATIONS FOR THERAPY	MONITORING PARAMETER(S)	DESIRED ENDPOINT(S)	MONITORING FREQUENCY
4/3	Insensate feet	Absence of infection trauma, ulcerations	Daily self-inspection Quarterly exam	Foot exam, Pt. interview	No complications	Inspect quarterly Interview q visit
	Not on daily ASA tx	↓ risk CV complications 2° to diabetes	Rec EC ASA 325 mg QD*	GI upset, dark tarry stools, MI	⊖SX ⊖ occult blood	SX — q visit Biannual fecal blood
	Poor control of cholesterol	Improve control, prevent complications	Refer for MNT Rec. cholestyramine 4 g BID[b]	TC, CDL, HDL, TG c/o constipation GI upset	TC<200 TG<200 CDL<100 HDL>45, ⊖ c/o AE	TC q visit Panel q 8 wks ⊗2 Sxs — q visit
	Not doing SMBG	Learn and perform regular SMBG	Instruct on SMBG	Observation of technique, SMBG log	Proper tech. Use of BGM daily	Observe tech 2x/yr Review log q visit
	No dilated retinal exam	Annual dilated retinal exam	Refer to ophthalmologist	Pt. interview -copy of consult report	Compliant with annual exam	Annually
	No recent dental exam	Dental exam q 6 months	Refer to dentist	Pt. interview Copy of consult report	Compliant with appts	q 6 mo
	liver dysfunction	monitor liver function	monitor LFTs	ALT, AST	<35	q 3-6 mo
6/17/98	pt complaint of constipation	Relieve constipation, return to normal bowel habits	Metamucil 1 tsp qd to bid as needed	Pt interview, abdominal cramps, diarrhea, constipation, bronchospasm.	↑ # and ease of BM, ⊖ AE	q visit

*Treatment began 4/8.   [b] cholestyramine ↑ to 8 g BID.

PHARMACIST'S CARE PLAN AMBULATORY MONITORING WORKSHEET (AMW)

Patient ___George Jones___

Page 1

Pharmacist ___John O'Malley___

Date ___3-3-98___

Pharmaco-therapeutic Goal	Monitoring Parameter	Desired Endpoint	Monitoring Frequency	3/3	3/18	3/23	3/30	4/3	4/8	4/10	4/22	5/6	5/20	6/17
1	Consult report	Rule in/out diabetes	q week until resolved				✓	Resolved						
2	BP	<130/85	q visit	152/98 140/90				140/84	140/85	138/85	138/85	136/84	140/86	136/82
	lisinopril AE: dizziness	⊖	q visits ↓ q 3 mo						⊖	⊖	⊖	⊖	⊖	⊖
	lisinopril AE: headache	⊖							⊖	⊖	⊖	⊖	⊖	⊖
	lisinopril AE: cough	⊖							⊖	⊖	⊖	⊖	⊖	⊖
	lisinopril AE: ↑K+	<5	2x year											
3	Pt. interview	adhere 4/5 days	q visit	⊖				⊕	⊕	⊕	⊕	⊕	⊕	⊕
	Weight	<160 lb	q visit	240				235	235	235	230	225	218	210
	BMI	<27	q visit	37				36	36	36	35	34	33	32
4	Profile and pt. interview	⊕	q visit	+/-				⊕	⊕	⊕	⊕	⊕	⊕	⊕
5	Profile and pt. interview	d/c furosemide ⊖ symptoms	q visit	+/-			✓		⊖	⊖	⊖	⊖	Resolved	
6	# cigs/day	Pt. currently refuses ∅	revisit quarterly	1 ppd				1 ppd						
7	Amt Etoh/wk	pt. currently refuses ∅	revisit quarterly	4 beers								4 beers		

PHARMACIST'S CARE PLAN AMBULATORY MONITORING WORKSHEET (AMW)

Patient ___George Jones___ Pharmacist ___John O'Malley___

Page ___2___ Date ___3-3-98___

Pharmaco-therapeutic Goal	Monitoring Parameter	Desired Endpoint	Monitoring Frequency	3/3	3/18	3/23	3/30	4/3	4/8	4/10	4/22	5/6	5/20	6/17
8	Pt. interview consult reports	(+)	q visit	+/⊖				(+)	(+)	(+)	(+)	(+)	(+)	(+)
9	Pt. interview	adhere 4/5 days	q visit	⊖				(+)	(+)	(+)	(+)	(+)	(+)	(+)
10	Observe technique	proper technique	2x; ↓ 2x/yr					√	√					
10	Review log	PFM w/o SX	q visit					√	√	√	√	√	√	√
11	Pt. interview/ consult report Pt. currently refuses	annually complete exam	revisit quarterly	⊖				⊖						⊖
12	Pt. interview Pt. currently refuses	complete test q 6 mos	revisit quarterly	⊖				⊖						⊖
13	FBG	<120	every visit			190				AVG 190	AVG 180	AVG 180	AVG 160	AVG 150
13	SMBG preprandial	<120		Random 244	Random 258					AVG 190	AVG 190	AVG 180	AVG 162	AVG 152
13	SMBG postprandial	<140								AVG 240 230	AVG 200 230	AVG 200	AVG 200	AVG 200
13	SMBG bedtime	100–140	↓							AVG 180	AVG 180 170	AVG 170	AVG 160	AVG 160
13	HbAlc	<7%	q 3 mo; ↓ q 6 mo					11.6						
13	SCr	<1.2	q 6 month				1.8							
13	U/A	⊖	annual				+prot +gluc -ket							

PHARMACIST'S CARE PLAN AMBULATORY MONITORING WORKSHEET (AMW)

Patient ___George Jones___
Page 3

Pharmacist ___John O'Malley___
Date ___3-3-98___

Pharmaco-therapeutic Goal	Monitoring Parameter	Desired Endpoint	Monitoring Frequency	3/3	3/18	3/23	3/30	4/3	4/8	4/10	4/22	5/6	5/20	6/17
13	urine microalbumin	<30	q 6 mo					35						
13	urine culture	(1)	prn			(1)								
13	EKG	received	annual					isch oldMI						
13	Foot screen	received	quarterly						✓	✓	✓	✓	✓	✓
13	skin screen	received	quarterly					✓						
13	symptoms of hyperglycemia -nocturia	(1)	q visit	(+)				(+)	(+)	(+)	(+)	(+/-)	(1)	(1)
	-polyuria	(1)	q visit	(1)				(1)	(1)	(1)	(1)	(1)	(1)	(1)
	-polydypsia	(1)	q visit	(1)				(1)	(1)	(1)	(1)	(1)	(1)	(1)
	-polyphagia	(1)	q visit	(1)				(1)	(1)	(1)	(1)	(1)	(1)	(1)
13	dilated retinal exam	received	annual					to schedule						
13	dental exam- Pt. refuses at this time	received	revisit quarterly						(1)					
13	Repaglinide AE- rash GI upset	(1)	q visit; ↓ q 3 mo							(1)	(1)	(1)	(1)	(1)
13	signs & symptoms of hypoglycemia	(1)	q visit							(1)	(1)	(1)	(1)	(1)

PHARMACIST'S CARE PLAN AMBULATORY MONITORING WORKSHEET (AMW)

Patient   George Jones

Page 4

Pharmacist   John O'Malley

Date   3-3-98

Pharmaco-therapeutic Goal	Monitoring Parameter	Desired Endpoint	Monitoring Frequency	3/3	3/18	3/23	3/30	4/3	4/8	4/10	4/22	5/6	5/20	6/17
14	Profile and pt. interview	d/c furosemide w/o symptoms	q visit					✓						
15	Foot inspection	⊖ sign of infx	q month ⊗ 3						⊖			⊖		⊖
16	Foot exam—sensation	10/10	quarterly					7/10				⊖		⊖
16	Pt. interview	no complications	q visit					⊖	⊖	⊖	⊖	⊖	⊖	⊖
17	ASA-AE GI upset	⊖	q visits ↓q 3 mo							⊖	⊖	⊖	⊖	⊖
17	ASA-AE dark, tarry stools	⊖	q visit; ↓q 2-3 mo							⊖	⊖	⊖	⊖	⊖
17	ASA-efficacy prevent MI	⊖	q visit							⊖	⊖	⊖	⊖	⊖
18	Total cholesterol	<200	q visit				290				215	220	210	198
18	LDL cholesterol	<100	q 8 wk ⊗2, ↓ 2-3 mo				229							135
18	HDL cholesterol	>45	↓				45							46
18	TG	<200	↓				80							84
18	Cholestyramine AE—constipation, GI upset	⊖	q visit; ↓q 3 mo						⊖/⊕	⊖/⊕	⊖/⊕	⊖/⊕		⊖/⊕

PHARMACIST'S CARE PLAN AMBULATORY MONITORING WORKSHEET (AMW)

Patient George Jones
Page 5

Pharmacist John O'Malley
Date 3-3-98

Pharmaco-therapeutic Goal	Monitoring Parameter	Desired Endpoint	Monitoring Frequency	3/3	3/18	3/23	3/30	4/3	4/8 4/10	4/22	5/6 5/20	6/7
19	Observe technique	proper technique	q 6 mo						✓	✓		
19	Review w SMBG log	completes log	q visit						✓	✓	✓ ✓	✓
20	Pt. interview, copy of report	receive exam	annual	⊖				⊖				⊕ S/13
21	Pt. interview, copy of report	receive exam	q 6 month	⊖				⊖				⊖
22	ALT	<35	q 3-6 mo				56					
22	AST	<35	q 3-6 mo				98					
23	# and ease of BM	normal	q visit									
23	AE of metamusil Abdominal cramps	⊖										
23	diarrhea	⊖										
23	constipation	⊖										
24	bronchospasm	⊖										

AMBULATORY PHARMACIST'S CARE PLAN

Patient __Sarah McLucas__ Pharmacist __Alexa Sheffield__ Date __4-23-98__

Page 1 of 2

DATE IDENTIFIED	PROBLEM (TPL)	PHARMACOTHERAPEUTIC AND RELATED HEALTH CARE GOAL	RECOMMENDATIONS FOR THERAPY	MONITORING PARAMETER(S)	DESIRED ENDPOINT(S)	MONITORING FREQUENCY
4/23/98	Poor control of diabetes	Improve control of diabetes; prevent complications	Refer to dietitian for meal planning*	FBG, SMBG, HbA1c Pt. symptoms SX of hypergly.	FBG<120 hsBG 100-140 HbA1c<7%	FBG and SMBG q visit HBA1c q 3 mo; then ↓ q 6 mo
"	Poor control of HTN	Improve control of HTN; prevent complications	Refer to dietitian for meal planning	BP	<130/85	q visit
"	Poor control of lipids	Improve control of hypercholesterolemia; prevent complications	d/c cholestyramine Rec fluvastatin 20 mg q PM	TC LDL, HDL, TG AE of fluvastatin	TC<200 LDL<100, HDL>45 TG <200 ⊖ AE	TC q visit; panel q 8 wks x2 LFTs baseline then 8 wks then q 6 mo AE q visit;
"	Postmenopausal w/o HRT	Eliminate post-menopausal SXs and ↓ assoc risks (CV and osteoporosis)	Rec. conj. estrogen 0.625 mg QD and medroxyprogesterone 2.5 mg QD	Vasomotor SX AE of HRT	⊖ symptoms and ⊖ AE	q visit
"	Not on ASA QD tx	Prevent cardiovascular complications	Rec Ec ASA 325 mg QD*	GI upset, bleeding, dark stools	⊖ SX or occult blood	SX q visit; occult blood 2x/yr.
"	PPA in Tavist-D may worsen BP & BG	Avoid worsened BP and BG control	D/C Tavist-D Rec loratadine* 10 mg QD w/ seasonal symptoms	Pt. profile	D/C w/o ↑ SX	q visit until resolved
"	Nonadherence to diet	Adhere to prescribed diet	Refer to dietitian	report of adherence to meal plan	Pt. report ↓ wt, ↓BMI	q visit
"	NSAID may ↑ BP	Avoid worsened BP control	D/C NSAIDs Rec acetaminophen up to 4 g QD*	Pt. profile	D/C w/o ↑ SX	q visit until resolved

*Treatment began 4/23.

AMBULATORY PHARMACIST'S CARE PLAN

Patient Sarah McLucas   Pharmacist Alexa Sheffield   Date 4-23-98

Page 2 of 2

DATE IDENTIFIED	PROBLEM (TPL)	PHARMACOTHERAPEUTIC AND RELATED HEALTH CARE GOAL	RECOMMENDATIONS FOR THERAPY	MONITORING PARAMETER(S)	DESIRED ENDPOINT(S)	MONITORING FREQUENCY
4/23/98	Taking Tavist-D year-round	Control seasonal allergic rhinitis SXs	D/C Tavist-D take loratidine only w/seasonal SX	hayfever SX	⊖ SX ⊖ AE	q visit
"	Taking Naprosyn and ibuprofen	Avoid duplicate tx	D/C Naprosyn and ibuprofen	Pt. report and profile	no increased pain	q visit until resolved
"	Poor control of OA pain	Control pain Preserve/increase functional status	Rec. Acetaminophen up to 4 g QD and re-evaluate	OA pain	pain<2/10 (per pt. report)	q visit
"	NSAID may ↑ SXs of GERD	Avoid SXs of GERD	D/C Naprosyn	Patient Profile	d/c w/o SX	q visit until resolved
"	Nonadherence to cholestyramine	Control hypercholest.	D/C cholestyramine Begin fluvastatin tx	Pt. report and profile	↑compliance to tx	q visit until resolved
"	No SMBG	Regular SMBG	Instruct on self-monitoring	Observation of technique -SMBG log	Proper technique Daily use of log	-Observe technique 2x/yr -Log→q visit
"	No exercise plan	Adhere to exercise plan	Daily walk	Report of adherence weight	Positive report wt and BMI ↓	q visit

PHARMACIST'S CARE PLAN AMBULATORY MONITORING WORKSHEET (AMW)

Patient Sarah McLucas

Page 1

Pharmacist Alexa Sheffield

Date 4/23/98

Pharmaco-therapeutic Goal	Monitoring Parameter	Desired Endpoint	Monitoring Frequency	Date 4/14	4/20	4/23	5/7	6/18	7/30				
1,6	FBG	<120	q visit	142	138		140	136	130				
↓	SMBG preprandial	<120	q visit				140	135	130				
↓	SMBG postprandial	<120	q visit				200	180	180				
↓	SMBG Bedtime	100-140	q visit				160	150	150				
↓	HBAlc	<7%	q 3 mo; ↓ q 6		9.4				8.8				
↓	SX of hyperglycemia -polyuria	(-)	q visit				(-)	(-)	(-)				
↓	-polydipsia	(-)	q visit				(-)	(-)	(-)				
↓	-polyphagia	(-)	q visit				(-)	(-)	(-)				
↓	Dialated retinal exam	received	annual					(+)					
↓	Dental exam	received	2x/yr			(+)							
↓	Skin screen/assess	received	quarterly			(+)							
↓	Foot screen	received	quarterly			(+)							
↓	SCr	<1.2	q 6 mo		0.8								

PHARMACIST'S CARE PLAN AMBULATORY MONITORING WORKSHEET (AMW)

Patient __Sarah McLucas__
Page 2

Pharmacist __Alexa Sheffield__
Date __4/23/98__

Pharmaco-therapeutic Goal	Monitoring Parameter	Desired Endpoint	Monitoring Frequency	Date 4/14	4/20	4/23	5/7	6/18	7/30
1	U/A	⊖	annual		⊖				
1	Urine microalbumin	⊖	annual		⊖				
1	EKG	received WNL	annual	WNL					
2	BP	<130/85	q visit	134/86		132/88	130/82	128/80	
3	Total cholesterol	<200	q visit	232		230	220	200	
3	LDL cholesterol	<100	q 8 wk (×2)	145					
3	HDL cholesterol	>45	→	30					
3	TG	<200	→	284					
3	AE of fluvastatin GI upset	⊖	q visit			⊖	⊖	⊖	
3	headache	⊖	q visit			⊖	⊖	⊖	
3	back or muscle pain or tenderness	⊖	q visit			⊖	⊖	⊖	
3	ALT	<35	Baseline; q 8 wk, q 6 mo	10				=	
3	AST	<35	→	9				9	

PHARMACIST'S CARE PLAN AMBULATORY MONITORING WORKSHEET (AMW)

Patient ___Sarah McLucas___

Pharmacist ___Alexa Sheffield___

Date ___4/23/98___

Page 3

Pharmaco-therapeutic Goal	Monitoring Parameter	Desired Endpoint	Monitoring Frequency	4/14	4/20	4/23	5/7	6/18	7/30
4	Vasomotor SX	⊖	q visit				⊖	⊖	⊖
4	AE of estrogen/progestin breast pain	⊖	q visit				refuses tx		
4	GI upset	⊖	q visit				→		
4	vaginal bleeding	⊖	q visit						
4	thromboembolic comp	⊖	q visit				→		
5	AE of ASA tx GI upset	⊖	q visit				⊖	⊖	⊖
5	dark, tarry stools	⊖	q visit				⊖	⊖	⊖
5	home fecal occult blood test	performed	2x/yr			✓			
6	Patient profile	dc PPA	every visit until d/c				d/c		
7	Pt. interview	adhere 4/5 days	q visit				+	+	+
7	Weight	<150	q visit			162	160	154	152
7	BMI	<27	q visit			27	27	26	26
8, 12	Patient profile	dc NSAIDs	every visit till d/c				d/c		

PHARMACIST'S CARE PLAN AMBULATORY MONITORING WORKSHEET (AMW)

Patient __Sarah McLucas__

Page 4

Pharmacist __Alexa Sheffield__

Date __4-23-98__

Pharmaco-therapeutic Goal	Monitoring Parameter	Desired Endpoint	Monitoring Frequency	4/14	4/20	4/23	5/7	6/18	7/30				
9	SX of seasonal allergic rhinitis	(-)	q visit				(-)	(-)	(-)				
	AE of loratadine: dry mouth	(-)	q visit				(-)	(-)	(-)				
	sedation	(-)	q visit				(-)	(-)	(-)				
10	Pt. profile	d/c w/o SXs	q visit				dc						
11	OA pain (knee)	pain <2/10	q visit				3/10	2/10	3/10				
13	Pt. profile	dc w/o SXs; ↑ compliance	q visit until resolved				dc						
14	Correct technique	(+)	q 6 mo.				(+)	(+)	(+)				
14	Completing log	(+)	q visit				(+)	(+)	(+)				
15	Pt. interview	adhere 4/5 days	q visit				(+)	(+)	(+)				

AMBULATORY PHARMACIST'S CARE PLAN

Patient **Sarah McLucas**   Pharmacist **Alexa Sheffield**   Date **4-23-98**

Page 1 of 2

DATE IDENTIFIED	PROBLEM (TPL)	PHARMACOTHERAPEUTIC AND RELATED HEALTH CARE GOAL	RECOMMENDATIONS FOR THERAPY	MONITORING PARAMETER(S)	DESIRED ENDPOINT(S)	MONITORING FREQUENCY
4/23/98	Poor control of diabetes	Improve control of diabetes; prevent complications	Refer to dietitian for meal planning*	FBG, SMBG, HbA1c, Pt. symptoms SX of hypergly.	FBG<120, hsBG 100-140, HbA1c<7%	FBG and SMBG q visit, HbA1c q 3 mo; then ↓q 6 mo Revised 7/30/98
"	Poor control of HTN	~~Maintain~~ Improve control of HTN; prevent complications	Refer to dietitian for meal planning	BP	<130/85	q visit Revised 7/30/98
"	Poor control of lipids	Improve control of hypercholesterolemia; prevent complications	b/c cholestyramine w/u Rec fluvastatin* 20 mg q PM	TC, LDL, HDL, TG, AE of fluvastatin	TC<200, LDL<100, HDL>45, TG <200 ⊖ AE	LFTs baseline, 8 wks @2 TC q visit; panel q 8 wks @2, AE q visit;
"	Postmenopausal w/o HRT	Eliminate post-menopausal SXs and ↓assoc risks (CV and osteoporosis)	Rec. conj. estrogen 0.625 mg QD and medroxyprogesterone 2.5 mg QD	Vasomotor SX, AE of HRT	⊕symptoms and ⊖ AE	q visit
"	Not on ASA QD tx	Prevent cardiovascular complications	Rec Ec ASA 325 mg QD*	GI upset, bleeding, dark stools	⊖SX or occult blood	SX q visit, occult blood 2x/yr.
"	PPA in Tavist-D w/u worsen BP & BG	Avoid worsened BP and BG control	D/C Tavist-D Rec loratidine 10 mg QD w/ seasonal symptoms	Pt. profile	D/C w/o ↑SX	q visit until resolved resolved
"	Nonadherence to diet	Adhere to prescribed diet	Refer to dietitian	report of adherence to meal plan	Pt. report ↓wt, ↓BMI	q visit
"	NSAID w/u ↑BP	Avoid worsened BP control	D/C NSAIDS Rec acetaminophen up to 4 g QD*	Pt. profile	D/C w/o ↑SX	q visit until resolved resolved

*Treatment began 4/23.

AMBULATORY PHARMACIST'S CARE PLAN

Patient __Sarah McLucas__   Pharmacist __Alexa Sheffield__   Date __4-23-98__

Page 2 of 2

DATE IDENTIFIED	PROBLEM (TPL)	PHARMACOTHERAPEUTIC AND RELATED HEALTH CARE GOAL	RECOMMENDATIONS FOR THERAPY	MONITORING PARAMETER(S)	DESIRED ENDPOINT(S)	MONITORING FREQUENCY
4/23/98	Taking Tavist-D year-round	Control seasonal allergic rhinitis SXs	D/C Tavist-D take loratidine only w/seasonal SX	hayfever SX	⊖SX ⊖AE	q visit
"	Taking naprosyn and ibuprofen	Avoid duplicate tx	D/C naprosyn and ibuprofen	Pt. report and profile	no increased pain	q visit → resolved
"	Poor control of OA pain	Control pain Preserve/increase functional status	Rec. Acetaminophen up to 4 g QD and re-evaluate	OA pain	pain<2/10 (per pt. report)	q visit
"	NSAID may SXs of GERD	Avoid SXs of GERD	D/C naprosyn	Patient Profile	d/c w/o SX	q visit until resolved
"	Nonadherence to cholestyramine	Control hypercholest.	D/C cholestyramine begin fluvastatin tx	Pt. report and profile	↑compliance to tx	q visit until resolved
"	No SMBG	Regular SMBG	Instruct on self-monitoring	Observation of technique -SMBG log	Proper technique Daily use of log	-Observe technique 2x/yr -Log→q visit
"	No exercise plan	Adhere to exercise plan	Daily walk	Report of adherence weight	Positive report ↓wt and BMI	q visit
7/30/98	not meeting goals for control of diabetes	improve control of diabetes; prevent complications	Acarbose 25 mg po ⊗ 1 week; ↑ to bid ⊗ 1 week; ↑ to tid and reevaluate	FBG/SMBG, HbA1c, abdominal pain diarrhea, flatulence, LFTs	FBG <120, PPBG <140, hsBG 100-140, HbA1c <7, ALT, AST <35, ⊖AE	All q visit except HbA1c q 3 months; LFTs q 6 months; q 6 months

PHARMACIST'S CARE PLAN AMBULATORY MONITORING WORKSHEET (AMW)

Patient ____Sarah McLucas____

Pharmacist ____Alexa Sheffield____

Date ____4/23/98____

Page 1

Pharmaco-therapeutic Goal	Monitoring Parameter	Desired Endpoint	Monitoring Frequency	4/14	4/20	4/23	5/7	6/18	7/30				
1,6	FBG	<120	q visit	142	138		140	136	130				
1	SMBG preprandial	<120	q visit				140	135	130				
1	SMBG postprandial	<120	q visit				200	180	180				
1	SMBG Bedtime	100-140	q visit				160	150	150				
1	HBAlc	<7%	q 3 mo; ↓ q 6		9.4				8.8				
1	SX of hyperglycemia -polyuria	(-)	q visit				(-)	(-)	(-)				
1	-polydipsia	(-)	q visit				(-)	(-)	(-)				
1	-polyphagia	(-)	q visit				(-)	(-)	(-)				
1	Dialated retinal exam	received	annual					(+)					
1	Dental exam	received	2x/yr			(+)							
1	Skin screen/assess	received	quarterly			(+)							
1	Foot screen	received	quarterly			(+)							
1	SCr	<1.2	q 6 mo	0.8					0.8				

PHARMACIST'S CARE PLAN AMBULATORY MONITORING WORKSHEET (AMW)

Patient __Sarah McLucas__

Page 2

Pharmacist __Alexa Sheffield__

Date __4/23/98__

Pharmaco-therapeutic Goal	Monitoring Parameter	Desired Endpoint	Monitoring Frequency	Date 4/14	4/20	4/23	5/7	6/18	7/30					
1	U/A	(−)	Annual		(−)									
1	Urine microalbumin	(−)	Annual		(−)									
1	EKG	received WNL	Annual	WNL										
2	BP	<130/85	q visit			134/ 86	132/ 88	130/ 82	128/ 80					
3	Total cholesterol	<200	q visit			232	230	220	200					
3	LDL cholesterol	<100	q 8 wk (×) 2		145									
3	HDL cholesterol	>45			30									
3	TG	<200	→↓		284									
3	AE of fluvastatin GI upset	(−)	q visit				(−)	(−)	(−)					
3	headache	(−)	q visit				(−)	(−)	(−)					
3	back or muscle pain or tenderness	(−)	q visit				(−)	(−)	(−)					
3	ALT	<35	Baseline; q 8 wk, q 6 mo		10			11						
3	AST	<35	→↓		9			9						

PHARMACIST'S CARE PLAN AMBULATORY MONITORING WORKSHEET (AMW)

Patient **Sarah McLucas**

Page **3**

Pharmacist **Alexa Sheffield**

Date **4/23/98**

Pharmaco-therapeutic Goal	Monitoring Parameter	Desired Endpoint	Monitoring Frequency	4/14	4/20	4/23	5/7	6/18	7/30
4	Vasomotor SX	⊖	q visit				⊖	⊖	⊖
4	AE of estrogen/progestin breast pain	⊖	q visit				refuses tx		
4	GI upset	⊖	q visit				→	→	→
4	vaginal bleeding	⊖	q visit						
4	thromboembolic comp	⊖	q visit				→	→	→
5	AE of ASA tx GI upset	⊖	q visit				⊖	⊖	⊖
5	dark, tarry stools	⊖	q visit				⊖	⊖	⊖
5	home fecal occult blood test	performed	2x/yr			✓			
6	Patient profile	dc PPA	every visit until d/c				d/c — RESOLVED →		
7	Pt. interview	adhere 4/5 days	q visit				+	+	+
7	Weight	<150	q visit			162	160	154	152
7	BMI	<27	q visit			27	27	26	26
8, 12	Patient profile	dc NSAIDs	every visit till d/c				d/c — RESOLVED →		

PHARMACIST'S CARE PLAN AMBULATORY MONITORING WORKSHEET (AMW)

Patient __Sarah McLucas__

Page 4

Pharmacist __Alexa Sheffield__

Date __4-23-98__

Pharmaco-therapeutic Goal	Monitoring Parameter	Desired Endpoint	Monitoring Frequency	4/14	4/20	4/23	5/7	6/18	7/30			
				Date								
9	SX of seasonal allergic rhinitis	(-)	q visit				(-)	(-)	(-)			
	AE of loratadine: dry mouth	(-)	q visit				(-)	(-)	(-)			
	sedation	(-)	q visit				(-)	(-)	(-)			
10	Pt. profile	d/c w/o SXs	q visit				dc — RESOLVED →					
11	OA pain (knee)	pain <2/10	q visit				3/10	2/10	3/10			
13	Pt. profile	dc w/o SXs; ↑ compliance	q visit until resolved				dc — RESOLVED →					
14	Correct technique	(+)	q 6 mo.				(+)	(+)	(+)			
14	Completing log	(+)	q visit				(+)	(+)	(+)			
15	Pt. interview	adhere 4/5 days	q visit				(+)	(+)	(+)			
16	AE of acarbose abdominal pain	(-)	q visit									
	diarrhea	(-)	→									
	flatulence	(-)										